T0329730

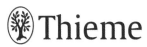

Eva Eberspächer-Schweda

AnaesthesiaSkills
in veterinary medicine

Perioperative management in small, companion and domestic animals

119 figures

Georg Thieme Verlag

Stuttgart • New York

Priv.-Doz. Dr. med. vet. habil.
Eva Eberspächer-Schweda
AnästhesieSkills
Unter den Linden 30/3/17
2000 Stockerau
Austria

Bibliographical data of the German National Library (Deutsche Nationalbibliothek)
The German National Library (Deutsche National-bibliothek) lists this publication in the German National Bibliography; detailed bibliographic information can be found on the Internet at http://dnb.d-nb.de.

Your opinion is important to us!
Please write to us at:
www.thieme.de/service/feedback.html

Georg Thieme Verlag KG
Rüdigerstraße 14, 70469 Stuttgart, Germany
www.thieme.com

Printed in Italy

Translated from the German 2nd edition "AnästhesieSkills. Perioperatives Management bei Klein-, Heim- und Großtieren", Georg Thieme Verlag 2020

Cover design: © Thieme
Image credits Cover: © Thieme/Photo: Priv.-Doz. Dr. med. vet. habil. Eva Eberspächer-Schweda, Großmugl
Graphics: From: "AnästhesieSkills. Perioperatives Management bei Klein-, Heim- und Großtieren", Georg Thieme Verlag 2020.
Translation (including graphics): Priv.-Doz. Dr. med. vet. habil. Eva Eberspächer-Schweda, Großmugl
Copyediting: Dr. med. vet. Stefanie Gronau, Haimhausen
Typesetting: Druckhaus Götz GmbH, Ludwigsburg
Printing: LEGO S.p.A, Vicenza

DOI 10.1055/b000000630

ISBN 978-3-13-245850-5   1 2 3 4 5 6

Also available as eBook:
eISBN (PDF) 978-3-13-244475-1
eISBN (epub) 978-3-13-244476-8

Important Note: Veterinary medicine is an ever-changing science undergoing continual development. Research and clinical experience are continually expanding our knowledge, in particular our knowledge of proper treatment and drug therapy. Insofar as this book mentions any dosage or application, readers may rest assured that the authors, editors, and publishers have made every effort to ensure that such references are in accordance with **the state of knowledge at the time of production of the book.**

Nevertheless, this does not involve, imply, or express any guarantee or responsibility on the part of the publishers in respect to any dosage instructions and forms of applications stated in the book. **Every user is requested to examine carefully** the manufacturers' leaflets accompanying each drug and to check, if necessary in consultation with a physician or specialist, whether the dosage schedules mentioned therein or the contraindications stated by the manufacturers differ from the statements made in the present book. Such examination is particularly important with drugs that are either rarely used or have been newly released on the market. **Every dosage schedule or every form of application used is entirely at the user's own risk and responsibility.** The authors and publishers request every user to report to the publishers any discrepancies or inaccuracies noticed. Prior to any use in food-producing animals the differing approvals and restrictions on the use that are in effect in the individual countries must be taken into account.

Some of the product names, patents, and registered designs referred to in this book are in fact registered trademarks or proprietary names, even though specific reference to this fact is not always made in the text. Therefore, the appearance of a name without a designation as proprietary is not to be construed as a representation by the publisher that it is in the public domain.

Thieme addresses people of all gender identities equally. We encourage our authors to use gender-neutral or genderequal expressions wherever the context allows.

Data protection: Where required by data protection laws, personal names and other data are edited and either removed or pseudonymized (alias names). This is always the case with patients, their relatives and friends, partly also with other persons, e.g. those involved in the treatment of patients.

Dedication

To my family

Foreword

This book was originally written in German. It was born out of my own need not to have a small compact book at hand where one can quickly find the most important facts about anaesthesia in pets. A book in which one can read up on standard values or drugs and their dosages or read about complications, the anaesthetic management of the most important diseases and the species that is only occasionally presented as a patient. This book in no way claims to be a textbook, but it is intended to be helpful in daily practice!

At seminars and CE courses I have been told time and again how nice it would be if the "AnästhesieSkills" were also available in English – after all, there are some countries where no textbook in the national language is available in such a small speciality as veterinary anaesthesia. Of course, there are excellent veterinary anaesthesia books in English from the USA or Great Britain, but the "cooking style" of how anaesthesia is done in these countries is somewhat different from the central European "cooking style". After all, anaesthesia is like cooking a good soup – for the soup to taste good and be easily digestible, the ingredients, their quantity and the preparation must be right. In different countries, even in different parts of countries, people cook differently, so everyone has their own tastes and favourite dishes. For this reason, the protocols and procedures presented in this book reflect my preferences and experiences, which have developed through many professional discussions and years of working in various international settings. The protocols in this book could be described as an internationally influenced central European "cooking style". I would like them to be used as a stimulus to critically analyse one's own routines, to consider other or new approaches and to adopt them where appropriate.

I did the translation myself and although I have a good command of English, I am sure that some expressions may not have been chosen optimally. I would appreciate your feedback to make it better next time!

I would like to thank Sandra Schmidt and Eva Wallstein from Thieme Publishing, who believed in this book and supported its realisation from the very beginning. I would also like to thank Stefanie Gronau, who put the finishing touches on the book.

Only the support and love of my family makes such an ambitious project possible – you are the greatest treasure in my life!

I am especially happy that Lilli, our dog, made it onto the cover.

Vienna, August 2023
Eva Eberspächer-Schweda

Contents

Basics

Contents

Anaesthesia practice

Contents

Contents

Contents

Contents

Appendix

Authors Introduction

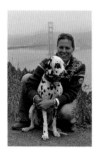

Priv.-Doz. Dr. med. vet. habil. Eva Eberspächer-Schweda

Eva Eberspächer-Schweda is a specialist in laboratory animal science and a Diplomate of the American College of Veterinary Anesthesia and Analgesia.

After studying veterinary medicine at the Justus Liebig University in Gießen, Germany, she worked as research assistant in the laboratory of the Department of Anaesthesiology at the Klinikum rechts der Isar of the Technical University in Munich, Germany. She then completed a residency in anaesthesia and intensive care medicine at the Veterinary Medical Teaching Hospital of the University of California in Davis, USA.

Since 2007 she has been a university assistant in the Department of Anaesthesiology and Perioperative Intensive Care Medicine, Department of Small Animals and Horses at the University of Veterinary Medicine Vienna, Austria.

In 2010 she habilitated in anaesthesiology and perioperative intensive care. She has been involved in student teaching for many years and has won several prizes such as the title "Senior Teacher of the Year", the students' "Oscar" for special commitment in teaching, and the "Vetucation Award" for her outstanding online training.

Since 2020, she has been Director of Education at the European School for Advanced Veterinary Studies and works independently in postgraduate education with her company "AnaesthesieSkills". She is a valued speaker at conferences and trains veterinarians and assistants in small and large animal anaesthesia in clinical and experimental settings.

Priv.-Doz. Dr. med. vet. habil. Eberspächer-Schweda is a member of more than 10 academic associations, including the German Society of Anaesthesiology and Intensive Care Medicine, the Veterinary Emergency and Critical Care Society and the European Academy of Sciences and Arts.

Part I
Basics

1 The Anaesthesia Machine

The Association of Veterinary Anaesthetists (AVA) defined several years ago the recommended requirements that a veterinarian must meet in order to perform general anaesthesia in a dog, cat or horse. Any veterinarian who performs general anaesthesia must be able to,

1. secure the animal's airway (e.g. by endotracheal intubation),
2. administer oxygen,
3. perform manually controlled ventilation (e.g. by using an Artificial Manual Breathing Unit (AMBU bag), an anaesthesia machine or, in case of horses, a demand valve),
4. administer drugs and infusion solutions intravenously, ideally via a venous catheter and
5. perform cardiopulmonary resuscitation (CPR).

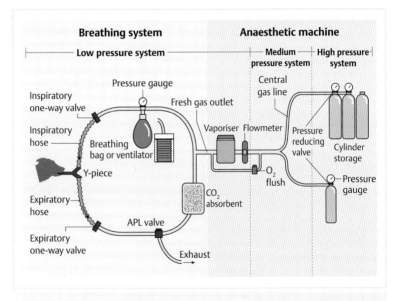

Fig. 1.1 Schematic overview of an anaesthesia machine with patient part (shown here as an example with a circle system as breathing system) and the actual machine part; APL valve: adjustable pressure limiting valve.

In order to fulfil these 5 requirements, the veterinarian must, on the one hand, have the necessary materials and equipment on site and, on the other hand, be proficient in the necessary techniques (e.g. intubation, catheterisation, manual ventilation).

With the help of a modern anaesthesia machine, inhalation anaesthetics and oxygen can be administered to the patient in a safe and dosed manner. Carbon dioxide (CO_2) can be removed from the exhaled air. Most anaesthesia machines can act as breathing monitor and be used for manual ventilation.

The anaesthesia machine generally consists of the patient part (= breathing system) and the actual machine part (▶ Fig. 1.1).

1.1 Patient part or breathing system

The patient part of the anaesthesia machine includes all parts of the breathing system that are downstream of the fresh gas outlet, i.e. usually the non-rebreathing system or the circle system as a rebreathing system.

1.1.1 Non-rebreathing system or rebreathing system?

The non-rebreathing system (or semi-open system) differs from the rebreathing system (or semi-closed and closed system) in the way it eliminates CO_2. In the **semi-open system**, this works by increasing the fresh gas flow, which flushes out the CO_2 with the exhaust air. In the **semi-closed** and **closed** system (= circle system, because of the constantly recirculating gas flow), the CO_2 is taken out of the system by the absorber lime. It is called semi-closed because the supply of O_2 and inhalation anaesthetic exceeds the consumption of the animal, i.e. the exhaust air continuously escapes via the pressure relief valve. A system is closed when the supply of O_2 and inhalation anaesthetic exactly covers the patient's needs and (despite the pressure relief valve being open) no more exhaust air escapes from the system.

The open system has a special position among the anaesthesia systems. This is classically the so-called Schimmelbusch mask with which patients were anaesthetised with ether at the beginning of gas anaesthesia. Nowadays, anaesthesia chambers, such as those used for the induction of anaesthesia in small pets/laboratory animals or exotics, are also included (▶ Fig. 1.2). There is no fixed definition, in short: "everyone gets something, including the anaesthetist". Consequently, it should only be used with excellent suction (e.g. under an exhaust hood). To work with an open system, one does not necessarily need an anaesthesia machine. Usually, the semi-open (non-rebreathing) system and the semi-closed (rebreathing) system are used in veterinary medicine because, among other things, the exposure of staff and the environment to hazards from

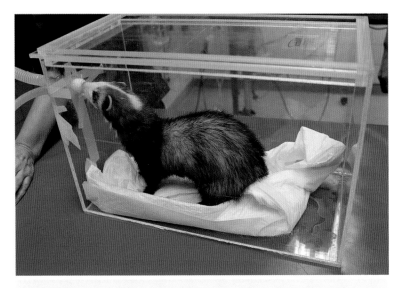

Fig. 1.2 Open system for anaesthesia induction in small mammals and exotics.

the use of the open system is too high and conditions for safely performing anaesthesia with the closed system are too difficult to fulfil under practice conditions.

1.1.2 Non-rebreathing system

There are many different non-rebreathing systems, all with slightly different set ups. One system commonly used is the so-called Bain system (▸ Fig. 1.3), which is also called Mapleson D system. It can be designed as a coaxial system, i. e. the inspiratory tube lies within the expiratory tube, which can be advantageous.

In non-rebreathing systems, the entire exhaled gas mixture is completely discharged from the system with the exhaust air. For this reason, the fresh gas flow must be at least as large as the respiratory minute volume, which is approx. 200–250 ml/kg/min.

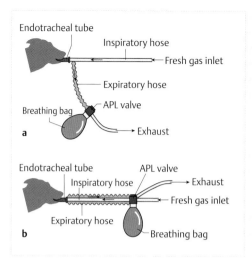

Fig. 1.3 Example for a non-rebreathing system (Bain or Mapleson D system); APL valve: adjustable pressure limiting valve.
a   Normal system.
b   Coaxial system (breathing hose within hose).

Definition

Minute ventilation

Minute ventilation is calculated from tidal volume (10–15 ml/kg) times respiratory rate (depending on the species, approx. 8–12 /min for small animals, up to 20 /min for small companion animals). The tidal volume is one of the few parameters that is constant in almost all animal species. The standard values for respiratory rate are listed in (▶ Table 2.1).

Due to the advantages of the Bain system (▶ Table 1.1), its use is recommended for **small mammals, cats and dogs under 5–8 kg.** It can also be used for larger animals without any problems, but then the waste and thus the costs increase disproportionately.

1.1.3 Rebreathing or circle system

The circle system can be described as semi-closed or closed depending on the amount of fresh gas flow. As mentioned above, in the semi-closed system the supply of O_2 and inhalation anaesthetic exceeds the consumption by the animal. Consequently, part of the exhaust air must continuously escape from the system through the pressure relief valve (hence "semi-closed"). If the circle sys-

Table 1.1 Advantages and disadvantages of the non-rebreathing system (e.g. Bain system)

Advantages	Disadvantages
Low dead space volume	High fresh gas flow (large quantities), inhalation anaesthetic and oxygen are wasted, i.e. discarded unused = more expensive and harmful for the environment
Little respiratory resistance	Loss of heat and moisture from the patient
Rapid changes in concentration (inhalation anaesthetic, oxygen) are possible, the system is very "direct"	Coaxial systems are difficult to clean and unrecognised disconnection of the inner tube may occur
Various sizes available, also coaxial systems where theoretically the exhaled air warms the inspiratory gases	An accidentally closed pressure relief valve can quickly lead to barotrauma
Little weight on the patient (tubes and adapters are lightweight)	In the case of poor/insufficient exhaust, possible contamination of the environment with waste gases

tem is used in such a way that supply and consumption by the patient are exactly the same, the system "closes". This means that even though the pressure relief valve is open, neither O_2 nor inhalation anaesthetic escapes. Under practical conditions, the semi-closed system is much more convenient, because the use and the safety range correspond better to the clinical requirements.

Clinical relevance

Closed system and low-flow anaesthesia
In order to work with a closed system, several conditions must be met:
1. The patient's oxygen requirement must be calculated (4–8 ml O_2/kg/min). To be able to administer these small amounts correctly, the flowmeter must have a particularly small scale and accuracy.
2. The circle system must be absolutely leak-free (perfect result in the leak test).
3. The vaporiser must still function accurately with very small carrier gas flow rates.
4. Multi-gas monitoring is absolutely recommended because there is a risk of using a hypoxic gas mixture. In addition, nitrogen (N) must be washed out of the patient and the system at the beginning of anaesthesia, i. e. up to 15 min high oxygen flow and subsequent control before the system is "closed".

5. The closed system is not recommended for ruminants and horses as they produce and exhale methane perioperatively which should be removed continuously from the system.

Because of these conditions and the low safety margin, the closed system is only recommended in the hands of a professional with the appropriate monitoring and equipment. A somewhat less complicated alternative is the so-called **low-flow anaesthesia**, in which the supply of O_2 and inhalation anaesthetic only slightly exceed the actual demand of the patient (e.g. 10 ml/kg/min O_2 demand plus 500 ml/min O_2 as a safety margin; for a 20 kg dog = 700 ml/min O_2). This option is relatively safe, very cost-effective by reducing oxygen and inhalation anaesthetic waste, much less harmful to staff and the environment, and maintains heat and humidity in the system.

It is important to note that this low-flow anaesthesia should only be applied when the concentrations of oxygen and inhalation anaesthetic are already equilibrated between the anaesthesia machine and the patient. In practice, this means that just induced patients attached to the anaesthesia machine are first provided with relatively high flow rates in order to quickly exchange nitrogen as part of the air in the lungs with oxygen and to quickly increase the concentration of the inhalation anaesthetic. Once a steady state has been reached (this can be checked with the multi-gas monitor), it is possible to turn the flow rate down to low-flow anaesthesia. Note that it takes a relatively long time to increase or decrease the concentration of the inhalation anaesthetic in the system now – if the concentration in the system is to be changed quickly, the flow rate must also be increased in parallel with the adjustment at the vaporiser.

Components that must always be present in a circle system (▶ Fig. 1.4):
- Expiratory and inspiratory breathing hoses, which are connected to the patient via the Y-piece
- Two one-way valves situated in the expiratory and inspiratory limb, which allow flow only in one direction
- Breathing bag
- Soda lime in a transparent canister
- Pressure relief or adjustable pressure limiting (APL) valve
- Exhaust hose
- Pressure gauge or manometer

The circle system is an example of the so-called patient part of the anaesthesia machine.

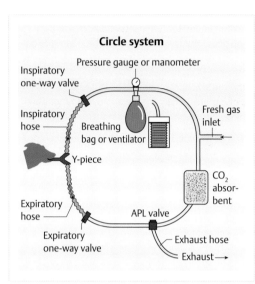

Fig. 1.4 Structure of a circle system; APL valve: adjustable pressure limiting valve.

Breathing hoses, Y-piece and one-way valves

The diameter of the breathing hoses should be chosen according to the size of the patient. For small animal patients up to 10 kg a small diameter hose (Ø 15 mm), for animals heavier than about 10 kg a large diameter hose (Ø 22 mm) is recommended. For large animals, hoses with a diameter of 2 inches (equivalent to about 50 mm) are used. A short hose with a large diameter will reduce breathing resistance.

Classic breathing hoses consist of separate inspiratory and expiratory hoses. In the coaxial system, on the other hand, the inspiratory hose is inside the expiratory hose. This simplifies handling (only one hose) and theoretically the inhaled gas is warmed by the exhaled gas. In practice, this usually only works to a limited extent, because the gases often flow too quickly to really exchange heat.

The Y-piece connects the breathing hoses to each other and the tube system to the patient (via the endotracheal tube or the laryngeal mask). The part of the Y-piece that is outside the circular gas flow is part of the apparatus dead space. The volume of the Y-piece should therefore be as small as possible.

The inspiratory and expiratory one-way or unidirectional valves allow the flow of respiratory gases in one direction and thus prevent rebreathing of the gases already exhaled (including CO_2). The valve disks should always be free to move, i. e. after prolonged anaesthesia the cover should be unscrewed and the disks dried.

One-way valve disks

Before using the anaesthesia machine, always check the presence and free movement of the valve disks (i. e. by blowing into the attached hoses). A missing expiratory valve disk or one that is stuck in the open position increases dead space and leads to massive CO_2 rebreathing and hypoxaemia (p. 378) (▶ Fig. 8.20). If a valve disk is lost or broken, a cut-out circle from an old X-ray film can be used temporarily.

Breathing bag

The breathing bag is the only expandable component of the anaesthesia machine. It serves as a fresh gas reservoir for the patient and allows the changing volumes in the system through inhalation and exhalation. The patient's spontaneous breathing can be recognised by deflation and inflation of the bag. The size of the breathing bag should be chosen according to the size of the animal and should be about 5 times tidal volume (this equals 5×10–15 ml/kg). A bag that is too large makes the system "slower", i. e. changes in concentration occur more slowly and waste gas fraction is increased. A bag that is too small impairs the patient's spontaneous breathing, because it limits the volume to be inspired (= danger that the bag collapses).

The animal can be ventilated manually via the breathing bag. To do this, the pressure relief valve must be closed and the pressure in the system increased by compressing the bag. The increase in pressure causes the lungs to expand. The average maximum pressure to be applied is 8–15 cmH_2O for small animals, and up to 20–30 cmH_2O for large animals which can be controlled with the manometer in the breathing system. It should not be forgotten that the pressure relief valve must be fully opened again after manual ventilation has ended.

If a ventilator is connected for mechanical positive pressure ventilation, the ventilator takes the place of the bag. The breathing bag must be removed for this and the pressure relief valve closed (these steps work automatically in many modern devices by diverting the gas flows after flipping a switch). Ventilators often have their own pressure relief valve that opens at a certain (relatively high) pressure in the system.

Good to know

Optimal filling of the breathing bag
Optimal filling of the breathing bag is such that the patient neither feels pressure in the airways due to excessive inflation of the bag (overpressure? is APL valve fully open?) nor that the bag collapses during a stronger inspiration and the breath has to be abruptly stopped due to a collapsing bag (leak in the system? not enough fresh gas flow?)

CO_2 absorbent or soda lime

The absorbent or soda lime in the anaesthesia machine binds the CO_2 exhaled by the patient and thus takes it out of the circle system. There are several types of absorbent. The most commonly used today is based on a mixture of calcium and sodium hydroxide. The granules are white when unused, of varying grain size and have a rough (enlarged) surface.

The binding of CO_2 is an **exothermic** chemical **reaction** in which, among other things, **water is required** and **acid** is produced.

- The heat released can easily be felt on the soda lime canister and can thus be interpreted as an indication of successful CO_2 absorption. If the soda lime is used up, the canister remains cold.
- No chemical reaction can take place with dried-out (old) soda lime, although no CO_2 has been bound yet. Unfortunately, it must still be discarded and replaced; subsequent moistening is not recommended.
- The acid that is produced enables the colour change of the added indicator ethyl violet from white to purple. If most of the soda lime has turned purple, it is used up and should be discarded and replaced.

Good to know

Colour change soda lime
The colour change from white to purple indicates the consumption of the CO_2 by the soda lime. Over time, the purple colour fades and the granules become white again. However, the lime is still used up and can no longer absorb CO_2. In case of doubt, the soda lime should always be discarded and replaced.

There is a newer (and more expensive) CO_2 absorbent with which the colour change to purple persists, i. e. the consumption can be seen even after days. For safety reasons, this lime may be recommended, especially if the anaesthesia machine is used only rarely.

When exhausted soda lime is used, CO_2 cannot be taken out of the circle system. There is a rebreathing of CO_2. CO_2 rebreathing can be easily recognised by an elevation of the baseline in the capnography waveform (= increase in inspiratory CO_2) (▶ Fig. 8.20).

Pressure relief or adjustable pressure limiting (APL) valve

The pressure relief or APL or pop-off valve is usually placed above or next to the breathing bag. It opens at a pressure in the system of about 1–2 cmH$_2$O. During spontaneous ventilation, the pressure relief valve should always be fully open. During manual ventilation it must be (at least partially) closed. Connected to the APL valve is the exhaust hose.

Exhaust hose

The exhaust hose discharges the excess gases in the anaesthesia system without contaminating ambient air. Gases are either removed via active or passive suction or passed through an activated carbon filter that absorbs inhalation anaesthetics and releases the remaining gases back into room air.

Sometimes (when active suction is used) holes are intentionally made in the exhaust hose close to the anaesthesia machine. These serve to prevent a vacuum (negative pressure) from building up in the system through active suction. Room air is drawn in through the holes and the vacuum is neutralized. These holes should not be closed. If the system is working correctly, no exhaust air escapes from these holes.

The advantages and disadvantages of the rebreathing system can be found in ▶ Table 1.2.

Table 1.2 Advantages and disadvantages of the rebreathing or circle system

Advantages	Disadvantages
Low flow rates are possible, less waste of inhalation anaesthetics and oxygen = cheaper and better for the environment	Higher breathing resistance due to unidirectional valves and soda lime
Humidification and warming of the respiratory gases through recycling	Slower system, i.e. concentration changes of inhalation anaesthetic or oxygen in the system take more time
Less contamination of the environment by exhaust gases, less stress on personnel	Higher purchase costs

Pressure gauge or manometer

The pressure gauge or manometer indicates the pressure in the breathing system in cmH_2O. When a patient is connected to the breathing system and breathing spontaneously, the pressure should range from slightly negative (to approx. $-2\,cmH_2O$, inspiration) to slightly positive (to approx. $+2\,cmH_2O$, expiration). Except for positive pressure ventilation, no pressure should build up in the system and thus in the lungs.

1.2 Anaesthetic machine

In addition to the patient part or breathing system, the anaesthesia machine consists of the actual machine part that produces the gas mixture. This machine part includes the oxygen source via central lines or cylinders (high-pressure system), the oxygen flush (medium-pressure system) and the vaporiser and flowmeter (low-pressure system) (▶ Fig. 1.5). Oxygen can also be produced by an oxygen concentrator.

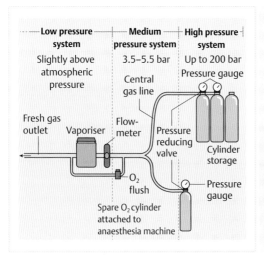

Fig. 1.5 Schematic overview of the machine part with the respective pressure systems.

1.2.1 High-pressure system

The high-pressure system includes the **oxygen source**, which is provided either by cylinders on the machine or centrally. The pressure is around 200 bar with a full cylinder, it can be read on the **pressure gauge** (also called manometer) and serves as an indicator of how much O_2 is still available in the cylinder. The pressure is reduced to the medium pressure with the aid of a pressure **reducing valve**. With a central gas supply, there is a lower pressure in the pipes (approx. 5 bar).

Oxygen source

Oxygen is often provided by means of tanks or cylinders. These are colour- and shape-coded, i.e. only the corresponding lines, couplings and cylinders match and can be connected easily. To connect the cylinder to the system, a 32 mm aluminium wrench is needed and should be attached to the anaesthesia machine for quick reaction in an emergency. Precautions must be taken when using gas cylinders:

- If the cylinders are to stand, they must be fixed absolutely tilt-proof. If this is not possible (e.g. after changing), the cylinder must be laid down, even if it is empty.
- Immediately mark empty cylinders so that they are not accidentally remounted on the unit.
- Observe storage instructions (store in a cool place, do not use grease or oil, no open fire, use protective cap)!

Practice tip

How long does O_2 in the cylinder last?
With a simple calculation you can work out the litres of oxygen that are still in the cylinder:

> Size of the cylinder (litres) × pressure (bar) = litres of oxygen in the cylinder

When a full 10 l cylinder of O_2 is mounted to the anaesthesia machine, the pressure gauge shows 200 bar. This means there are 2000 l of compressed O_2 in the cylinder. If one would continuously supply all patients with 2 l/min O_2, the O_2 would last for 1000 min, which is almost 17 h. The pressure decrease in the cylinder correlates linearly with the volume of O_2, i.e. if there is still 50 bar in the cylinder, there is still approx. 500 l of O_2 available.

Oxygen concentrator: O_2 from room air

Another way of providing oxygen that is quite suitable for small animal practice is "self-production" with the help of an oxygen concentrator. They are available at reasonable cost in veterinary supply stores and are practically maintenance- and wear-free. With a little skill, it can be connected to the anaesthesia machine or used for the permanent supply of hypoxaemic patients (via nasal probe or O_2 cage). Oxygen concentrators work with low pressure (flow rate of max. 5 or 10 l/min) and, depending on the device and flow rate, can extract up to a maximum of 95% O_2 from the room air, which is sufficient for the vast majority of patients and indications.

1.2.2 Medium pressure system

The medium pressure system (3–5 bar) includes central oxygen lines and the oxygen flush or bypass.

Oxygen flush or bypass

The oxygen (O_2) flush or bypass button is usually marked in an obvious way because it must be found quickly in emergency situations. It belongs to the so-called medium or working pressure system of the anaesthesia machine (with a pressure of up to 5 bar) and should therefore be operated with care when a patient is connected to the system. To be on the safe side, the patient can be disconnected from the system beforehand to avoid accidental barotrauma of the lungs. If the oxygen flush is used without first disconnecting the patient from the system, it must be ensured that no pressure builds up in the system: the pressure gauge in the breathing system should show no or hardly any pressure increase and the breathing bag, while inflating, should remain loosely filled.

When the button is pressed, pure oxygen flows into the breathing system of the anaesthesia machine at a rate of 25–75 l/min.

The oxygen flush is used to quickly
- fill the system, e.g. during a leak check or in case of a collapsed breathing bag,
- "wash out" inhalation anaesthetic, i. e. quickly reduce the anaesthetic gas concentration, e.g. in the event of an anaesthetic overdose.

Careful!

O_2 flush to fill the breathing bag
It can happen that the breathing bag collapses so much during anaesthesia that the patient can no longer take a breath (the reason is often a leak in the system, is the cuff properly inflated?).

In this case, the O_2 flush can be used to quickly fill the system. It is important to note that there is NO inhalation anaesthetic mixed with the oxygen, so the concentration in the system decreases rapidly. To prevent the patient from being too lightly under anaesthesia, it is often necessary to deepen the level of anaesthesia with IV anaesthetics, e.g. propofol (small animals), thiopental or ketamine (large animals).

1.2.3 Low pressure system

Vaporiser

The commonly used volatile anaesthetics isoflurane, sevoflurane and desflurane are liquid at standard conditions (temperature, air pressure). They must be vaporised in order to be administered by inhalation.

There are basically two types of vaporisers used for this purpose:

The **precision vaporisers** (▶ Fig. 1.6a), which are specifically calibrated to a particular anaesthetic (colour-coded), have a bypass, compensate for heat loss through vaporisation as well as ambient pressures and are placed outside the anaesthetic system (out-of-circuit). This has the advantage that they are relatively independent of the patient's fresh gas flow, temperature and breathing or ventilation modalities. Depending on their age, condition and maintenance, these vaporisers are still relatively expensive. Precision vaporisers can be operated with air, oxygen (always > 33%) and nitrous oxide as carrier gas.

The **universal vaporisers** (▶ Fig. 1.6b) are neither calibrated nor compensated for temperature or pressure. They can be used universally for all volatile anaesthetics and are placed in the inspiratory limb within the respiratory system (in-circuit). They are relatively simple in construction and therefore much cheaper than a precision vaporiser. Because of their (real and supposed) advantages, they are sometimes praised and still used in veterinary medicine. They should only be used by experienced anaesthetists on spontaneously breathing animals, as life-threatening high anaesthetic gas concentrations can quickly develop during manual or mechanical ventilation. Anaesthetic gas concentration, inspiratory and expiratory O_2 and CO_2 should always be monitored to

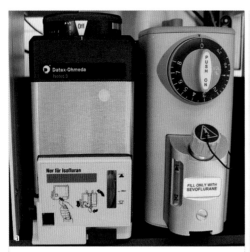

Fig. 1.6 Comparison of vaporisers.
a Precision vaporiser.
b Universal vaporiser.

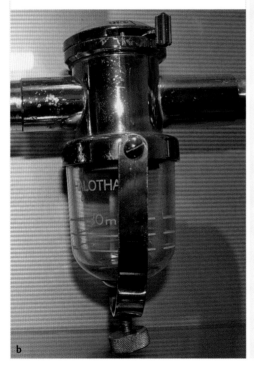

avoid complications. For safety reasons, only 100% oxygen should be used as a carrier gas. This type of vaporiser (e.g. Ohio 8, Komesaroff and Stephens) is no longer up-to-date today and is therefore no longer recommended.

Clinical relevance

Precision vaporiser for isoflurane or sevoflurane
- Operate with an accuracy of approx. 10% at an ambient temperature of 10 to 40 °C
- Are calibrated with air as the carrier gas. If 100% oxygen is used as the carrier gas, the concentration of the volatile anaesthetic (e.g. isoflurane) increases
- If a higher flow rate is used (e.g. 4 l/min instead of 1.5 l/min O_2), significantly more inhalation anaesthetic is used, although the concentration in the system is the same at both flow rates
- The carrier gas should always be at least 33% O_2

Desflurane Vaporiser
- Is temperature-compensated and is warmed up to 39 °C with the help of a power connection
- Operating temperature is reached after approx. 5–10 min. This is necessary to ensure uniform evaporation despite the special physical properties of desflurane

Good to know

Zero or off position, when not in use
If the vaporiser is not in operation or if no anaesthetic gas is to reach the patient, the adjusting wheel must be locked in the "zero" or "off" position. As long as it is not locked, a small amount of anaesthetic gas can enter the system even if the vaporiser is set to "0".

Practice tip

When the vaporiser is or was tilted ...

If the vaporiser tips over, the inhalation anaesthetic runs into the fresh gas by-pass in the vaporiser, where there should be no anaesthetic. This means that the anaesthetic can no longer be diluted and there is a risk of a massive over-dose in the next patient. Actually, in such a case, the vaporiser should be profes-sionally serviced before reuse. If this is not possible, one can help oneself (not state-of-the-art and only in an emergency!) by flushing the vaporiser for a few hours with a high flow of fresh gas (and of course without a patient on the sys-tem) and then have it serviced at the next opportunity.

Flowmeter

Gas flow of the carrier gas is adjusted via the flowmeter (or rotameter). In prin-ciple, the gas flows through a conical tube and moves the vertically movable float inside up and down depending on the mass flow. There are different types of floats which are read differently (▶ Fig. 1.7):
• A float in the shape of a ball is read at the equator.
• A float in the shape of a cylinder or hourglass is read at the upper edge.

Each flowmeter on the anaesthesia machine is calibrated for one carrier gas (oxygen, air or nitrous oxide). Oxygen should always be mounted last in the direction of flow, which minimises possible complications in case of breakage or malfunction of the other flowmeters.

The vaporiser and flowmeter belong to the so-called low-pressure system, which operates at a pressure just above atmospheric pressure. The gas mixture is then delivered to the breathing system via the **fresh gas outlet**.

1.3 Checking the anaesthesia machine

Before using the anaesthesia machine, the most important points should be checked:
• How much of oxygen (p. 31) is in the cylinder?
• Is there enough inhalation anaesthetic in the vaporiser (p. 33)?
• Is the soda lime (p. 28) functional?
• Is the exhaust functional or has the activated carbon filter (p. 29) been weighed to see if it is full?
• Have the hoses been cleaned and hung up to dry?

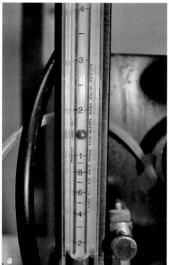

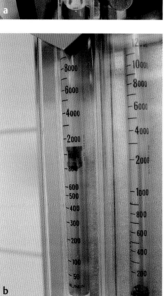

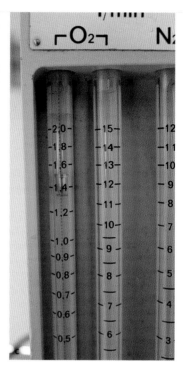

Fig. 1.7 Flowmeter with different floats, all set to 1.5 l/min flow rate.
a Ball.
b Cylinder without stabiliser.
c Cylinder with stabiliser.

1.3.1 Leak check

Before each use, the breathing system of the anaesthesia machine should be checked for leaks. In addition, the tightness should be checked if parts have been replaced, e.g. new CO_2 absorbent has been added or the oxygen cylinder has been changed. The anaesthesia machine must be completely assembled for the test.

1. Close the Y-piece. Most modern anaesthesia machines have a "parking place" which is used to attach and close the Y-piece.
2. Close the pressure relief valve. Do not use force, always close and open carefully.
3. Press the oxygen flush button until a pressure of 20 cmH$_2$O (small animals) or 30 cmH$_2$O (large animals) is reached on the pressure gauge – the flowmeter must not be turned on!
4. The pressure should be maintained for at least 10 seconds.
5. If there is no leak, the pressure relief valve is opened (quickly) and the pressure should immediately drop back to 0 cmH$_2$O.
6. However, if the pressure decreases during this time, the system has a leak. To determine how big the leak is, the flowmeter can be turned on to the point where the target pressure on the pressure gauge becomes constant again. The setting on the flowmeter then shows how much O_2/min is needed to compensate for the loss due to the leakage.

The leak is often found around the sealing rings of the unidirectional valves, at the soda lime canister or at the breathing bag. If you can't find it by listening, it may help to coat the suspect areas with liquid soap or soapy water. If the system is under pressure, bubbles will form at the leak.

If there is a leak in the system during anaesthesia with a patient, the cuff of the endotracheal tube (p. 153) is often not inflated far enough to seal the trachea. The cuff should always be inflated just enough to seal the trachea, but no further to avoid damaging the tracheal mucosa.

1.4 Literature

[1] Bednarski RM. Anesthetic breathing systems. Semin Vet Med Surg Small Anim 1993; 8:82–89
[2] McGowan LS, Macksey LF. Reducing the Carbon Footprint of Anesthesia: Low-Flow Anesthesia and Other Techniques. AANA J 2022; 90: 253–262. Erratum in: AANA J. 2022; 90: 386
[3] Muret J, Kelway C; Members of the SFAR's Sustainability Group French Society of Anaesthesia; Intensive Care. Why should anaesthesiologists and intensivists care about climate change? Anaesth Crit Care Pain Med 2019; 38: 565–567
[4] O'Shaughnessy SM, Mahon P. Compliance with the automated machine check. Anaesthesia 2015; 70: 1005–1006
[5] Wicker P, Smith B. Checking the anaesthetic machine. J Perioper Pract 2006; 16: 585–590

2 Monitoring

Monitoring during anaesthesia is extremely important to be able to assess the patient's condition. The correct interpretation of the monitored parameters helps to perform the anaesthesia safely, without too many fluctuations or even complications.

A differentiation can be made between non-apparatus and apparatus monitoring.

Clinical relevance

I have never had any problems and suddenly a patient dies on me!

Unfortunately, it can happen that an animal dies during or shortly after anaesthesia. The search for the cause is often unsatisfactory. However, a first question to ask oneself in all honesty is: Were there really no signs beforehand or did I simply not look and therefore overlook the looming complication? A critical evaluation of one's own monitoring routines can help to answer this question. Which monitoring (pulse oximetry, capnography, electrocardiography, blood pressure and temperature measurement) and which staff with which level of training are available to me? How often do I really look? What consequences or therapeutic measures follow if deviations are detected?

If necessary, management can be improved so that complications can be recognised and treated early on, so that life-threatening situations do not occur in the first place.

2.1 Non-apparatus monitoring

Non-apparatus monitoring includes the assessment of all parameters that can be detected with one's own senses, e.g. eyes, hands, ears and fingers.

2.1.1 Respiration, pulse and circulation

Respiration

Breathing should be evaluated by adspection (raising and lowering of the chest) and auscultation. Parameters that the experienced anaesthetist constantly assesses, almost subconsciously, are **respiratory rate** and **depth**, as well as **respiratory effort** and **sounds** (▶ Table 2.1). Any change gives clues to the depth of anaesthesia (e.g. an increasing respiratory rate often means that the anaesthesia is becoming more superficial) and the patient's condition (e.g. if the work of breathing increases, this often means problems!).

Table 2.1 Physiologic values respiratory rate and pulse rate

Species	RR/min	PR/min
Dog	10–40	80–120
Cat	20–30	108–132
Rabbit	32–100	120–330
Guinea pig	100–130	150–280
Ferret	30–60	120–260
Rat	70–150	200–500
Mouse	100–160	310–840
Hamster	35*–135	200*–500
Horse	10–14	28–40
Cattle	10–30	60–80
Sheep	16–30	60–80
Goat	10–30	60–80
Llama	10–30	60–80
Alpaca	10–30	60–90
Pig	15–30	70–120

RR respiratory rate, PR pulse rate
*during hibernation

An example: The work of breathing increases due to hypoxaemia, which can be caused, for example, by
a) Obstructed endotracheal tube
b) Pneumothorax with thoracic surgery
c) Increased dead space

The thoracic excursions or the movements of the breathing bag on the anaesthesia machine are assessed. The breathing type (costal vs. abdominal) or abnormal thoracic movements (e.g. flail chest) can also give an indication of deviations from the norm.

Pulse

By **palpating a peripheral artery**, the pulse rate, quality and regularity can be assessed (▶ Table 2.1). The rhythm should also be evaluated, arrhythmia can be an indication of cardiac problems. Filling and tension of the vessel provide information about the patient's volaemic status.

Heart and pulse rate should always both be assessed and compared with each other. If the heart rate is higher than the pulse rate, this is called a pulse deficit. A classic example of an arrhythmia causing a pulse deficit is bigeminy (p. 362) (every normal beat is followed by a ventricular extrasystole, which often does not lead to a cardiac contraction [= pulse]) after the administration of thiopental (p. 140).

Practice tip

Peripheral pulse palpable?

As a rule of thumb, if the peripheral pulse (e.g. at the metatarsal artery or the lingual artery) can still be felt, the mean arterial blood pressure (MAP) is probably still above 60 mmHg. If the peripheral pulse is no longer palpable, it can be assumed that the patient is severely hypotensive and the vital autoregulated organs (kidneys, heart and brain) are no longer perfused adequately. This evaluation is more reliable in the awake animal and can be influenced by anaesthetics.

Circulation/perfusion

Other clinical perfusion parameters besides **heart rate** and **pulse quality** are **capillary refill time**, which should be less than 2 sec, and **mucous membrane colour**. Any deviation from the physiological (pale) pink mucosal colour in non-pigmented animals is usually not physiological:

• Pale pink to white = vasoconstriction, hypoperfusion to shock, anaemia
• Red = vasodilation, (local) congestion, endotoxaemia
• Bright red = suspected carbon monoxide poisoning
• Blue-grey = cyanosis, hypoxaemia
• Yellow = jaundice, potentially liver damage

Temperature of the extremities is also a perfusion parameter. In the non-anaesthetised animal, the **state of consciousness** can also be evaluated. **Blood pressure**, also a perfusion parameter, must be measured using a blood pressure monitor.

Indirect clues of perfusion status may be provided by the surgical site: Tissue colour, colour and intensity of bleeding and the pressure in the vessels.

2.1.2 Reflexes and other non-apparatus monitoring

Reflexes

The **palpebral reflex** is one of the most commonly used reflexes for monitoring the depth of anaesthesia. It involves gently touching the medial canthus of the eye and observing whether the upper lid closes or not, or how fast the reaction is. In horses, you can also gently stroke the upper or lower eyelid along the lashes and assess the reaction.

The **corneal reflex** should not be part of the standard monitoring repertoire, as constant contact with the cornea can cause damage. Testing of this reflex should be reserved for emergencies, or when one wants to determine death (eyeball becomes "soft" in deceased animals).

The **pupillary reflex** is the reflexive adaptation of pupil width to different light conditions (bright/much light = pupil narrows/miosis; little light = pupil widens/mydriasis). There are anaesthetics that affect pupil size, in which case testing this reflex is not meaningful (e.g. opioids cause miosis in dogs and mydriasis in cats and horses). In animals that are very deeply anaesthetised, this reflex may be severely weakened or no longer present, even though the animal is still alive.

The **toe pinch reflex** is a classic reflex used in anaesthesia for small mammals. One gently pinches the interdigital space without causing injury and assesses the retraction of the limb. This reflex seems to stop first in the forelimbs and then in the hindlimbs in most species with the induction of anaesthesia.

The **anal reflex** is a good sign, e.g. after performing an epidural local anaesthesia, whether the local desensitisation works or not. If the sphincter muscle relaxes after injection of local anaesthetics into the epidural space, it can be assumed that the analgesic effect has begun. If the sphincter muscle contracts on contact, the analgesic effect has not (yet) set in. The anal reflex can also be evaluated in general during anaesthesia.

Response to stimuli

Reactions to painful stimuli can be varied: Increase in respiratory or heart rate, deeper breaths, increase in blood pressure or spontaneous movements are all signs of light anaesthesia.

Muscle tone

Muscle relaxation is one of the three components of general anaesthesia, along with **hypnosis** and **analgesia**. Increased muscle tone is therefore a clear sign that the depth of anaesthesia is too shallow. In small animals it is easy to test by evaluating the jaw tone (by opening and closing the jaw). In large animals, especially horses, the tone of the neck muscles is a good indicator. At the latest when an animal under general anaesthesia shows spontaneous movements, the muscle tone is definitely not as relaxed as it should be.

Ocular changes

The position of the eye (bulb position) is a good indicator of the stage of anaesthesia (p. 60).

Protrusion of the third eyelid is also a sign in anaesthesia. The third eyelid protrudes extremely in dogs and cats when acepromazine (p. 64) is used. You can practically tell from a distance that acepromazine has been administered.

In horses, tearing of the eyes is a sign of shallow anaesthesia. Often a strong palpebral reflex can be triggered at the same time.

2.2 Apparatus monitoring

2.2.1 Oesophageal stethoscope

The oesophageal stethoscope (▶ Fig. 2.1) is a tube with a membrane in a balloon that can be advanced over the oesophagus to above the base of the heart while listening to respiratory and cardiac sounds. Among the different tube sizes, it is necessary to choose so that the membrane lies against the oesophageal membrane. At the end of the tube there is an earpiece, like a conventional stethoscope, through which heart rate, rhythm, sounds and murmurs as well as respiratory rate, depth and sounds can be heard very well. The oesophageal

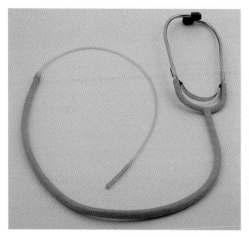

Fig. 2.1 Oesophageal stethoscope.

stethoscope performs well, especially when patients are completely draped for surgery and there is no longer access for auscultation of the heart. It can also be connected to a loudspeaker and expanded to perform electrocardiography and temperature measurement.

▶ Advantages
- Non-invasive and very easy to apply
- Cost effective
- Different sizes available (very thin tubes for cats, medium and thicker tubes for larger dogs)
- Easy to clean

▶ Disadvantages
- Should not be used in procedures on the head, in the oral cavity or in oesophageal surgery
- Cannot be used in large animals

2.2.2 Pulse oximeter

Pulse oximetry non-invasively and continuously determines the arterial (not capillary!) oxygen saturation (O_2 saturation) of haemoglobin by measuring the absorption of light in two (or more) different wavelengths.

On one side of the clip, (at least) two light-emitting diodes emit red (640 nm) and infrared (940 nm) light; on the other side, a photodetector picks up the light that has not been absorbed by tissue and blood. Oxyhaemoglobin (i. e. haemoglobin loaded with oxygen) mainly absorbs light with the wavelength 660 nm, deoxygenated haemoglobin (haemoglobin without oxygen) mainly absorbs light with the wavelength 940 nm. The absorption of static tissue is subtracted as "background noise" from the pulsatile (therefore **pulse** oximeter) absorption.

The ratio between the absorbed light of both wavelengths results in the O_2 saturation of the haemoglobin in the arterial (pulsatile) blood in percent (%). **Normal values in healthy animals are between 98 and 100%.**

In addition to oxygen saturation, the pulse oximeter indicates the pulse quality and rate and, if displayed plethysmographically, the waveform can provide information about the volaemic status of the animal: if the pulse wave is "compressed" during inspiratory positive pressure ventilation, this indicates hypovolaemia. No statement can be made about the "strength" of the pulse, as the devices improve the graphic representation so that even small (weak) waveforms are clearly visible.

The pulse oximeter sensor can be clamped basically anywhere an artery runs under hairless skin or non-pigmented mucous membrane: Tongue, lips, nasal septum, ear, prepuce, vulva, tail or knee folds, metatarsal or toe bones, interdigital fold, etc.

For small mammals (i. e. rodents), devices are needed that can measure pulse rates of up to 500 /min and also detect small pulse amplitudes. It is important to know the relationship between the oxygen saturation (%) measured with the pulse oximeter and the arterial oxygen partial pressure (p_aO_2) (most important values ▶ Table 2.2). This relationship can be represented by the oxyhaemoglobin dissociation curve (▶ Fig. 2.2). P_aO_2 is the actual value to be as-

Table 2.2 Corresponding values: Pulse oximetry (%) to arterial partial pressure of O_2 (p_aO_2 in mmHg) and their clinical significance

Value on pulse oximeter, oxygen saturation (%)	O_2 partial pressure in arterial blood* (mmHg)	Clinical significance
98–100	about 100	Normoxaemia
95	about 80	Hypoxaemia
90	about 60	Severe hypoxaemia

* at 21% inspiratory O_2 and at sea level

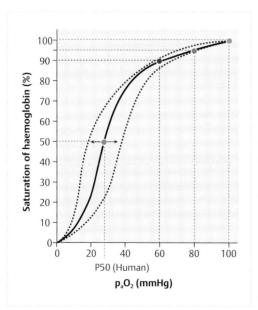

Fig. 2.2 Oxyhaemoglobin dissociation curve.

sessed. Based on the sigmoidal curve, a value of 90% on the pulse oximeter already corresponds to severe hypoxaemia, corresponding to an arterial O_2 partial pressure of 60 mmHg!

Clinical relevance

P50 value

The P50 value corresponds to the arterial pO_2 in mmHg (human: 27) at which 50% of the haemoglobin is saturated. It indicates where the curve is located and varies according to animal species; e.g. llamas are adapted to life at high altitude, the erythrocytes have a very high affinity for O_2, therefore their curve is shifted to the left.

The curve can be shifted to the right by

- ↑ Temperature
- ↑ CO_2 partial pressure
- ↑ H^+ ions (= ↓ pH)
- ↑ 2,3-BPG (biphosphoglycerate, an enzyme that influences the binding of O_2 to haemoglobin)

Right shift of the curve occurs e.g. through physical exercise. Right shift facilitates the unloading of O_2 into the tissue, which is useful during exercise and supports the supply of the tissue with oxygen.

Good to know

Inaccurate measurement with the pulse oximeter is possible due to

- Compression of the tissue by the sensor (partial compression of the artery); cause: sensors are often taken from human medicine and exert too much pressure on the tissue
- Pigmentation (light cannot freely penetrate the tissue, too much of the light is absorbed)
- Pulse is not detected (e.g. due to tremors, vasoconstriction, or hypotension)
- Drugs (e.g. alpha2 agonists cause strong vasoconstriction)
- Methaemoglobin (tends to measure towards 85% saturation, but is a false measurement)
- Carboxyhaemoglobin (COHb), which is carbon monoxide bound to haemoglobin, tends to show a reading of 98% even though the animal is oxygen deficient:

- COHb prevents the unloading of oxygen from haemoglobin into the tissues
- Oxygen is therefore there (hence the high reading) but cannot be made available to the tissues
- An animal with smoke inhalation can therefore suffer from severe hypox-aemia even though the pulse oximeter shows 98%
- Co-oximetry could be used to measure the proportion of COHb and O_2Hb

Careful!

Oxygen saturation does not equal oxygen content

IMPORTANT: **Oxygen saturation** does NOT give you any information about **oxygen content** in the blood! Oxygen content must be calculated using the following formula:

Oxygen content = (Haemoglobin [g/dl] × 1.36 × oxygen saturation [%])
+ (0.0031 × p_aO_2 [mmHg])

This means, among other things, that the tissue of a patient who displays an oxygen saturation of 100% is not automatically sufficiently supplied with oxygen. For this, there must also be sufficient transport capacity in the form of enough haemoglobin!

Complications or deviations from the norm are discussed in the chapter on "Hypoxaemia" (p. 378).

2.2.3 Non-invasive and invasive blood pressure measurement

Blood pressure measurement (in mmHg) is one of the most important and in-formative clinical monitoring parameters to assess the cardiovascular status of a patient. One can measure arterial blood pressure non-invasively (more practical, but not as reliable and meaningful) or invasively (not very practical, as it is costly, but continuous and reliable). In small mammals, measurement is often difficult or not possible at all. In dogs and cats as well as in large animals, especially horses under inhalation anaesthesia, perioperative blood pressure measurement should be part of the standard monitoring. This is especially true if longer procedures are planned.

The measurement should always be taken at the level of the base of the heart.

Non-invasive blood pressure measurement

There are two different methods to non-invasively measure arterial blood pressure:
• Oscillometric method
• Doppler sonography

Both methods work according to the **Riva-Rocci principle**, in which the blood flow in an extremity is occluded with a cuff and the return of the blood flow is detected.

Oscillometric method

The oscillometric method works according to the **Riva-Rocci principle** with an automatically inflating and deflating cuff fitted around an extremity. The width of the cuff should be about **30–40% of the limb circumference** and should be selected appropriately depending on the device (see instruction manual!) and animal species. The inflatable part should be placed over an artery.

Actually, only the mean arterial pressure (MAP) is measured, the systolic and diastolic blood pressure is then calculated with complicated (and secret) algorithms. That is (among other reasons) why MAP is probably the most reliable of the three values.

Good to know

Potential causes for incorrect values in oscillometric blood pressure measurement
• Too small cuff: falsely overestimates the blood pressure, thus shows falsely high values
• Too large cuff: falsely underestimates the blood pressure, thus shows falsely low values
• Incorrect positioning of the cuff (inflatable part not over the artery)
• Severe hypo- or hypertension of the patient
• Strong vasoconstriction (e.g. due to alpha2 agonists or hypothermia)
• Severe arrhythmia, extreme bradycardia or tachycardia
• Thick fur coat on the extremities
• "Dachshund legs": with short and thickly muscled extremities, the measurement does not always seem to be reliable
• Movement, tremors, spasms or vibration
• Strongly bent or too tightly bound limbs

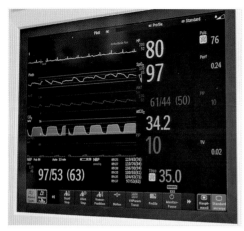

Fig. 2.3 Discrepancy between invasive (61/44 (50) mmHg) and non-invasive blood pressure measurement (97/53 (63) mmHg) in a clinical situation.

The readings obtained with the oscillometric method must always be assessed in the overall context and with clinical judgement. It may happen that the displayed values appear real but are far from the actual values (▶ Fig. 2.3).

Taping the cuff – yes or no?

It is important for a valid measurement that the cuff lies flat on the limb and that it does not "slip down" over a joint, which can easily happen especially with short muscled legs. A short piece of tape may be able to prevent this. However, the tape must never be so tight that the cuff can no longer inflate or the vessels underneath are occluded.

Doppler sonography

In this method, the **Doppler crystal** is applied directly distal to a **cuff** over an extremity artery (▶ Fig. 2.4). For this, one should clip the fur and use lubricant gel. The Doppler crystal is fixed to the limb with tape over the artery. Proximal to the crystal, a cuff with the appropriate size and with attached sphygmomanometer (pressure gauge) is attached around the limb and inflated until the sound caused by erythrocytes flowing past the crystal stops. Then the pressure is slowly released from the cuff. As soon as the blood flow returns (= recurring

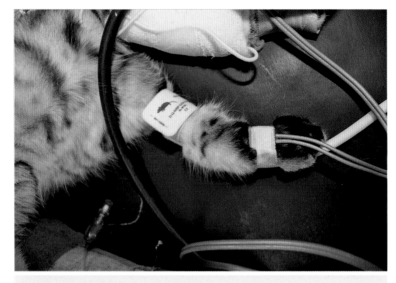

Fig. 2.4 Typical position of Doppler crystal and cuff in a cat.

sound) is heard again, the systolic blood pressure can be read on the pressure gauge. The Doppler can cause disturbing noises, in which case it is recommended to use headphones.

You can measure as often as you like, so the method is conditionally continuous. However, one **should not measure more frequently than every 2.5 to 3 min** with either method in order not to jeopardise adequate perfusion of the limb.

The measurements are quite reliable, even in cases of hypo- or hypertension and in case of doubt with the oscillometric device, the Doppler method should be used for re-measurement. In cats, the Doppler method underestimates the true systolic blood pressure, the measured pressure is therefore more similar to the mean arterial blood pressure.

In addition to measuring blood pressure, the Doppler crystal can also be used to measure the heart rate of exotic animals such as reptiles, birds or small mammals. To do this, the crystal is placed over an artery or directly over the heart. The sound itself provides additional information about changing haemodynamic conditions.

With both non-invasive blood pressure measurement techniques, **the trend of the blood pressure over time is more meaningful than the individual value**.

Invasive blood pressure measurement

The invasive method is also called direct blood pressure measurement and is more expensive and more complex than non-invasive methods. However, it is considered the "gold standard".

A fluid-filled catheter and tubing system transmits the pulse wave, which is taken directly through a catheter in a peripheral artery, to the pressure transducer (▶ Fig. 2.5). The transducer then "translates" the mechanical pressure wave into an electrical signal and transmits this to the monitor. The blood pressure waveform is continuously displayed graphically on the monitor. The infusion bag (usually filled with heparinised 0.9% NaCl), which is pressurised with the help of an inflatable pressure bag, prevents the arterial blood from running back into the tubing system. The tubing system has particularly rigid walls so that the pulse wave is not buffered by the system and thus partially lost. It is available as a set including the transducer.

With the invasive blood pressure measurement, the systolic and diastolic blood pressure can be measured exactly and the mean arterial blood pressure is calculated. The result is continuously displayed graphically as a blood pressure curve (▶ Fig. 2.6, orange).

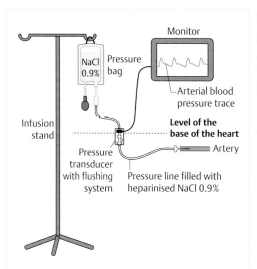

Fig. 2.5 Set-up for invasive blood pressure measurement.

Monitor

NaCl 0.9% | Pressure bag

Arterial blood pressure trace

Infusion stand

Level of the base of the heart

Artery

Pressure transducer with flushing system

Pressure line filled with heparinised NaCl 0.9%

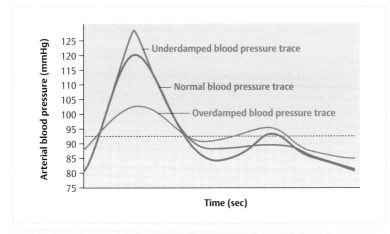

Fig. 2.6 Blood pressure curves: normal (orange), overdamped (green) and underdamped (blue).

Before starting the measurement, the system must be "zeroed" against ambient pressure. To do this, the 3-way stopcock on the transducer needs to be turned so that the transducer is open to the environment. Then "zero" on the monitor has to be pressed until the monitor shows (0), i. e. zero. The transducer must be positioned at the level of the base of the heart.

There is a risk of infection when a catheter is placed in an artery and connected to a system. For this reason, special attention must be paid to cleanliness and asepsis. The access can be used for taking arterial blood samples for blood gas analysis as part of perioperative management. However, the catheter should be removed after 3 days at the latest, or earlier if there are signs of infection.

Good arterial accesses in small animals are the dorsal metatarsal, palmar and auricular arteries. In large animals, the lateral metatarsal artery, facial artery, transverse facial artery and auricular artery have proven effective. The arterial catheter must be clearly marked and labelled to prevent accidental injection of drugs or similar.

Invasive blood pressure measurement should be used in
- Emergency or high-risk patients
- Longer, complicated procedures in small animals
- Longer procedures under inhalation anaesthesia in large animals

Good to know

Potential causes for incorrect measurement during invasive blood pressure measurement:

- Overdamping (curve looks damped and soft) due to e.g. an air bubble, blood, thrombus or kink in the tubing system: systolic blood pressure is underestimated, diastolic pressure is overestimated, MAP remains the same (▶ Fig. 2.6, green)
- Underdamping (curve looks exaggeratedly jagged and sharp) due to e.g. the use of tubing systems with soft walls that cause a vibration in the fluid column: systolic blood pressure is greatly overestimated, diastolic pressure is underestimated, MAP again remains relatively the same (▶ Fig. 2.6, blue)
- Transducer is not at the level of the base of the heart
- Incorrect calibration to ambient pressure ("zeroing")
- Vasoconstriction

If the measurement is incorrect, it often helps to flush the arterial catheter by hand (not with the transducer system, which also has a flushing function, but which flushes fluid into the artery quite uncontrollably and with high pressures), recalibrate to the ambient pressure and reposition the transducer to the level of the base of the heart.

2.2.4 Electrocardiography

The **electrocardiogram** (ECG) continuously displays the electrical activity at the heart and the heart rate (▶ Fig. 2.7). It should be noted that no information about the actual contraction of the heart muscle is provided. An animal can in fact be pulseless (= dead) for minutes and the ECG still looks more or less normal.

Using the ECG as a perioperative cardiac monitoring tool is not about being able to perform a professional ECG assessment like a cardiologist. Rather, it is about being able to

1. Distinguish a physiological or "normal" ECG from a pathological or "non-normal" ECG, and possibly to know the cause of the pathological ECG
2. Decide whether the pathological ECG requires treatment
3. Initiate appropriate therapy if necessary

The ECG electrodes are placed on the patient via **needle electrodes** (small pets), **adhesive ECG pads** (small animals), **alligator** or **flat clips** (small and large animals) or highly elegant with an **oesophageal probe** (which may also

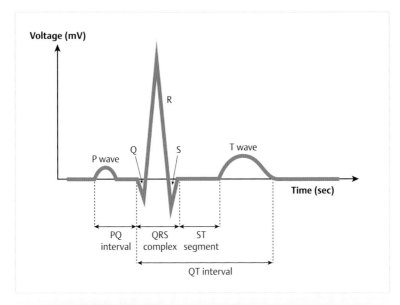

Fig. 2.7 Physiological ECG lead.

include a thermometer, small animals). In veterinary medicine, 3-electrode conduction is sufficient for perioperative monitoring, emergency and intensive care medicine. The positioning is specified by colour coding.

Good to know

Colour coding of ECG leads
- Red electrode = Right forelimb
- Yellow electrode = Left forelimb
- Green or black electrode = Left hindlimb

If the limbs are not available or it is impractical to place the electrodes accordingly, a comparable position can also be chosen (e.g. the right neck or chest area instead of the right forelimb). The transoesophageal ECG is available for some monitoring devices, which is advanced through the oesophagus to above the base of the heart and so does not need to be attached to the exterior of the animal at all.

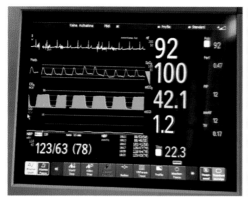

Fig. 2.8 ECG artefact (irregular spikes) caused by use of monopolar cautery.

Unfortunately, ECG monitoring is relatively susceptible to interference and artefacts occasionally occur (▶ Fig. 2.8). With a little routine, however, you can recognise many of these artefacts and eliminate the cause.

Good to know

Artefacts in the ECG can be caused by:
- Detached electrodes or electrodes that do not have sufficient contact with the animal; the contact of clamps can be improved e.g. with alcohol on the fur
- The "crossing" of cables or interference with nearby electrical equipment; the alternating current can cause the so-called 50 Hertz interference, which looks similar to atrial flutter
- Muscle tremors, spasms or movement of the patient
- Electrical interference with other devices such as monopolar cautery (▶ Fig. 2.8)

Normal ECG traces as well as some of the most important arrhythmias that are common during anaesthesia can be found under "Arrhythmias" (p. 354).

2.2.5 Capnography

Capnography can be used to measure the CO_2 partial pressure (pCO_2 in mmHg) in respiratory gases and respiratory rate, and depending on the technical equipment of the device, possibly additional parameters such as O_2 and volatile

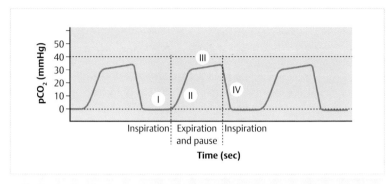

Fig. 2.9 Normal capnography waveform. I = inspiration, II = start expiration, III = plateau phase, IV = start inspiration.

anaesthetic concentrations, airway pressures and tidal volume (multi-gas analysers).

A distinction is made between **capnography**, in which the values are shown graphically with a curve on a display over time (▶ Fig. 2.9), from **capnometry**, where only the end-tidal CO_2 value (**etCO₂**) is displayed as a number.

The normal capnography waveform has four different phases:

- **Phase I:** Inspiration, baseline, zero pCO_2
- **Phase II:** Start of expiration, pCO_2 rises rapidly
- **Phase III:** Plateau phase, expiration of alveolar air, pCO_2 rises only very slightly until the end of expiration is reached: the highest pCO_2 value corresponds to the **end-tidal CO_2 value** (**etCO₂**), which is similar to the alveolar and thus the arterial value (but slightly lower)
- **Phase IV:** Beginning of inspiration, pCO_2 decreases rapidly; examples of variations from the normal waveform and their interpretation can be found in the chapter "Abnormal waveforms in capnography" (p. 375).

A requirement for a good measurement is endotracheal intubation, a laryngeal mask airway or a fixed mask over the mouth/snout/nose. This non-invasive measurement technique provides valuable information about gas exchange or ventilation and indirectly about the circulatory status of the patient.

Good to know

False measurements of multi-gas analysers in horses and ruminants
Particularly in ruminants, methane gases can develop during digestion. In infrared multi-gas analysers, methane cannot be distinguished from inhalation anaesthetics. Therefore, a "measurement" of non-real high values of the inhalation anaesthetics occurs.

The **normal value of CO_2** (= **normocapnia**) defines **normoventilation** and varies from animal to animal and is **about 30–45 mmHg** in arterial blood (= p_aCO_2, ▸ Table 2.3). In venous blood, the pCO_2 is approx. 5–10 mmHg higher (= p_vCO_2), in exhaled air it is approx. 5–10 mmHg lower than in arterial blood (▸ Table 2.3).

A **low etCO$_2$** (= **hypocapnia**) is defined as **hyperventilation** (p. 373). If the etCO$_2$ is low, it can also be a sign of impending circulatory failure (the blood is no longer transported to the lungs, CO_2 remains in the tissues, less is exhaled although it accumulates in the body). A low etCO$_2$ can also be a sign of a pulmonary embolism or a blocked endotracheal tube.

An **increased etCO$_2$** (= **hypercapnia**) is defined as **hypoventilation** (p. 369), i.e. the animal breathes out too little CO_2 and the partial pressure increases. CO_2 is often (slightly) elevated in anaesthetised animals due to the nature of general anaesthesia and for other reasons, which can be tolerated to some extent in most cases. If etCO$_2$ rises during anaesthesia above a certain level, intermittent positive pressure ventilation must be considered. If it increases for unexplained reasons, malignant hyperthermia (p. 384) must be considered as a (rare but existing) differential diagnosis. Besides hyperthermia, an increased etCO$_2$ is one of the first signs of this disease.

Table 2.3 Reference values partial pressure CO_2 in mmHg

	Cat	Dog	Horse
Arterial	28–32	36–44	45–50
Venous	34–38	32–49	about 5–10 mmHg higher than arterial values
Endtidal	Arterial values minus 5–10	Arterial values minus 5–10	Arterial values minus 5–10*

* Gradient can increase significantly under inhalation anaesthesia.

2.2.6 Temperature measurement

The measurement of core body temperature in °C is easy to perform via a rectal or oesophageal probe (▶ Table 2.4). Clinically useful are digital thermometers that display a reading within 10 seconds. For continuous measurement of small animal patients under anaesthesia, a temperature probe can be permanently inserted into the oesophagus or the rectum, protected by a plastic cover, and taped to the tail (▶ Fig. 2.10). This would also avoid disturbing the awake animal to measure temperature, e. g. in intensive care patients.

Good to know

Incorrect temperature measurement is possible if ...
- the probe has slipped out unnoticed,
- there is a lot of faeces in the rectum during a rectal measurement,
- the measurement is taken rectally after a rectal lavage,
- the oesophageal probe is in the stomach and the abdomen is opened and/or lavaged with irrigation solutions.

Table 2.4 Physiologic values for core body temperature

Species	°C
Dog	38.0–39.0
Cat	38.0–39.3
Rabbit	38.5–40.0
Guinea pig	37.2–39.5
Ferret	37.8–40.0
Rat	37.0–39.5
Mouse	35.0–39.0
Hamster	37.0–38.0
Horse	37.5–38.0
Cattle	38.3–38.8
Sheep	38.5–39.5
Goat	38.3–39.0
Llama	37.5–38.9
Alpaca	36.4–37.8
Pig	38.3–39.0

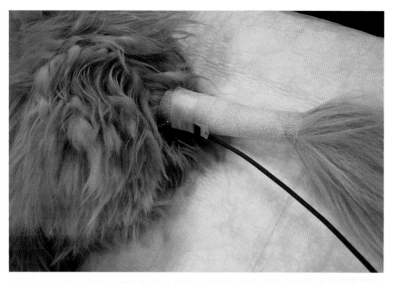

Fig. 2.10 Permanently rectally inserted temperature probe in an intensive care patient.

2.3 Literature

[1] Caulkett NA, Cantwell SL, Houston DM. A comparison of indirect blood pressure monitoring techniques in the anesthetized cat. Vet Surg 1998; 27: 370–7

[2] Grandy JL, Dunlop CI, Hodgson DS, Curtis CR, Chapman PL. Evaluation of the Doppler ultrasonic method of measuring systolic arterial blood pressure in cats. Am J Vet Res 1992; 53: 1166–9

[3] Grandy JL, Steffey EP, Miller M. Arterial blood pO_2 and pCO_2 in horses during early halothane-oxygen anaesthesia. Equine Vet J 1987; 19: 314–318

[4] Oblouk Darovic G, Vanriper S, Vanriper J. Fluid filled monitoring systems. In: Hemodynamic monitoring – invasive and noninvasive clinical application. Oblouk Darovic G (Ed.), Philadelphia: Saunders 2002; 149–175

[5] Wagner AE, Brodbelt DC. Arterial blood pressure monitoring in anesthetized animals. J Am Vet Med Assoc 1997; 210: 1279–85

3 Stages of general anaesthesia

During anaesthesia, the depth of anaesthesia should be continuously assessed and adjusted: "As light as possible, as deep as necessary". This prevents on the one hand "waking up" or movement due to a too light level of anaesthesia and on the other hand cardiovascular and respiratory collapse in case of overdose. Four stages of general anaesthesia can be distinguished; each stage has characteristic features.

All stages of anaesthesia are passed through from 1 to 4 if high doses are used. The length of time the animal is in each stage depends partly on the type and dose of drugs used, or the type or speed of application. Ideally, the anaesthetist should be able to **stabilize the animal quickly in stage 3.2** which represents a level of anaesthesia adequate for painful procedures.

When waking up from (deep) anaesthesia, all stages are passed through again in reverse order. Here, it is desirable to go through stage 2 as quickly as possible in order to avoid unattractive excitation phases with vocalisations or dangerous moments with uncontrolled movements in the recovery phase (especially important in horses and other large animals).

3.1 Stage 1 or analgesia stage

All reflexes are preserved, but possibly delayed. Intubation, for example, is still absolutely impossible because the coughing reflex is still present. The bulb is central, the pupils are dilated, but this also depends on the anaesthetics administered. Clinically, a prolapse of the third eyelid, yawning or whimpering is seen in dogs and cats. In large animals, the head lowers, movement of the ears decreases and the lower lip becomes relaxed. Although the stage is called "analgesia stage", animals may still feel pain (depending on what medication has been administered). The patient's appearance depends to a large extent on its temperament.

3.2 Stage 2 or excitation stage

In stage 2, the animal loses its voluntary control and the reactions to external stimuli are uncontrolled, unpredictable and unexpected. Reflexes begin to be delayed. The bulb is still central, pupils are very dilated (as already mentioned, this also depends on the medication given), sometimes nystagmus is visible (very obvious in the horse). Muscles may begin to twitch or become stiff. Animals may suffer from nausea.

Good to know

Good induction of and recovery from general anaesthesia = short stage 2
In the process of a good, calm induction of and recovery from anaesthesia, stage 2 is passed through very quickly, practically undetectable. There is never any nystagmus or muscle rigidity, nor is the patient uncontrolled or uncontrollable. Good and adequate preanaesthetic sedation is usually the decisive factor for this.

3.3 Stage 3 or surgical stage

Stage 3 is again divided into three stages, which are passed through fluidly as the anaesthesia deepens.

3.3.1 Stage 3.1: Light anaesthesia

If patients are not stimulated at this stage (pain, movement, noise), they lie still and relaxed. Often this stage is sufficient for diagnostic procedures such as an ultrasound examination or computer tomography. The respiratory and heart rate slows down, the bulb is central or begins to rotate down and the pupils are normally wide or constricted. Muscle tone is potentially decreased but not necessarily relaxed yet. Palpebral reflex is positive.

3.3.2 Stage 3.2: Surgical tolerance

At this stage, intubation can be performed and most surgical procedures or other painful stimuli are tolerated. There is no response to a painful or unpleasant stimulus. All other characteristics are basically the same but even more pronounced than in stage 3.1. The bulb is rotated down or begins to rotate in a central position again. The pupils are normally wide or constricted. Muscles are completely relaxed. Palpebral reflex is negative.

3.3.3 Stage 3.3: Deep anaesthesia

In this stage, there is a complete lack of reflex response. The bulb is in a central position and the pupils are dilated. Breathing becomes shallow, irregular and slow. Heart rate decreases. Mucous membranes slowly become cyanotic, vital organs are not sufficiently supplied with oxygen. Muscles are completely relaxed.

3.4 Stage 4 or asphyxia

Basically, an animal that is at this stage is overdosed and aiming straight for cardiovascular and respiratory collapse. The overdose causes maximum depression of the central nervous system. Respiratory depression can lead to respiratory arrest. The circulation deteriorates to the point of shock. Pulses are weak, blood pressure is low and the heart rate continues to decrease. The bulb is in a central position, pupils are maximally dilated and pupillary reflex is weak or can no longer be triggered. If the level of anaesthesia is not immediately reduced and resuscitation procedure started, the animal will die.

4 Drugs

This chapter lists a selection of drugs used in veterinary anaesthesia in **alphabetical order**. In addition to the pharmacokinetics, the effects and indications for use, as well as contraindications, precautions and adverse effects are briefly described. Other important information is summarised under "Miscellaneous". For each drug, the recommended dosages for the treated species are presented in tabular form. The clinical use in the individual animal species is additionally described under "Species-specific anaesthesia" (p. 150).

Country-specific laws and licensing must be complied with at all times.

4.1 Basic information on pharmacotherapy

Drugs should always be selected and dosed individually for the patient. The drug itself, the desired effect and the patient more or less dictate the mode of application.

Some basic rules apply to the dosage:
- A higher dose per kg is usually required in
  - excited compared to calm animals,
  - healthy compared to sick animals,
  - young and middle-aged compared to very young and old animals,
  - small compared to large animals and
  - patients in which you want a stronger effect.
- Subcutaneous (SC) and intramuscular (IM) dosing is often slightly higher than intravenous (IV) dosing.
- Different animal species and even different breeds of an animal species may require significantly different dosages.
- When anaesthetics are combined, one can usually reduce the respective dose.

In addition, there are **patient-dependent factors** that influence the dosage and choice of medication, these are e.g.:
- **Hypoproteinaemia**
  - Many drugs are bound to proteins and are then inactive; less protein in the plasma also means a higher free (active) fraction of the drug.
- **Core body temperature**
  - For every 1 °C loss in temperature from physiological body temperature, the minimum alveolar concentration (MAC) of isoflurane (p. 102) decreases by 5%, i.e. one needs 5% less inhalation anaesthetic to reach the same endpoint.

Definition

Effect, potency and affinity of anaesthetics using the example of opioids

The **effect** is usually understood as the desired effect, i. e. analgesia or sedation in case of opioids.

The **potency** indicates how much (i. e. what dose per kg) is needed to obtain the (maximum) desired effect.

The higher the **affinity** of a drug to its receptor, the more tightly it binds. This gives an indication of 1. which drug will ultimately exert the effect at the receptor and 2. how long the duration of action is.

For example, buprenorphine (p. 76) is significantly less analgesic than morphine (i. e. has a lesser effect). However, it is more potent (i. e. you need a lower dose per kg to achieve the maximum effect). And finally, it has a higher affinity to the receptor, so it would displace morphine from it and has a longer duration of action.

Each syringe into which a drug is drawn up must be clearly **labelled** with the name of the drug. For diluted or mixed drugs (but better for all drugs), the **concentration** and **date** must also be written on the syringe.

4.2 Acepromazine

- **Phenothiazine derivative**
- **Neuroleptic, tranquiliser**

▶ Pharmacokinetics
- Alpha1 receptor antagonist (vasodilation)
- Dopamine2 receptor antagonist (hypothermia, antiemetic effect)
- Histamine1 receptor antagonist (calming down)
- **Onset of effect:** IV 15 min, IM 20 min, SC 30 min, PO 1 h or longer (takes a very long time, no emergency drug!)
- **Duration of effect:** 3–6 h

▶ Effects
- Calming down, sedation (dampening of the CNS without hypnotic effect; "pink cloud")
- Antiemetic
- Anxiolytic
- Antiarrhythmic

▶ **Indications**
- Calming down, sedation (resolving defensive movements during examinations, etc.)
- Calming in stressful situations, transport or similar
- Premedication
- In combination with local anaesthesia for minor procedures
- In combination with opioids (= neuroleptanalgesia) as premedication
- Antiemetic in the context of anaesthesia, travel sickness (**dog**, **cat**)

▶ **Contraindications/precautions**
- Hypotensive or hypovolaemic patients (e.g. after severe blood loss)
- Shock
- Impaired liver function

Careful!

Breed specific sensitivity
(White) Boxer dogs of a breeding line from Great Britain seem to react very sensitively with severe hypotension and shock to the administration of even low-dose acepromazine. However, there is no scientific proof yet.

▶ **Adverse effects**
- Hypotension due to vasodilation
- Hypothermia due to vasodilation and inhibition of temperature regulation
- Paradoxical effect in very aggressive animals (disinhibition)
- Decreases platelet aggregation without affecting homeostasis
- Adrenalin reversal (= reduction instead of increase in blood pressure after adrenalin administration)
- Low risk of priapism (= penile prolapse) in **stallions** (a recent study shows that it is okay to use acepromazine in stallions as well)

▶ **Miscellaneous**
- Temporarily decreases haematocrit by accumulating erythrocytes in the spleen; however, it seems to be a suitable drug for laparoscopic surgery (spleen size is relatively small compared to other protocols)
- **No analgesic effect!**
- No attenuation of respiratory function (possibly initial panting) at low doses
- No change in heart rate, possibly reflex tachycardia at higher doses

Table 4.1 Dosages for acepromazine (mg/kg)

Species	IV	IM/SC	PO
Dog	0.01–0.05	0.01–0.05, up to 0.5	1–2
Cat	0.05–0.2	0.05–0.2	1–2
Rabbit	–	0.1–0.5 (up to 2)	–
Ferret	0.05–0.3	0.1–0.3	–
Horse	0.01–0.05	0.01–0.05	–
Sheep/goat	0.03–0.05	0.05–0.1	–

IV intravenous, IM intramuscular, SC subcutaneous, PO orally

- Contrary to earlier opinion, it does not lower seizure threshold or trigger seizures in patients with a history of seizures, but is even able to suppress seizure activity
- Can be wonderfully combined with opioids (butorphanol, methadone) as premedication for anxious dogs and cats

▶ Dosages
- Dosages are listed in ▶ Table 4.1
- **Observe maximum dosages** regardless of the route of administration:
  - **Dog** 3 mg/animal
  - **Cat** 1 mg/animal
  - **Horse** 20 mg/animal

▶ Literature

[1] Driessen B, Zarucco L, Kalir B, Bertolotti L. Contemporary use of acepromazine in the anaesthetic management of male horses and ponies: a retrospective study and opinion poll. Equine Vet J 2011; 43: 88–98
[2] Eberspächer E, Baumgartner C, Henke J, Erhardt W. Invasive Blutdruckmessung nach intramuskulärer Verabreichung von Acepromazin als Narkoseprämedikation beim Hund. Tierärztl Prax (K) 2005; 33: 27–31
[3] Tobias KM, Marioni-Henry K, Wagner R. A retrospective study on the use of acepromazine maleate in dogs with seizures. J Am Anim Hosp Assoc 2006; 42: 283–9
[4] Wilson DV, Evans AT, Carpenter RA, Mullineaux DR. The effect of anesthetic protocols on splenic size in dogs. Vet Anaesth Analg 2004; 31: 102–108

4.3 Alfaxalone

- **Steroid anaesthetic, neurosteroid**
- **Hypnotic**

▶ Pharmacokinetics
- Interacts with the GABA$_A$ receptor, enhances GABAergic neurotransmission
- Further mechanisms of action are suspected
- **Onset of effect:** IV within 1–2 min, IM 5–10 min (licenced only for IV use)
- **Duration of effect:** IV bolus about 10 min

▶ Effects
- Hypnosis
- Muscle relaxation

▶ Indications
- Intramuscular sedation/premedication of aggressive or older, sick **cats**; good in combination with midazolam and/or butorphanol
- Good **alternative to propofol** for IV induction of anaesthesia in cats for anaesthesia that has to be repeated daily (e.g. for dressing changes, radiotherapy or similar) or **anaemic cats** (does not cause Heinz bodies, p. 183)
- Anaesthesia induction of **foals, sheep, goats** (observe legal regulations!)

▶ Contraindications/precautions
- **Caution with rapid IV administration of high doses:** risk of apnoea, should be able to intubate

▶ Adverse effects
- Fewer cardiovascular effects than e.g. propofol
- Peripheral vasodilation, resulting in hypotension
- Respiratory depression, after rapid IV application also apnoea
- Overall restless recovery phases, possibly vocalisations, it helps when benzodiazepines are also administered during induction
- Muscle twitching, body movements, opisthotonos in the induction or recovery phase, especially without premedication and in a noisy environment

▶ Miscellaneous
- Very well suited for **"exotic"** and **wild animals**
- Disadvantage of off-label IM application for larger cats and dogs is the large volume and the high price

Table 4.2 Dosages for alfaxalone (mg/kg)

Species	IV	IM
Dog	1–2 (5)	1–5
Cat	1–2 (5)	1–5
Rabbit	2–3	5
Guinea pig	2–3	5
Ferret	2–3	5
Small rodents	2–3	5
IV intravenous, IM intramuscular		

▶ **Dosages**
- Dosages are listed in ▶ Table 4.2
- Titrate slowly to effect intravenously over 60 s
- Can be administered as continuous rate infusion in **dogs** and **cats**: 6–8 mg/kg/h
- It does not really accumulate in the body and is easy to titrate

▶ **Literature**

[1] Kalchofner Guerrero KS, Reichler IM, Schwarz A, Jud RS, Hässig M, Bettschart-Wolfensberger R. Alfaxalone or ketamine-medetomidine in cats undergoing ovariohysterectomy: a comparison of intra-operative parameters and post-operative pain. Vet Anaesth Analg 2014; 41: 644–653

[2] Maney JK, Shepard MK, Braun C, Cremer J, Hofmeister EH. A comparison of cardiopulmonary and anesthetic effects of an induction dose of alfaxalone or propofol in dogs. Vet Anaesth Analg 2013; 40: 237–44

[3] Muir W, Lerche P, Wiese A, Nelson L, Pasloske K, Whittem T. Cardiorespiratory and anesthetic effects of clinical and supraclinical doses of alfaxalone in dogs. Vet Anaesth Analg 2008; 35: 451–62

[4] Warne LN, Beths T, Whittem T, Carter JE, Bauquier SH. A review of the pharmacology and clinical application of alfaxalone in cats. Vet J 2015; 203: 141–148

4.4 Amantadine

- **NMDA receptor antagonist**
- **Dopamine receptor agonist**

▶ **Pharmacokinetics**
- Originally used as a drug against influenza caused by influenza A viruses and in the treatment of Parkinson's disease
- Acts as a weak NMDA receptor antagonist similar to ketamine and increases dopamine concentration in the brain
- It reduces central sensitisation

- **Onset of effect:** Soon initial effect, but takes long (days to weeks) for maximum effect
- **Duration of effect:** Should be administered as a long-term medication in chronic pain patients, at least 21 days

▶ Effects
- Antihyperalgesia (caused by neuropathic pain)

▶ Indications
- Can be a component in multimodal analgesia for small animal patients with chronic neuropathic pain, e.g. osteoarthritis or tumour pain

▶ Contraindications/precautions
- Few clinical studies are available in companion animals
- Do not use in untreated glaucoma patients (human medicine)
- Caution in patients with impaired liver or kidney function and congestive heart failure

▶ Adverse effects
- Little known; possible side effects are agitation, soft faeces and diarrhoea

▶ Miscellaneous
- **Amantadine is primarily not an analgesic!** It reduces the central sensitisation caused by chronic pain; this is an important component of pain that should be treated as part of a multimodal approach; it therefore works best in combination with "real" analgesics
- Works particularly well in combination with NSAIDs for pain caused by osteoarthritis
- Can also be combined well with opioids
- May cause less weakness in the hindlimbs than gabapentin in long-term administration

▶ Dosages
- Dosages are listed in ▶ Table 4.3
- Pharmacokinetically, splitting the dose into two doses per day seems to be better than the previously recommended single dose
- The duration of treatment should be long in order to permanently reduce central sensitisation; 21 days would be good, longer would be better; some patients may benefit from lifelong administration
- After discontinuation of amantadine, the effect lasts for about 24 hours

Table 4.3 Dosages for amantadine (mg/kg)

Species	PO
Dog	3–5 SID-BID
Cat	3–5 SID-BID
PO orally, SID 1 × daily, BID 2 × daily	

▶ **Literature**

[1] Bleidner WE, Harmon JB, Hewes WE, Lynes TE, Hermann EC. Absorption, distribution and excretion of amantadine hydrochloride. J Pharmacol Exp Ther 1965; 150: 484–90

[2] Lascelles BD, Gaynor JS, Smith ES, Roe SC, Marcellin-Little DJ, Davidson G, Boland E, Carr J. Amantadine in a multimodal analgesic regimen for alleviation of refractory osteoarthritis pain in dogs. J Vet Intern Med 2008; 22: 53–9

[3] Siao KT, Pypendop BH, Stanley SD, Ilkiw JE. Pharmacokinetics of amantadine in cats. J Vet Pharmacol Ther 2011; 34: 599–604

4.5 Atipamezole

- **Alpha2 receptor antagonist**

▶ **Pharmacokinetics**
- Selective and specific **alpha2 antagonist** with high affinity to the receptor
- **Onset of effect:** IV 2–3 min, IM/SC 3–10 min; **IM application is recommended** because the onset of action after IV administration can be very rapid with vocalisation, agitation, rowing motion and aggression
- **Duration of effect:** 2–3 h

▶ **Effects**
- Reversal of all effects (sedation/analgesia/muscle relaxation and cardiovascular side effects) of a selective alpha2 agonist (medetomidine, dexmedetomidine, detomidine, romifidine)

▶ **Indications**
- Discontinuation of sedation/anaesthesia
- Overdose of the agonist
- Partial antagonisation to combat (cardiovascular) side effects of alpha2 agonists, one may use half of the used volume of the alpha2 agonist and administer SC or IM

► **Contraindications/precautions**
• Breeding animals (according to package insert)
• Liver and kidney damage

► **Adverse effects**
• Hypotension
• May cause gastrointestinal side effects such as vomiting and diarrhoea
• May cause hyperactivity and agitation

► **Miscellaneous**
• In the usual commercial preparations, the **volume of the antagonist corresponds to that of the agonist**; the concentration is increased 5-fold
• For partial antagonisation of the effect of xylazine (a non-specific alpha2 agonist), a dose of 0.2 mg/kg (dog, cat) and 0.05–0.1 mg/kg (horse, only in emergencies) is described
• **IV application not recommended in daily routine,** but apply slowly IV in case of emergency

► **Dosages**
• Dosages are listed in ► Table 4.4

Table 4.4 Dosages for atipamezole (mg/kg)

Species	IV slowly	IM/SC
Dog	5 times medetomidine or 10 times dexmedetomidine dose (= **same volume!**)	
Cat	2.5 times medetomidine or 5 times dexmedetomidine dose (= **half the volume!**)	
Rabbit	0.3–0.7	0.5–1
Guinea pig	–	2.5–5 times medetomidine or 10 times dexmedetomidine dose (= **same volume!**)
Ferret	–	0.4–1
Small rodents	2.5 times the medetomidine dose (= **half the volume!**)	
Horse	0.1–0.2	–
South American camelids	0.125	–

IV intravenous, IM intramuscular, SC subcutaneous

4.6 Atropine

- **Parasympatholytic**

▶ Pharmacokinetics
- Competitive **antagonist of acetylcholine** (has an anticholinergic effect) and peripherally blocks the muscarinic receptors at the parasympathetic post-ganglionic synapses
- **Onset of effect:** IV 30 s, IM/SC 5–15 min
- **Duration of effect:** About 30 min

▶ Effects
- After a short **initial phase of bradycardia and bradyarrhythmia**, which is particularly pronounced at lower doses or slow administration, **tachycardia** occurs due to reduction of the vagal influence on the sinus node

▶ Indications
- Therapy of arrhythmias (p. 350)
- Sinus bradycardia (especially if caused by vagal stimulation, e.g. by opioids)
- 1st, 2nd and 3rd degree AV block
- Supraventricular and vagal bradyarrhythmia
- Sinuatrial block
- Preanaesthetic reduction of bronchial secretion (under discussion, as secretion also thickens)
- Bronchospasm

▶ Contraindications/precautions
- Tachycardia
- Glaucoma
- Obstructive disease of the gastrointestinal tract, paralytic ileus, ulcerative colitis
- Obstruction of the urinary tract
- Horse: reduced motility of the gastrointestinal tract may lead to colic – use only in emergency situation!
- Bovine: may lead to inappetence and rumen immotility

▶ Adverse effects
- Reduction of the motility of the gastrointestinal and urogenital tract
- Drying of the oral mucous membrane
- Intestinal paralysis, colic
- Urinary retention

- Agitation or drowsiness, ataxia, central nervous seizures
- Initial bradycardia (often with late treatment of high vagal tone and/or low dose)
- Excess tachycardia (often after administration of high doses because the effect was not waited for)

▶ Miscellaneous
- Mydriasis
- Bronchodilatation
- Penetrates blood-brain and placental barriers (may be beneficial before Caesarean section with bradycardic foetuses)
- Some breeds of rabbits and other herbivores have atropine esterases, enzymes that metabolise atropine very rapidly; therefore, the effect is very short
- Subcutaneous absorption is very irregular, for this reason IM or IV application is preferred

▶ Dosages
- Dosages are listed in ▶ Table 4.5

Table 4.5 Dosages for atropine (mg/kg)

Species	IV	IM/SC
Dog	0.02–0.04	0.02–0.04
Cat	0.01–0.04	0.02–0.04
Rabbit	0.05	0.05–0.1
Guinea pig	0.05–0.1	0.05–0.1
Ferret	0.04	0.02–0.05
Small rodents	–	0.1–0.4
Horse	0.005–0.01*	–
Cattle	–	0.06–0.12*
Sheep/goat	–	0.15–0.3*
South American camelids	–	0.15–0.3*
Pig	0.02–0.05	0.02–0.05

IV intravenous, IM intramuscular, SC subcutaneous, *use not recommended

4.7 Azaperone

- Butyrophenone
- Neuroleptic
- Brand name, licenced for pigs: Stresnil

▶ Pharmacokinetics
- Blocks dopamine2 receptors in the brain, thereby inhibiting dopamine release
- Blockade of alpha1 receptors
- **Onset of effect:** IV within 1–2 min, IM 5–10 min, maximum effect after 15–30 min
- **Duration of effect:** After IM injection about 120 min, after IV injection about 30–60 min

▶ Effects
- Sedation
- Antiemetic
- Antiarrhythmic
- Decreases motor activity
- Antiadrenergic, anticholinergic, antihistaminic, antidopaminergic

▶ Indications
- **Used exclusively in pigs!**
- Sedation
- Before regrouping, inhibits aggressive behaviour
- For sows that do not accept their piglets
- Before transport
- For sows before giving birth for the first time
- For clinical examination or blood sampling (made easier by vasodilation)
- To reduce the risk of malignant hyperthermia (p. 384) in animals at risk
- Premedication before injection or inhalation anaesthesia
- Induction of anaesthesia in combination with ketamine

▶ Contraindications/precautions
- Hypovolaemia, shock
- History of seizures
- Prior to myelography

Table 4.6 Dosages for azaperone (mg/kg)

Pig	IM
Sedation	0.25–1.0
Premedication/reduction of aggressive behaviour	2.0–2.5
Sedation and (light) anaesthesia	2.5–8
IM intramuscular	

▶ Adverse effects
- Vasodilation, resulting in hypotension
- Hypothermia (uncoupling of central thermoregulation, vasodilation)
- In high doses, **penis prolapse** in boars, risk of injury
- Crosses placental barrier, causes depression in piglets (when used during Caesarean section)

▶ Miscellaneous
- **No analgesic effect**
- Leads to increased prolactin secretion
- The calmer the environment, the better the sedative effect

▶ Dosages
- Dosages are listed in ▶ Table 4.6
- **IV administration** is sometimes performed under field conditions (into the lateral ear vein), but may cause severe excitation
- No more than 1 mg/kg should be used in **adult animals**, higher doses may be used in **younger pigs**

▶ Literature

[1] Brodbelt DC, Taylor PM. Comparison of two combinations of sedatives before anaesthetising pigs with halothane and nitrous oxide. Vet Rec 1999; 145: 283–287

[2] Heinonen ML, Raekallio MR, Oliviero C, Ahokas S, Peltoniemi OA. Comparison of azaperone-detomidine-butorphanol-ketamine and azaperone-tiletamine-zolazepam for anaesthesia in piglets. Vet Anaesth Analg 2009; 36: 151–157

4.8 Bupivacaine

- **Local anaesthetic (amide type)**
- **Analgesic**

▸ Pharmacokinetics
- Blocks Na channels (in higher doses also the K channels) in the neuronal membrane and thus prevents transmission of the action potential
- **Onset of effect:** Different data from 5 up to 15 min, epidural up to 1 h
- **Duration of effect:** About 3 to 6 h

▸ Effects
- Local analgesia, dose-dependent sensory and motor blockade

▸ Indications
- Surface or infiltration anaesthesia, epidural and spinal anaesthesia, intraarticular application
- Local and regional anaesthesia for surgical procedures
- Pain therapy

▸ Contraindications/precautions
- **Never give IV!** Aspirate before injection
- Local infection at the site of local anaesthesia
- Systemic infection, sepsis

▸ Adverse effects
- In vitro wound healing disorders could not be confirmed in vivo
- Neurotoxic and cardiotoxic at higher doses, especially with accidental IV administration
- With overdose, central nervous signs initially, with increasing dosage:
  - Muscle tremors, ear twitching
  - Generalised convulsions
  - Unconsciousness and respiratory arrest
  - Cardiovascular symptoms (changes in ECG) are seen

▸ Miscellaneous
- „Antagonisation" of the effect in case of overdose with lipid injection possible: treatment in case of overdose or accidental IV injection see chapter "Local anaesthesia" (p. 413)

▸ Dosages
- Dosages are listed in ▸ Table 4.7

Table 4.7 Dosages for bupivacaine (mg/kg)

Species	Tissue	Epidurally
Dog	1–2	0.5–1
Cat	1–2	0.5–1
Rabbit	1–2	–
Guinea pig	1–2	–
Ferret	1–2	–
Small rodents	5	–
Horse	1 (intraarticular)	–

Dosages are **maximum doses in 24 h**.

4.9 Buprenorphine

- **Opioid, partial μ receptor agonist**
- **Analgesic**
- **Scheduled drug** – comply with legal regulations!

▶ Pharmacokinetics
- Very **strong affinity to the μ receptor**, cannot be completely displaced from binding site either by other μ receptor agonists or by the opioid antagonist naloxone
- Desired **effect** (= analgesia) **is lower** than that of pure μ receptor agonists (e.g. morphine, methadone)
- **Potency** of buprenorphine **is greater** than that of pure μ receptor agonists, which means that a lower dose is needed for the maximum desired effect
- **Onset of effect:** Slow, sedation after approx. 15 min, analgesia after approx. 30 min, strongest effect approx. 1–1.5 h after IV administration, IM even slower; SC application not recommended due to significant loss of effect
- **Duration of effect:** Long, 4–6 h, potentially up to 8 h

▶ Effects
- Analgesia, in **cats** almost as effective as pure μ receptor agonists

▶ Indications
- (Postoperative) analgesia
- Enhances the sedative effect of CNS depressant drugs

▶ **Contraindications/precautions**

• Preoperative use can be problematic as effect cannot be topped up by other opioids as these cannot bind to the μ receptor

▶ **Adverse effects**

• Fewer cardiovascular (bradycardia) and respiratory (respiratory depression) side effects than pure μ receptor agonists
• Salivation
• Hypothermia, but also hyperthermia, especially in recovery when not painful (**cat, horse**)
• Movement, restlessness (**dog, horse**), euphoria (**cat**)
• Allotriophagia, **small rodents** show Pica behaviour (eating disorder)
• Postoperative administration in still anaesthetised **rabbits** may cause severe respiratory and circulatory depression

▶ **Miscellaneous**

• **Cat, horse**: Mydriasis
• **Dog**: Miosis
• Is very well absorbed by the cat via the oral transmucosal route, is a very suitable application option (not in dogs!), formulation without preservative seems to taste better than multi-dose buprenorphine, see also "Anaesthesia protocols cat" (p. 184)
• Combination with other opioids makes little sense due to its high affinity to the μ receptor

▶ **Dosages**

• Dosages are listed in ▶ Table 4.8

Table 4.8 Dosages for buprenorphine (mg/kg)

Species	IV	IM	OTM
Dog	0.01–0.03	0.01–0.03	–
Cat	0.01–0.02	0.01–0.02	0.01–0.04
Rabbit	0.01–0.05	0.01–0.05	–
Guinea pig	0.01–0.05	0.01–0.05	–
Ferret	0.01–0.05	0.01–0.05	–
Small rodents	0.03–0.1	0.03–0.1	–
Horse	0.005–0.01	0.005–0.01	–
Cattle	0.001–0.01	0.001–0.01	–
Pig	0.01–0.05	0.05–0.1	–
IV intravenous, IM intramuscular, OTM oral transmucosal			

► Literature

[1] Bortolami E, Slingsby L, Love EJ. Comparison of two formulations of buprenorphine in cats administered by the oral transmucosal route. J Feline Med Surg 2012; 14: 534–539

[2] Martinez EA, Hartsfield SM, Melendez LD, Matthews NS, Slater MR. Cardiovascular effects of buprenorphine in anesthetized dogs. Am J Vet Res. 1997; 58: 1280–1284

[3] Robertson SA, Taylor PM, Sear JW. Systemic uptake of buprenorphine by cats after oral mucosal administration. Vet Rec 2003 31; 152: 675–8

[4] Robertson S, Taylor P, Lascelles B, Dixon M. Changes in thermal threshold response in eight cats after administration of buprenorphine, butorphanol and morphine. Vet Rec 2003; 153: 462–465

4.10 Butorphanol

- **Opioid, κ receptor agonist, μ receptor antagonist** (according to recent data it also has agonistic activity at the μ receptor)
- **Analgesic (moderate, mainly visceral)**
- **Sedative**

► Pharmacokinetics
- Butorphanol has an agonistic effect on the κ receptor (sedation) and an antagonistic effect on the μ receptor (analgesia)
- Effect is highly dependent on animal species, breed, age, temperament, site of application and pain status of the patient
- **Onset of effect:** IV 5 min, IM 15 min
- **Duration of effect: Dog, horse** 1.5 to 2 h; **cat** with visceral pain apparently up to 6 h, with somatic pain significantly shorter

► Effects
- Primarily sedation especially in combination with other sedatives (e.g. alpha2 agonists)
- Good **visceral analgesia**, but only short-acting and weaker than pure μ receptor agonists such as methadone or morphine
- Antitussive (especially in **dogs**, not in cats)

► Indications
- Premedication
- Sedation (especially in combination with alpha2 agonists and ketamine)
- Pre-, intra- and postoperative analgesia (weak and short-acting)

► Contraindications/precautions
- Do not use in case of productive cough (**dog**)
- **Caution** with constipation, colic, faecal impaction (**horse**)

▶ Adverse effects
- Less cardiovascular and respiratory depression compared to pure μ receptor agonists
- **Dog**: Transient ataxia, anorexia and diarrhoea
- **Horse**: Transient ataxia, head twitching and tremors possible

▶ Miscellaneous
- Ceiling effect, e.g. in **dogs** at 0.4 mg/kg IV, does not make sense to use higher doses
- Mydriasis (**cat**)

▶ Dosages
- Dosages are listed in ▶ Table 4.9
- In **horses**, successful postoperative use after colic surgery (p. 336) has been described: Butorphanol as continuous rate infusion with 0.013 mg/kg/h

Clinical relevance

Ceiling effect (= saturation effect)
This effect describes the property of some active substances (e.g. butorphanol, buprenorphine) in which there is no increase in the (desired) effect despite an increase in dose. However, side effects may increase further. A further increase in dose can even lead to a kind of antagonisation of the (desired) effects.

Table 4.9 Dosages for butorphanol (mg/kg)

Species	IV	IM
Dog	0.2–0.4	0.2–0.4
Cat	0.2–0.4	0.2–0.4
Rabbit	0.2	0.2–0.5 to 1
Guinea pig	0.2	0.2–0.5
Ferret	0.2	0.2–0.5
Small rodents	0.2	0.2–0.5
Horse	0.01–0.05	0.01–0.05
Cattle	0.05	0.05
Sheep/goat	0.05	0.05–0.2
South American camelids	0.05	0.05–0.2
Pig	–	0.2
IV intravenous, IM intramuscular		

4.11 Carprofen

- **Non-steroidal anti-inflammatory drug**
- **Analgesic (inflammatory pain)**

▶ Pharmacokinetics
- Inhibition of cyclooxygenase (COX2 selective)
- Inhibition of phospholipase A2 and thus of prostaglandin synthesis
- **Onset of effect:** After 30 min
- **Duration of effect:** 12 up to max. 24 h

▶ Effects
- Analgesic
- Antipyretic
- Anti-inflammatory
- Antiendotoxic
- Antithrombotic
- Antihyperalgesic

▶ Indications
- Postoperative pain (soft tissue and orthopaedic pain)
- Inflammatory pain (all "-itis" diseases)
- Chronic pain (e.g. degenerative joint diseases, tumour and tooth pain)

▶ Contraindications/precautions
- Heart, liver or kidney damage
- Gastrointestinal ulcers or bleeding
- **Dogs** < 10 months of age, **cats** < 5 months of age
- Patients with bleeding tendencies or surgery with large blood loss
- Dehydrated or hypotensive animals
- **Caution** in geriatric animals with chronic diseases
- **Not recommended in cats**, as metabolism is very irregular
- Do not use as a long-term drug

▶ Adverse effects
- Gastrointestinal problems (vomiting, diarrhoea, ulceration [especially **cat**], protein loss enteropathy, haemorrhage)
- Lethargy
- Kidney problems (acute renal failure especially in hypotensive animals or patients with impaired renal function)
- Liver problems (hepatocellular toxicosis)
- Embryotoxic, premature closure of the ductus arteriosus Botalli, delays birth

Table 4.10 Dosages for carprofen (mg/kg)

Species	IV	SC	PO
Dog	4	4	4 SID or 2 BID
Cat	4	4	4
Rabbit	4	4	1.5
Guinea pig	4	4	4
Ferret	4	4	4
Small rodents	4–10	4–10	4–10
Horse	0.7	–	–
Cattle	0.7 (up to 1.4)	–	–
Sheep/goat	0.7	–	–

IV intravenous, SC subcutaneous, PO orally, SID 1 × daily, BID 2 × daily

- Causes cartilage damage
- Toxic to bone marrow
- Local swelling

▶ Miscellaneous
- Interactions with other NSAIDs and/or glucocorticoids (give 24 h apart, gastric protection), but can be combined well with metamizole
- **Labrador Retrievers** seem to be particularly **sensitive**

▶ Dosages
- Dosages are listed in ▶ Table 4.10
- Due to the risk of side effects, especially in **dogs** with chronic pain, always try to titrate the dose as low as possible and as high as necessary; there are dogs that are pain-free with less than half the dose (2 mg/kg, 1 × daily)

4.12 Cimicoxib

- **Non-steroidal anti-inflammatory drug, COX2 selective**
- **Analgesic**

▶ Pharmacokinetics
- Inhibition of cyclooxygenase, which mediates the transformation of arachidonic acid to prostaglandins, prostacyclin and thromboxane
- Has a **COX2 selective effect** and is therefore also called a COX2 inhibitor; COX1 is not inhibited
- **Onset of effect:** Within 2 h
- **Duration of effect:** About 10–14 h, should not be used longer than 90 days

▶ Effects
• Analgesic
• Antipyretic
• Anti-inflammatory

▶ Indications
• Peri- and postoperative pain management after orthopaedic and soft tissue surgery in **dogs**
• Chronic pain and inflammation in osteoarthritis in **dogs**

▶ Contraindications/precautions
• Gastrointestinal ulcers or bleeding
• Bleeding tendency
• **Puppies** < 8 weeks
• Do not use in patients that are dehydrated, hypovolaemic or hypotensive
• **Caution** in pregnant or lactating animals
• **Caution** in animals with reduced cardiac or hepatic function

▶ Adverse effects
• Mild, transient gastrointestinal disturbances (vomiting, diarrhoea), weight loss
• Rarely anorexia, lethargy
• Very rarely renal toxicity with increase in renal parameters

▶ Miscellaneous
• Interacts with other NSAIDs and glucocorticoids, therefore concomitant use is not recommended
• Can be administered with or without food
• In case of long-term use, regular veterinary control including blood testing is recommended

▶ Dosages
• Target dose is 2 mg/kg, dose range can be 1.8–2.7 mg/kg depending on the weight of the dog and tablet size used (▶ Table 4.11)

Table 4.11 Dosages for cimicoxib (mg/kg)

Species	PO
Dog	2 SID, 1 BID
PO orally, SID 1 × daily, BID 2 × daily	

4.13 Detomidine

- **Alpha2 agonist, imidazole derivative**
- **Sedative, analgesic for large animals**

▶ Pharmacokinetics
- Stimulates the central alpha2 receptors, thereby inhibiting nerve impulses in the CNS; duration and intensity strongly dose-dependent
- Detomidine binds relatively non-specifically to the alpha2 receptor and to some extent also to the (undesirable) alpha1 receptor, which can be seen in the alpha1 to alpha2 ratio (1:260)
- Antagonisable by atipamezole
- **Onset of effect:** 1 min, max. effect within 5 min, IM 10–15 min, max. after 30 min, gel sublingual (**horse**) up to 45 min
- **Duration of effect:** Up to 2 h

▶ Effects
- Sedation and analgesia (stimulation of the central alpha2 receptors)
- Muscle relaxation (inhibition of conduction in the spinal cord)

▶ Indications
- Sedation to facilitate clinical examination and treatment
- In combination with local anaesthesia painful interventions (i. e. dental treatments) in **large animals**

▶ Contraindications/precautions
- Hypovolaemia
- Existing AV block and severe coronary insufficiency
- Respiratory diseases, especially upper airway obstruction (causes relaxation of the upper airways)
- Exhaustion, shock
- Chronic renal insufficiency
- Use with caution in patients with intestinal obstipation
- Newborn, sick foals
- **Not suitable for sedation for transport (ataxia!)**

▶ Adverse effects
- Biphasic effect on blood pressure: initial severe vasoconstriction leads to hypertension, then the baroreceptor reflex causes bradycardia with return to normotension, possibly hypotension
- Bradycardia can become severe, 1st and 2nd degree AV blocks are possible

- Cardiac output is drastically reduced
- Respiratory depression, bradypnoea, but sometimes also tachypnoea with apnoea phases
- Diuresis, increased urine volume (due to inhibition of antidiuretic hormone, ADH)
- Hyperglycaemia (due to inhibition of insulin synthesis)
- Reduction in motility of the intestine (**horse**) and rumen (**cattle**)
- Ataxia, staggering, falling over (dose-dependent, especially after IV injection)
- Muscle tremors
- Profuse sweating, sometimes pilierection and urticaria (self-limiting)
- Hypothermia
- Increased uterine contractility in **pregnant animals** (without causing miscarriage)
- Increased sensitivity to touch
- Decreases haematocrit

▶ Miscellaneous
- Combination with sulphonamide-trimethoprim preparations can lead to sudden death
- Subcutaneous injection leads to localised inflammation

▶ Dosages
- Dosages are listed in ▶ Table 4.12
- **Intravenous administration** should be done slowly
- Dose-dependent effect, **horse**:
  ○ Mild sedation 0.01–0.02 mg/kg
  ○ Moderate sedation 0.02–0.04 mg/kg
  ○ Prolonged sedation and analgesia 0.04–0.08 mg/kg
  ○ Premedication anaesthesia 0.01–0.03 mg/kg
  ○ Continuous rate infusion e.g. for standing sedation 0.005–0.015 mg/kg/h

Table 4.12 Dosages for detomidine (mg/kg)

Species	IV	IM	OTM
Horse	0.01–0.04	0.01–0.08	0.04
Cattle	0.005–0.01	0.02–0.04	–
Sheep/goat	0.02–0.04	0.02–0.04	–

IV intravenous, IM intramuscular, OTM oral transmucosal

4.14 Dexmedetomidine

- **Selective alpha2 agonist, imidazole derivative, active stereoisomer of the racemic mixture medetomidine** (levomedetomidine has no pharmacological effect)
- **Sedative, analgesic for small animals**

▶ Pharmacokinetics
- Stimulates central alpha2 receptors, resulting in inhibition of nerve impulses in the CNS; duration and intensity are highly dose-dependent
- Alpha1 to alpha2 ratio is 1:1620
- Completely antagonisable by atipamezole
- **Onset of effect:** IV 2–3 min, IM up to 15–20 min
- **Duration of effect:** Dose-dependent 1–2 h

▶ Effects
- Sedation and analgesia (stimulation of the central alpha2 receptors)
- Muscle relaxation (inhibition of impulse conduction in the spinal cord)

▶ Indications
- Sedation to facilitate clinical examination and treatment
- Premedication before induction of anaesthesia
- Anaesthesia when used in combination with e.g. opioid and ketamine
- Postoperative sedation and analgesia, e.g. well suited as continuous rate infusion for continuous sedation for ventilator patients (small animals)
- Perioperative MAC reduction (= less inhalation anaesthetic is needed), see also chapter on "Isoflurane" (p. 102)

▶ Contraindications/precautions
- **Dog puppies** <6 months, **kittens** <5 months
- Pregnant animals
- **Do not use** in **dogs** with cardiovascular disease: "Dilated cardiomyopathy" (p. 279) or "Mitral valve insufficiency" (p. 285)!

▶ Adverse effects
- Similar to that of the racemic mixture medetomidine (p. 111), but shorter and less pronounced
- Biphasic effect on blood pressure: Initial severe vasoconstriction (pale mucous membranes) leads to hypertension, then the baroreceptor reflex causes bradycardia with return to normotension, possibly hypotension
- Bradycardia can become severe, 1st and 2nd degree AV blocks are possible

Cardiac output and therefore perfusion is drastically reduced
Decrease in respiratory rate without change in blood gas values; increases respiratory depressive effect of other anaesthetics
Sheep, goat: May cause **severe hypoxaemia**
Diuresis, increased urine volume (due to inhibition of antidiuretic hormone, ADH)
Hyperglycaemia (due to inhibition of insulin synthesis)
Vomiting
Reduction of intestinal motility
Ataxia, staggering, falling over (dose-dependent, especially after IV injection)
Hypothermia
Increased uterine contractility in pregnant animals
Temporary increase, subsequent decrease in intraocular pressure

▸ Miscellaneous
Combination with atropine not recommended; causes serious cardiac arrhythmias, increase in blood pressure and heart rate
Can cause a local anaesthetic effect, e.g. when administered intraarticularly

▸ Dosages
Dosages are listed in ▸ Table 4.13
As dexmedetomidine is commercially available at half the concentration of medetomidine, the volume to achieve a comparable effect is the same; the volume of the commercial preparation with the antagonist atipamezole also is the same
Can be administered intravenously, intramuscularly, subcutaneously, epidurally or intraarticularly (**dog**: 0.001–0.005 mg/kg dexmedetomidine in combination with 0.1 mg/kg morphine and 0.1–1 mg/kg bupivacaine)

Table 4.13 Dosages for dexmedetomidine (mg/kg)

Species	IV	IM/SC	OTM
Dog	0.002–0.02	0.005–0.02	–
Cat	0.002–0.01	0.005–0.02	0.02
Rabbit	–	0.04–0.08	–
Guinea pig	–	0.04–0.08	–
Ferret	–	0.04–0.08	–
Small rodents	–	0.05–0.1	–
Horse	0.0035 (Pony)	–	–

IV intravenous, IM intramuscular, SC subcutaneous, OTM oral transmucosal

- **Cat**: Can also be administered orally transmucosally, effect comparable to intramuscular administration
- Continuous rate infusion is very suitable for continuous sedation: 0.001–0.005 mg/kg/h, possibly in combination with opioids

Careful!

Attention arousal!
Animals may be aroused or startled from deep sedation by loud noise or change of position if dexmedetomidine is not used in combination with e.g. an opioid.

4.15 Diazepam

- **Benzodiazepine**
- **Central muscle relaxant**
- **Lipid soluble:** Contains **propylene glycol** as a solvent, as it dissolves poorly in water

▶ Pharmacokinetics
- Enhances the effect of the inhibitory neurotransmitter GABA at its receptor
- Antagonisable with flumazenil
- **Onset of effect:** IV within 2 min, IM approx. 10 min, oral and rectal transmucosal route up to 30 min
- **Duration of effect: Dog** shorter (1–2 h) than **cat** (2–5 h)

▶ Effects
- Dose-dependent
- Muscle relaxation (central)
- Anxiolytic
- Anticonvulsive
- Sedation
  - Very much dependent on animal species, age and health status
  - No real sedation in healthy, young animals
  - Good sedation in **neonatal**, **geriatric** or **very sick dogs** and **cats**, preferably in combination with butorphanol or very low-dose ketamine with only minor cardiovascular or respiratory side-effects
  - Good sedation in **foals** up to 4 weeks
- Appetite stimulant (especially **cat**, but also **dog**, **horse**)
- Anterograde amnestic (**human**, **animal?**)

▶ Indications
- Sedation and premedication before induction of anaesthesia (in combination with other sedatives or analgesics), desired effect only in "*very, very old, very, very young and/or very, very sick*" **small animals**
- Epilepsy, tetanus
- Appetite stimulation
- Functional urethra obstruction
- Behavioural problems (urine marking in **cat**)
- Muscle tension due to e.g. pain

▶ Contraindications/precautions
- Diazepam is excreted in milk in lactating animals and may cause CNS depression in the newborn offspring
- **Caution** in highly **agitated animals**: Diazepam may cause paradoxical states of excitation
- **Caution** in animals with **liver and/or kidney disease**: Duration of action may be greatly prolonged
- **Caution** in animals in the **first trimester of pregnancy**: May cause malformations

▶ Adverse effects
- Occur especially when diazepam is administered alone; when combined with other more sedating drugs (e.g. alpha2 agonists or ketamine), side effects are largely masked
- Healthy **dogs**, **cats**, **horses** that are not neonatal, geriatric or very sick: agitation, paradoxical states of arousal, possibly aggression and excitation
- **Horse**: Severe ataxia, muscle relaxation when used alone may lead to panic states
- **Propylene glycol** solvent: Pain on injection, muscle necrosis, haemolysis, cardiovascular side effects (arrhythmias, bradycardia, hypotension)
- May cause acute hepatocellular necrosis and failure in the cat after repeated administration over several days

▶ Miscellaneous
- No analgesic effect
- Diazepam can precipitate, therefore diazepam should not be mixed with other anaesthetics in one syringe. The only exception is ketamine!
- The solvent **propylene glycol** is highly irritating to veins, so slow application is necessary!

Table 4.14 Dosages for diazepam (mg/kg)

Species	IV	IM/SC	OTM/RTM
Dog	0.1–0.5	0.1–0.5	0.2–1
Cat	0.1–1	0.1–1	0.5–1
Rabbit	0.5–2	0.5–5	–
Guinea pig	–	0.5–5	2.5–5
Ferret	0.2–1	1–3	–
Small rodents	–	1–5	2.5–5
Horse	0.05–0.2	–	–
Cattle	0.2–0.5	–	–
Sheep/goat	0.2–0.5	–	–
South American camelids	0.1–0.2	0.2–0.3	–
Pig	1–2	1–2 (up to 5)	–

IV intravenous, IM intramuscular, SC subcutaneous, OTM oral transmucosal, RTM rectal transmucosal

▶ Dosages
- Dosages are listed in ▶ Table 4.14
- Very rapid and reliable absorption after IV, oral and rectal transmucosal administration
- SC and IM application painful and only incomplete absorption or poor bioavailability
- Intranasal application possible (status epilepticus), > 80% bioavailability
- Effects with increasing doses: Increase in appetite (0.05 mg/kg) < anxiolysis < muscle relaxation, sedation < interruption of status epilepticus (up to 1 mg/kg)
- Pigs seem to require very high doses

▶ Literature

[1] Center SA, Elston TH, Rowland PH, Rosen DK, Reitz BL, Brunt JE, Rodan I, House J, Bank S, Lynch LR, Dring LA. Fulminant hepatic failure associated with oral administration of diazepam in 11 cats. JAVMA 1996; 209: 618–25

4.16 Etomidate

- **Imidazole derivative**
- **Hypnotic (ultra-short acting) for anaesthesia induction**

There are two different preparations: an emulsion (active substance dissolved in fat) and one in which the active substance is dissolved in **propylene glycol**. **Caution**: Side effects as with propylene glycol in diazepam (p. 89)

▶ Pharmacokinetics
- Exact mechanism of action not yet known, indirectly increases the effect of the inhibitory neurotransmitter GABA
- **Onset of effect:** IV very fast, within 30 s to 1 min
- **Duration of effect:** 5–10 min

▶ Effects
- Hypnosis/unconsciousness with minimal effect on cardiovascular and respiratory systems (perfect for cardiac patients)
- Decreases intracranial pressure in a dose-dependent manner, lowers both O_2 consumption and blood flow in the brain, neuroprotective

▶ Indications
- Anaesthesia induction
  - ◦ in patients with cardiovascular insufficiency
  - ◦ in pregnant dogs with reduced general condition for Caesarean section (passes the placental barrier only incompletely)
  - ◦ for neurosurgical procedures or patients with increased intracranial pressure
  - ◦ in patients with trauma
  - ◦ in patients with liver insufficiency (is nevertheless metabolised quickly)

▶ Contraindications/precautions
- Patients with adrenal insufficiency (Addison's disease); a single initial dose seems to be ok in an emergency situation, but continuous rate infusion increases morbidity and mortality; corticosteroids may need to be substituted (see below)

▶ Adverse effects
- Due to solvent **propylene glycol**: pain on injection, muscle necrosis, haemolysis (**caution renal patient!**), cardiovascular side effects: arrhythmias, bradycardia, hypotension

Table 4.15 Dosages for etomidate (mg/kg)

Species	IV
Dog	0.5–2
Cat	0.5–2
Rabbit	0.5–2
Guinea pig	0.1–0.5
Ferret	0.5–2
Small rodents	1–10
IV intravenous	

- **Decreases cortisol and aldosterone levels**, in **dogs** not below the normal range, in **cats** levels return to normal range only after hours
- Myoclonia, twitching and muscle rigidity during induction of anaesthesia, especially if no or little premedication has been given; this can be prevented by simultaneous administration of midazolam or diazepam 0.2 mg/kg IV
- Possibly vomiting

▶ Miscellaneous
- **No analgesic effect**

▶ Dosages
- Dosages are listed in ▶ Table 4.15
- Administration **only IV**!

4.17 Fentanyl

- **Opioid, pure µ receptor agonist**
- **Analgesic**
- **Scheduled drug** – comply with legal regulations!

▶ Pharmacokinetics
- Pure µ receptor agonist
- Completely antagonisable by naloxone (should only be used in an emergency situation because all opioids, including endogenous opioids, are antagonised and acute pain may occur)
- **Onset of effect:** Fast, IV 1–3 min, max. effect after 5 min, IM 5–8 min
- **Duration of effect:** After IV bolus about 20–30 min

▶ **Effects**
- Analgesia, very effective
- Sedation, little effect

▶ **Indications**
- Excellent perioperative analgesia
- Postoperative analgesia
- Can be used well in the context of premedication or induction of anaesthesia (e.g. in combination with midazolam) in multimorbid patients

▶ **Contraindications/precautions**
- **Caution** in patients with **increased intracranial pressure**: they must be monitored closely! Hypoventilation should be avoided by positive pressure ventilation!

▶ **Adverse effects**
- Vagally mediated bradycardia
- Respiratory depression (by increasing CO_2 threshold)
- Hypothermia
- Panting (in the awake, non-painful **dog**)

▶ **Miscellaneous**
- Control of vagally mediated bradycardia by atropine (p. 72) or glycopyrrolate (p. 99)
- **Dog, cat**: Approximately 10 min before bolus administration or start of high-dose continuous rate infusion (CRI), atropine (0.04 mg/kg) or glycopyrrolate (0.02 mg/kg) IM can be administered to gently counteract bradycardia (prevention rather than therapy); this should only be done if no alpha2 agonist has been administered
- **Be prepared to ventilate** the patient after bolus administration or in case of high-dose continuous rate infusion

▶ **Dosages**
- Dosages are listed in ▶ Table 4.16
- **Postoperatively**, possibly together with other analgesics for severe pain use continuous rate infusion with approx. 6 µg/kg/h (= 0.1 µg/kg/min)

Table 4.16 Dosages for fentanyl

Species	IV bolus (µg/kg)	CRI (µg/kg/h)	IM/SC (µg/kg)
Dog	1–10	12–36	–
Cat	1–5	6–30	–
Rabbit	–	–	20*
Guinea pig	–	–	25*
Ferret	1–5	6–30	–
Small rodents	–	–	5–50*

IV intravenous, CRI continuous rate infusion, IM intramuscular, SC subcutaneous
*as part of fully antagonisable anaesthesia in combination with medetomidine and midazolam

▶ Transdermal application (fentanyl patch)
- Can be used in **dogs**, **cats** and **horses**, among other species
- Educate owners or use only when animal is hospitalised
- Do not cut the patch (there is one kind of patch that can actually be cut)
- Another transdermal application method is a **spot-on solution**, which causes effective plasma levels in **dogs** for up to 4 days
- **Onset of effect:** Varies greatly from species to species and from individual to individual (**dog** up to 24 h, **cat** up to 8 h, **horse** a few hours); in some patients very irregular and unreliable absorption
- **Duration of effect:** Up to 3 days, analgesic effect must be evaluated regularly, as an effective plasma level may not be reached
- **Application site:**
  - **Dog, cat:** Thoracic side and neck on a "flat" part of the skin
  - **Horse/foal:** Above the elbow medially on the front limb
  - Preparation of the skin: Clip the skin (do not shave, because microlesions of skin can increase absorption), clean with water only, dry, stick patch on (only on healthy skin areas)
  - Secure well with bandage and adhesive tape
  - Write the date and time of application and the name of the person responsible on the dressing
- **Adverse effects:**
  - Ataxia
  - Fatigue
  - Inappetence
  - Local skin irritation (remove patch!)

Table 4.17 Dosages for fentanyl patches in dogs, cats and foals

Weight	Dosage
< 5 kg	12 µg/h
5–10 kg	25 µg/h
10–20 kg	50 µg/h
20–30 kg	75 µg/h
30 kg	100 µg/h
Foal	100 µg/h

- **Contraindications:**
  - Fever, hyperthermia (indication of too high resorption rate – remove patch!)
  - Sedation
  - Renal or hepatic insufficiency
- **Dosages:**
  - Dosages are listed in ▶ Table 4.17
  - If the patch is to be used as a permanent medication, a new patch must be applied in an overlapping period of time to avoid a therapy gap

▶ Literature

[1] Aguado D, Benito J, Gomez de Segura IA. Reduction of the minimum alveolar concentration of iso-flurane in dogs using a constant rate of infusion of lidocaine-ketamine in combination with either morphine or fentanyl. Vet J 2011; 189: 63–66
[2] Eberspächer E, Stanley SD, Rezende M, Steffey EP. Pharmacokinetics and tolerance of transdermal fentanyl administration in foals. Vet Anaesth Analg 2008; 35: 249–55
[3] Freise KJ, Newbound GC, Tudan C, Clark TP. Pharmacokinetics and the effect of application site on a novel, long-acting transdermal fentanyl solution in healthy laboratory Beagles. J Vet Pharmacol Ther 2012; 35 Suppl 2: 27–33

4.18 Flumazenil

- **Benzodiazepine antagonist**

▶ Pharmacokinetics
- As an antagonist, competitively inhibits the benzodiazepine binding site at the GABA receptor
- **Onset of effect:** After IV administration 1–2 min, max. effect after 6–10 min
- **Duration of effect:** About 60 min

▶ Effects
- Antagonises benzodiazepine effects

▶ Indications
- Antagonising unwanted benzodiazepine effects

▶ Contraindications/precautions
- Relatively short half-life (50–60 min), therefore re-sedation may occur

▶ Adverse effects
- Nausea, vomiting
- Pain sensation may be increased

▶ Miscellaneous
- **Administer slowly**: It can lead to central arousal and, especially in horses, to very rapid recovery phases

▶ Dosages
- Should be administered **slowly IV**
- Dosages are listed in ▶ Table 4.18

Careful!

Pre-treatment of patient's **seizures** with benzodiazepines and using them as part of premedication or induction of anaesthesia makes a lot of sense. Seizures could recur with the use of flumazenil!

Table 4.18 Dosages for flumazenil (mg/kg)

Species	IV
Dog	0.01–0.08
Cat	0.01–0.08
Rabbit	0.01–0.08
Guinea pig	0.01–0.08
Ferret	0.05
Small rodents	0.01–0.08
Horse	0.01–0.02
IV intravenous	

4.19 Gabapentin

- **GABA analogue**
- **Ca^{2+} channel blocker**
- **Anticonvulsant**

▶ Pharmacokinetics
- Site of action not completely understood
- Antagonist at the NMDA receptor but no action on the GABA receptor, although the structure is similar to that of the inhibitory neurotransmitter GABA
- **Onset of effect:** Over a few hours, but it takes days to weeks for stable effect levels
- **Duration of effect:** Hours to days, should not be discontinued suddenly but tapered down like steroids to minimise side effects

▶ Effects
- Antiepileptic, anticonvulsive
- Antihyperalgesic (neuropathic pain)

▶ Indications
- Epilepsy (in higher dosage)
- Neuropathic pain
- Polyneuropathy, phantom pain
- Stress reduction in the cat (e.g. before a visit to the vet)
- Therapeutic attempt in the case of idiopathic headshaking in horses
- Therapeutic attempt in foals with hypoxaemic-ischaemic encephalopathy

▶ Contraindications/precautions
- Administer antacids at least 2 h apart (recommended in human medicine)
- Dose reduction in case of renal insufficiency

▶ Adverse effects
- Tiredness
- Dizziness, headache
- Vomiting
- Ataxia, unsteady gait, difficulty standing up
- Rarely acute pancreatitis

▶ Miscellaneous
- Opioids enhance the effect of gabapentin

Table 4.19 Dosages for gabapentin (mg/kg)

Species	PO (antihyperalgesic)	PO (anticonvulsive)
Dog	5–15 BID–TID	20–50 BID–TID
Cat	5–15 BID–TID	20–50 BID–TID
Rabbit	10 BID	–
Horse	2.5–5 BID–TID	8 BID–TID
PO orally, BID 2 × daily, TID 3 × daily		

- Works very well **in combination** with other analgesics, especially NSAIDs
- At the end of therapy, administration should be slowly tapered down over a period of days, otherwise there is a risk of **withdrawal symptoms**(anxiety, sleeplessness, pain, nausea, sweating)

▶ **Dosages**
- Dosages against neuropathic pain are far below those of the anticonvulsant dosage (▶ Table 4.19)
- There is evidence that doses in **dogs** should be administered at shorter intervals (every 6 h, i. e. 4 × daily)

Clinical relevance

Gabapentin for stress reduction in cats
Highly stressed and even aggressive cats become much more relaxed and manageable by the veterinarian if they are given 20–30 mg/kg gabapentin PO about 2–3 hours before transport. In practice, this means that the owner mixes the contents of a 100 mg capsule (or a 300 mg capsule in case of high doses or large cats) with a small amount of tasty wet food, which the cat then eats. Side effects are mild: sedation, ataxia, hypersalivation and occasional vomiting. All effects disappear after approx. 8 h.

▶ **Literature**
[1] Kukanich B, Cohen RL. Pharmacokinetics of oral gabapentin in greyhound dogs. Vet J 2011; 187: 133–5
[2] Van Haaften KA, Eichstadt Forsythe LR, Stelow EA, Bain MJ. Effects of a single preappointment dose of gabapentin on signs of stress in cats during transportation and veterinary examination. J Am Vet Med Assoc 2017; 251: 1175–81
Comment: Here you can read exactly how to turn stressed, aggressive cats into manageable pets for transport to and treatment by the vet

4.20 Glycopyrrolate

I

- **Parasympatholytic agent**

▶ Pharmacokinetics

- Competitive **antagonist** of **acetylcholine** (has an anticholinergic effect): peripherally blocks the muscarinic receptors at the parasympathetic postganglionic synapses
- **Onset of effect:** IV 1–5 min, IM 5 min (max. effect after 20 min), SC 15–20 min (max. effect after 30–45 min); takes longer than atropine
- **Duration of effect:** About 60 min (vagolytic effect), up to 7 h reduced glandular secretion; longer-acting than atropine

▶ Effects

- Low-dose or slowly administered glycopyrrolate causes (initial) bradycardia either by acting on the sinoatrial node or by its effects on **central** muscarinic receptors increasing vagal activity (less effect than with atropine)
- Central muscarinic effects of high-dose glycopyrrolate on heart rate are masked by **peripheral muscarinic blockade** at the sinoatrial node, which causes **tachycardia**

▶ Indications

- Therapy of arrhythmia (p. 350)
- Sinus bradycardia
- 1st, 2nd and 3rd degree AV block
- Supraventricular and vagal bradyarrhythmia
- Sinuatrial block
- Commonly used with opioids to counteract bradycardia caused by opioids
- Preanaesthetic reduction of bronchial secretion (usefulness is debated, as secretion also thickens)
- Therapy of bronchospasm

▶ Contraindications/precautions

- Tachycardia
- Glaucoma
- Obstructive disease of the gastrointestinal tract, paralytic ileus, ulcerative colitis
- Obstruction of the lower urinary tract
- **Horse:** Reduced motility of the gastrointestinal tract can lead to colic – use only in an emergency situation!
- **Cattle:** May lead to inappetence and rumen immmotility

Table 4.20 Dosages for glycopyrrolate (mg/kg)

Species	IV	IM/SC
Dog	0.005–0.02	0.01–0.02
Cat	0.005–0.02	0.01–0.02
Rabbit	0.005–0.02	0.01–0.02
Guinea pig	–	0.01–0.02
Ferret	0.01–0.02	0.01–0.02
Small rodents	–	0.01–0.02
Horse	0.005	–
Pig	–	0.002–0.004

IV intravenous, IM intramuscular, SC subcutaneous

▶ **Adverse effects**
- Reduction of the motility of the gastrointestinal and urogenital tract (longer than atropine!)
- Dry oral mucosa
- Intestinal paralysis, colic
- Urinary retention
- Agitation or drowsiness, ataxia, central nervous seizures
- Excess tachycardia after initial bradycardia (less frequent than with atropine)

▶ **Miscellaneous**
- Mydriasis
- Bronchodilation
- Does not penetrate blood-brain and placental barrier
- Significantly more expensive than atropine

▶ **Dosages**
- Dosages are listed in ▶ Table 4.20

4.21 Grapiprant

- EP4 receptor antagonist, similar to NSAIDs
- Piprant

▶ **Pharmacokinetics**
- Non-steroidal, but non-cyclooxygenase inhibiting, anti-inflammatory agent
- Selective antagonist of the EP4 receptor, blocking it highly specifically for prostaglandin E_2

- **Onset of effect:** Few hours, clinical response to treatment within 7 days
- **Duration of effect:** 6–10 h

▶ Effects
- Analgesia (osteoarthritis pain in **dogs**)

▶ Indications
- Analgesia associated with mild to moderate osteoarthritis in dogs
- As part of a multimodal therapeutic approach

▶ Contraindications/precautions
- Do not use in pregnant or lactating animals
- **Caution** in patients with hepatic or renal impairment, cardiovascular dysfunction or gastrointestinal disease
- Avoid co-administration with other anti-inflammatory drugs

▶ Adverse effects
- Mostly mild and transient gastrointestinal side effects such as vomiting, soft-formed faeces, diarrhoea and inappetence

▶ Miscellaneous
- Administer on an empty stomach and at least 1 h before the next feeding, bioavailability is then much greater (89% vs. 33%)
- Maximum treatment duration is 28 days, longer treatment should be carefully considered

▶ Dosages
- Target dose is 2 mg/kg, dose range can be 1.5–2.9 mg/kg depending on the weight of the dog and tablet size used (▶ Table 4.21)

Table 4.21 Dosages for grapiprant (mg/kg)

Species	PO
Dog	2 SID

PO orally, SID 1 × daily

► Literature

[1] Giorgi M. CJ-023,423 (Grapiprant) a potential novel active compound with antihyperalgetic properties for veterinary patients. Am J Anim Vet Sci 2015; 10: 53–56

[2] Kirby Shaw K, Rausch-Derra LC, Rhodes L. Grapiprant: an EP4 prostaglandin receptor antagonist and novel therapy for pain and inflammation. Vet Med Sci 2015; 21: 3–9

[3] Neudeck S. Osteoarthritis beim Hund – Grapiprant als neue Therapieoption. Kleintier konkret 2019; 22: 47–50

[4] Rausch-Derra LC, Huebner M, Rhodes L. Evaluation of the safety of long-term daily oral administration of grapiprant, a novel drug for treatment of osteoarthritic pain and inflammation, in healthy dogs. Am J Vet Res 2015; 76: 853–9

[5] Rausch-Derra L, Huebner M, Wofford J, Rhodes L. A prospective, randomized, masked, placebo-controlled multisite clinical study of grapiprant, an EP4 prostaglandin receptor antagonist (PRA), in dogs with osteoarthritis. J Vet Intern Med 2016; 30: 756–763

4.22 Isoflurane

- **Hypnotic**
- **Inhalation anaesthetic**

► **Pharmacokinetics**
- Halogenated hydrocarbon whose mode of action is only partially understood; CNS depressant
- Should be administered by inhalation using a precision vaporiser
- **Onset of effect:** Dose-dependent within seconds to a few minutes
- **Duration of effect:** Rapid recovery phase in a few minutes after the end of the intake

► **Effects**
- Hypnosis, unconsciousness
- Muscle relaxation
- Anticonvulsive effect

► **Indications**
- Maintenance of general anaesthesia
- Also rarely used for the induction of general anaesthesia for special indications
- Most commonly used inhalation anaesthetic in veterinary medicine

► **Contraindications/precautions**
- Predisposition to malignant hyperthermia (p. 384)
- Should not be used alone for patients with increased intracranial pressure
- Should not be used alone for painful procedures due to severe respiratory and cardiovascular depressant effect and **no analgesic effect**

▶ **Adverse effects**
- Dose-dependent **cardiovascular depression**
  - Myocardial depressant, negative inotropic effect
  - Severe vasodilation
- Dose-dependent **respiratory depression** (CO_2 tolerance is increased)
- Hypothermia
- Mucosal irritation, pungent odour, bronchoconstriction possible with mask induction without premedication (particularly pronounced in **guinea pigs**), salivation
- Nausea, vomiting

▶ **Miscellaneous**
- Almost no metabolisation via the liver (0.3%), this means that virtually all isoflurane inhaled by the patient is exhaled again (and could be reused in a low-flow circle system)
- Can trigger malignant hyperthermia
- Dramatically contributes to the greenhouse effect in the environment

▶ **Dosages**
- MAC values are listed in ▶ Table 4.22

Table 4.22 MAC values for isoflurane (%)

Species	MAC value
Dog	± 1.3
Cat	1.6–1.7
Rabbit	2.0–2.1
Guinea pig	1.15
Ferret	1.3–1.5
Small rodents	1.3–1.6
Horse	1.3
Cattle	1.1–1.3
Sheep/goat	1.3–1.6
South American camelids	± 1.1
Pig	1.45–1.75

MAC minimum alveolar concentration

Definition

MAC value

The MAC value is the minimum alveolar concentration of isoflurane (or any other inhaled anaesthetic agent) at which 50% of patients will not respond to a supramaximal stimulus with movement. This applies to young, healthy patients with no other sedatives/anaesthetics "on board". The MAC value is a measure of the potency of an inhalation anaesthetic and gives an indication of the dose required. It is influenced by many factors. The end-tidal measurement of the inhalation anaesthetic, i. e. the measurement at the end of expiration, is close to the alveolar concentration.

Clinical relevance

Which MAC value (what dose) do I need?

- 0.3 × MAC → unconsciousness
- 1.0 × MAC → 50% of patients show surgical tolerance
- 1.5–2 × MAC → all patients show surgical tolerance
- 1.7 × MAC → intubation possible

Example: Isoflurane in the dog

If no other anaesthetics/analgesics were used, an alveolar concentration of 1.5–2 × MAC (1 × MAC isoflurane in dogs is about 1.3%), i. e. 2 to 2.6% (!), would be needed for an anaesthetic depth with surgical tolerance. The cardiovascular side effects at such high doses are considerable, therefore one should always try to reduce the MAC value for example by premedication with other anaesthetics/analgesics.

Good to know

Environmental effects of inhalant anaesthetics

Anaesthesia and critical care in industrialised countries contribute to about 4% or more of all greenhouse gas emissions worldwide. Inhalation anaesthetics account for the largest share of this. Inhalation anaesthetics of the flurane group (isoflurane, sevoflurane) are fluorinated or fluorochlorinated hydrocarbons and remain in the atmosphere for years. Here they cause relevant effects on global warming. For this reason, efforts should be made to reduce the use of inhalation anaesthetics. This can be achieved by, among other things:

- Low flow anaesthesia
- Leak free anaesthesia machine
- Balanced anaesthesia technique

4.23 Ketamine/S-ketamine

- **Phencyclidine, dissociative anaesthetic**
- Ketamine is a **racemic mixture** of the enantiomers S-ketamine and R-ketamine, whereby S-ketamine has a stronger anaesthetic and analgesic effect and shows fewer side effects (e.g. hallucinations, states of confusion)

▶ **Pharmacokinetics**

- Sites of action are not fully understood; ketamine acts at several different receptors: it is mainly a **non-competitive NMDA receptor antagonist**, but also acts at **GABA** and **opioid receptors** and inhibits peripheral reuptake of catecholamines (noradrenalin, dopamine)
- The limbic system is stimulated, the thalamo-cortical system is inhibited
- **Onset of effect:** IV within a few minutes, IM 3–5 min (max. effect after about 15 min)
- **Duration of effect:** About 20–40 min anaesthetic effect, dissociative or depressive effect can last much longer

▶ **Effects**

- Dose-dependent mild to deep sedation, dissociative anaesthesia
- Pronounced somatic analgesia with higher doses
- Antihyperalgesic effect with lower doses
- Indirect stimulation of the sympathetic nervous system with stabilisation in blood pressure and heart rate, stabilisation of heart rhythm and increase in cardiac output

▶ **Indications**
- Component of premedication, especially in wild, aggressive animals; effectively induces and reinforces sedation
- Induction of anaesthesia
- Component of maintenance of anaesthesia
- Component of postoperative analgesia due to antihyperalgesic effect, especially after orthopaedic surgery

▶ **Contraindications/precautions**
- Hyperthyroidism
- Traumatic brain injury (because it increases intracranial pressure and cerebral O_2 demand)
- Increased intraocular pressure, glaucoma (but ok in low doses without increase in blood pressure)

▶ **Adverse effects**
- Increased skeletal muscle tone, catalepsy, may lead to hyperthermia
- Increased salivation and secretion in the respiratory tract
- Direct depression of the myocardium (only in very high doses)
- Eyes remain open (cornea therefore needs protection with eye ointment)
- Hallucinations and "bad dreams" in the recovery phase
- All adverse effects can be effectively suppressed when ketamine is combined with alpha2 agonists!

▶ **Miscellaneous**
- Reflexes are not completely abolished, but are no longer protective
- Should not be used as monoanaesthetic (causes catalepsy, hallucinations, insufficient analgesia, strong salivation)
- **Intramuscular injection is painful** and may cause muscle necrosis; should be avoided especially in small mammals, but is acceptable for IM mixed injection of anaesthetics for premedication
- Initial transient decrease in respiratory rate, followed by an **apneustic breathing pattern** (pause after deep gasping inspiration rather than expiration, followed by brief expiration)
- The first metabolite **norketamine** still has approx. 10–30% of the activity of ketamine (important e.g. in cats (p. 179), which metabolise ketamine more slowly compared to other mammals)
- When administered to an already anaesthetised animal, it acts primarily as an anaesthetic: It further deepens anaesthesia and may cause cardiovascular and respiratory depression. It should therefore be administered slowly and in low doses perioperatively when the animal is already anaesthetised

Table 4.23 Dosages for ketamine (mg/kg)

Species	IV	IM/SC	Intraperitoneally
Dog	1–5	1–10	–
Cat	1–8	2–12	–
Rabbit	5–15	5–40	–
Guinea pig	–	10–50	15–40
Ferret	2–10	5–20	–
Small rodents	–	4–100*	40–100
Horse	2–2.2	–	–
Cattle	2–5	4–10	–
Sheep/goat	2–5	2–10	–
South American camelids	–	5–10	–
Pig	2–5	Up to 15	–

IV intravenous, IM intramuscular, SC subcutaneous
* should not be injected IM in animals with less than 100 g body weight

▶ Dosages
- Dosages are listed in ▶ Table 4.23
- Ketamine should never be administered alone, but **always in combination with sedating and muscle-relaxing drugs**! Numerous possible combinations are described under "Species-specific anaesthesia" (p. 150), often ketamine is used in combination with benzodiazepines or alpha2 agonists
- Ketamine can be used very well as a **continuous rate infusion peri- and/or postoperatively**; ideally, a bolus should be administered beforehand (e.g. as part of the induction of anaesthesia)
  - **Dog, cat:** Perioperatively: 0.01–0.03 mg/kg/min; postoperatively: 0.002–0.005 mg/kg/min
  - **Horse:** Perioperatively: 0.01-0.03 mg/kg/min; postoperatively: 0.002–0.005 mg/kg/min

S-ketamine – the effective isomer

The dextrorotatory isomer of ketamine is about 2–3 × more potent than the rac-emic mixture (so you need about ½ to ⅓ of the dose of ketamine), has a stronger desired effect (sedation, analgesia) and fewer side effects (hallucinations, catalepsy). It is approved for human use (Ketanest S 25 mg/ml) and may be used for special cases.

Careful!

Caution with/in

- Cardiac diseases like hypertrophic cardiomyopathy in the cat (p. 290) or hypertension! Ketamine can also increase O_2 consumption when heart rate is increased
- Liver and kidney insufficiency!
- Patients with predisposition to epilepsy or myopathy/spasticity, e.g. breed-related (p. 181): potentially Devon Rex, Cornish Rex and Sphinx cats, or special interventions (myelogram)!

4.24 Lidocaine

- **Local anaesthetic** (amide type)
- **Analgesic** (local and systemic)

A variety of formulations are available: Injection solution, ointment, gel, pump spray and patch

▶ Pharmacokinetics
- Lidocaine blocks Na channels on the membrane inside the cell and thus prevents Na influx during depolarisation phase; transmission of action potentials on the nerve is interrupted
- **Onset of effect:** 1–3 min, up to 15 min depending on type of application
- **Duration of effect:** Dose-dependent 30 to 120 min, up to 3 h by addition of a vasoconstrictor (adrenalin)

▶ **Effects**
- Analgesia (locally and systemically)
- Antiarrhythmic (antiarrhythmic agent class 1B)
- Prokinetic on the gastrointestinal tract
- Anti-inflammatory
- Possibly radical scavenger
- Reduces the MAC value of inhalation anaesthetics (but rather ineffectively compared to e.g. opioids)

▶ **Indications**
- Local anaesthesia (infiltration, regional and superficial anaesthesia)
- Systemic analgesia, part of maintenance anaesthesia (IV bolus or continuous rate infusion)
- Postoperative analgesia (as local anaesthesia or systemic continuous rate infusion)
- Antiarrhythmic agent
  ○ Premature ventricular extrasystoles/arrhythmias associated with gastric torsion
  ○ Ventricular tachyarrhythmia: Bolus administration can/may need to be repeated; it is recommended to have midazolam or diazepam IV on hand for the central nervous side effects that may appear at high doses
  ○ Ventricular fibrillation, ventricular flutter
- Prokinetic effect in **horses**: Prophylaxis and therapy of postoperative ileus after colic surgery

▶ **Contraindications**
- Sinuatrial, AV or high degree heart block (with escape rhythm)
- Adam-Stokes syndrome (brief periods of unconsciousness due to temporary arrest of the sinus node), other diseases of the sinus node
- Congestive heart failure, shock, hypovolaemia, hypotension, bradycardia
- Severe respiratory depression, hypoxia

▶ **Adverse effects**
- Wound healing disorders (controversially discussed, proven in vitro, not in vivo)
- In case of overdose: CNS symptoms (dose-dependent): Drowsiness, depression, ataxia, paraesthesia, convulsions, vomiting, apathy
- Hypotension

▶ **Miscellaneous**
- If the formula contains **adrenalin as an additive** (vasoconstrictive agent), it **must not be given IV**!

- In tissues with low pH (e.g. inflammation) the effect is significantly reduced
- With hypokalaemia the effect is reduced
- Cats are particularly sensitive to the central nervous effects and should therefore be well monitored for side effects; they are the first to show muscle fasciculations and trembling with the ears/whiskers

▶ Dosages
- Dosages are listed in ▶ Table 4.24
- **Maximum doses** are described for administration within 24 hours; the toxic dose is approx. 3 × higher
- **Continuous rate infusions** should be preceded by a slow bolus of 1–2 mg/kg

In case of **epidural administration**, the following must be considered
- that motor function is also blocked when the corresponding nerves are reached (paralysis of the hindlimbs) and
- that the local anaesthetic does not migrate too far cranially, as this would
  ○ lead to massive vasodilation with hypotension and/or
  ○ to respiratory depression or apnoea

Table 4.24 Dosages for lidocaine (mg/kg, if not stated otherwise)

Species	IV	Tissue	CRI (mg/kg/min)	Epidurally
Dog	1–2 (bolus)	max. 8	0.01–0.08	0.2 ml/kg (2%)*
Cat	0.5–1 (bolus)	max. 4–6	0.01–0.06	0.2 ml/kg (2%)
Rabbit	–	max. 4	–	–
Guinea pig	–	max. 4	–	–
Ferret	–	max. 4–6	–	–
Small rodents	–	max. 4 (10 mouse)	–	–
Horse	1 (bolus)	max. 6	0.05	5–8 ml total (2%)
Cattle	–	max. 9	–	–
Sheep/goat	4	max. 6	–	0.2 ml/kg (2%)*
South American camelids	–	max. 6	–	0.2 ml/kg (2%)*
Pig	–	max. 6	–	–

IV intravenous, CRI continuous rate infusion, max. maximum, *reduce dose in very large animals

Clinical relevance

Vasoconstriction prolongs effect – adrenalin as additive
The addition of adrenalin or noradrenalin to local anaesthetics causes local vaso-constriction. This delays systemic absorption and thus prolongs the effect of short-acting local anaesthetics on the one hand and reduces the risk of toxic maximum concentrations in the blood on the other. The most effective dose of adrenalin (additive) is 1:200,000 (which corresponds to 5 µg/ml).

Of course, local anaesthetics with adrenalin as an additive are **not suitable for IV administration!**

4.25 Medetomidine

- **Selective alpha2 agonist, imidazole derivative**
- **Sedative, analgesic**

▶ Pharmacokinetics
- Stimulates central alpha2 receptors, thereby inhibiting nerve impulses in the central nervous system (CNS); duration and intensity highly dose-dependent
- Alpha1 to alpha2 ratio is 1:1620
- Completely antagonisable by atipamezole (p. 70)
- **Onset of effect:** IV 1 min, IM 5–15 min
- **Duration of effect:** Sedative effect dose-dependent up to 3 h, analgesic effect only about 30–45 min

▶ Effects
- Sedation and analgesia (stimulation of the central alpha2 receptors)
- Muscle relaxation (inhibition of stimulus transmission in the spinal cord)
- Anxiolytic (through reduced release of stress hormones)

▶ Indications
- Sedation to facilitate clinical examination and treatment
- Premedication before induction of anaesthesia
- Anaesthesia when used in combination with e.g. opioid and ketamine
- Postoperative sedation and analgesia
- Perioperative MAC reduction (reduces requirement for inhalation anaes-thetic)

▶ **Contraindications/precautions**
- Shock
- **Puppies** < 6 months, **kittens** < 5 months of age
- Pregnant animals
- Animals with diabetes mellitus (p. 333)
- Obstruction of the urinary tract (if it is not certain that the obstruction can be removed)
- **Caution** in dogs with cardiovascular disease, especially "Dilated cardiomyopathy (DCM)" (p. 279) and/or "Mitral valve insufficiency" (p. 285)!
- **Caution** in very old patients

▶ Adverse effects
- Biphasic effect on blood pressure: initial severe **vasoconstriction** (pale mucous membranes) causes **hypertension**; then the baroreceptor reflex causes **bradycardia** with return to **normotension**, possibly hypotension
- Bradycardia can become severe, 1st and 2nd degree AV blocks are possible
- **Cardiac output is drastically reduced**
- IV catheterisation can become difficult due to vasoconstriction
- Decrease in respiratory rate without change in blood gas values; increases respiratory depressant effects of other anaesthetics
- **Sheep**, **goat**: May cause severe hypoxaemia
- Diuresis, increased urine output (due to inhibition of antidiuretic hormone, ADH)
- Hyperglycaemia (due to inhibition of insulin synthesis), glucosuria
- Vomiting (**cat**, but also in approx. 20% of **dogs**)
- Reduction of intestinal motility
- Ataxia, staggering, falling over (dose-dependent, especially after IV injection)
- Hypothermia
- Increased uterine contractility in pregnant animals
- Transient increase, subsequent decrease in intraocular pressure

▶ Miscellaneous
- **Arousability!** Animals may be aroused from deep sedation or startled (by loud noise or change of position) if not used in combination with e.g. an opioid
- Mydriasis
- Very good in combination with ketamine
- Combination with **atropine is not recommended**, serious cardiac arrhythmias, severe increase in blood pressure and heart rate will occur

- The volume of the commercial preparations of the antagonist atipamezole is identical to the administered volume of the commercial preparations of medetomidine
- Partial antagonisation is also possible, e.g. if the (cardiovascular) side effects of medetomidine become too severe; administer atipamezole IM with half the volume of medetomidine used

▶ **Dosages**
- Dosages are listed in ▶ Table 4.25
- Above a certain dose (approx. 0.03–0.04 mg/kg in **dogs** and **cats**), there is no longer an increase in the desired effect, but a prolongation of the duration of action with simultaneous increase in side effects (the rationale for recommending higher dosages in dogs and cats is not clear)
- With the right indication (e.g. very agitated patient), it can also be used in very low dosages (0.001–0.003 mg/kg) in sick and old animals; in such a case, the combination with benzodiazepines and opioids is particularly suitable
- Can also be administered **sublingually/orally transmucosally**, is very well absorbed
- Can be administered **epidurally**: 0.01–0.015 mg/kg, possibly in combination with opioid or local anaesthetic

Table 4.25 Dosages for medetomidine (mg/kg)

Species	IV	IM/(SC)	OTM
Dog	0.005–0.02	0.01–0.04	–
Cat	0.005–0.02	0.01–0.04	0.04
Rabbit	–	0.08–0.12	–
Guinea pig	–	0.08–0.12	–
Ferret	–	0.08–0.1	–
Small rodents	–	0.08–0.15	–
Horse	0.007	0.01	–
Cattle	0.005	–	–
Sheep/goat	0.005	0.015–0.03	–
South American camelids	–	0.01–0.03	–
Pig	0.04	0.01–0.05; 0.08	–

IV intravenous, IM intramuscular, SC subcutaneous, OTM oral transmucosal

Good to know

What is Zenalpha?

Zenalpha is a combination preparation of medetomidine and vatinoxan, a peripheral alpha2 antagonist. It is approved for intramuscular administration alone in healthy dogs to induce sedation for e.g. clinical examination or for minor surgical procedures. Among other things, vatinoxan antagonises the peripheral circulatory effects of medetomidine: there is no vasoconstriction! This ensures better perfusion, which facilitates a higher O_2 delivery to the tissues. While heart rate and cardiac output are reduced even with Zenalpha, the effect is less pronounced than with medetomidine alone.

Off-label, Zenalpha has been used successfully as a premedication before general anaesthesia and in combination with other anaesthetics, as well as in very young and sick dogs.

▶ Literature

[1] Sinclair MD. A review of the physiological effects of alpha2-agonists related to the clinical use of medetomidine in small animal practice. Can Vet J. 2003; 44: 885–897

4.26 Meloxicam

- **Non-steroidal anti-inflammatory drug, highly COX2 selective**
- **Analgesic (inflammatory pain)**

▶ Pharmacokinetics
- Inhibition of the enzyme cyclooxygenase, which mediates the metabolism of arachidonic acid to prostaglandins, prostacyclin and thromboxane
- **Onset of effect: Cat:** SC/PO about 1–2 h, **dog:** SC about 2–3 h, PO 6–9 h
- **Duration of effect:** About 24 h

▶ Effects
- Analgesic
- Anti-inflammatory
- Antipyretic
- Antiexsudative
- Antiphlogistic

▶ **Indications**
- Acute and chronic pain, especially in musculoskeletal/chronic joint disorders; accumulates particularly well in inflamed joint fluid
- Peri- and postoperative pain relief
- Acute diseases of the respiratory tract, acute mastitis (**cattle**)
- **Pig:** Non-infectious diseases of the musculoskeletal system, puerperal septic-aemia and toxaemia
- **Dog, cat, horse:** Acute and chronic pain of the musculoskeletal system, uveitis, ocular inflammation, after ophthalmological operations, fever
- **Horse:** Colic pain

▶ **Contraindications/precautions**
- Acute or chronic diseases of the gastrointestinal mucosa, shock
- Acute or chronic renal insufficiency
- Heart failure (because it reduces renal perfusion)
- Coagulation disorders (e.g. Von Willebrand factor deficit)
- **Calves** under 1 week of age, **foals**, **dog puppies** and **kittens** with less than 6 weeks of age
- Pregnant or lactating animals (not approved according to the package insert, but may well be used in clinics in lactating animals)
- **Caution** in geriatric patients
- **Caution** in patients with chronic liver insufficiency
- **Caution** in hypotensive patients

▶ **Adverse effects**
- In general, NSAIDs have a variety of adverse effects; the most important ones are
  ○ Gastrointestinal irritation, ulceration and perforation, inappetence, diarrhoea, vomiting, haemorrhagic gastroenteropathy
  ○ Nephrotoxicity, especially in hypovolaemic patients
  ○ Blood coagulation disorders (but only little inhibition of platelet aggregation)

▶ **Miscellaneous**
- Should not be administered concurrently with other NSAIDs or steroids (24 h interval)
- Inhibits the migration of leukocytes into the area of inflammation

Table 4.26 Dosages for meloxicam (mg/kg)

Species	IM/SC	PO
Dog	0.2	0.2
Cat	0.05–0.2	0.05–0.2
Rabbit	0.4–0.6	0.4–0.6
Guinea pig	0.5–1	0.5–1
Ferret	0.2–0.3	0.2–0.3
Small rodents	1–5 (only SC)	1–5
Horse	0.6	0.6
Cattle	0.5	–
Sheep/goat	0.5	–
South American camelids	0.2–0.5	–
Pig	0.4	–
IM intramuscular, SC subcutaneous, PO orally		

▶ Dosages
- Dosages are listed in ▶ Table 4.26
- Older literature suggests relatively high doses for **cats** (0.3 mg/kg); these are considered outdated and should not be used or should only be used after critical consideration
- In **cats**, the highest dose should be given initially (0.1–0.2 mg/kg) and then the following doses reduced (0.05–0.1 mg/kg), for a maximum of 5 days (according to package insert)
- Meloxicam is not approved for IV administration, but can be given slowly IV, preferably diluted

Careful!

Meloxicam comes in different concentrations!
It is (**always!**) worth looking at the multidose vial and knowing the concentration of the drug used. Meloxicam is an example of this, there are very low concentration commercial preparations e.g. Metacam 0.5 mg/ml for **cats**, as well as a preparation for **large** and **small animals** with 5 mg/ml to the preparation for large animals with 20 mg/ml. Confusion can easily lead to serious overdose or ineffectiveness due to too low a dose.

4.27 Metamizole

- **Pyrazolone derivative**
- **Non-acidic non-opioid analgesic**

▶ Pharmacokinetics
- Inhibition of the enzyme cyclooxygenase COX3 (peripheral prostaglandin synthesis), which mediates the metabolism of arachidonic acid to prostaglandins, prostacyclin and thromboxane, but also of central prostaglandin synthesis
- Suspected to also act at cannabinoid, opioid and NMDA receptors
- Exact mechanism of action unclear
- **Onset of effect: Small rodents** after PO administration approx. 10–30 min (oral bioavailability in small mammals very good, therefore very effective), **cat, dog** after SC administration approx. 15 min, **horse** after IV administration 10–15 min, after IM administration approx. 30 min
- **Duration of effect:** About 4–6 h

▶ Effects
- Analgesic
- Antipyretic
- Spasmolytic on smooth muscle cells
- Antiphlogistic (in higher doses)

▶ Indications
- Acute and chronic pain
- Peri- and postoperative pain management
- Reduction of fever
- Infectious enteritis (**calf**), mastitis, pharyngitis, arthritis, neuralgia, tendovaginitis (**cattle**)
- **Pig**: Mastitis, metritis and agalactia (MMA) syndrome, influenza infection, osteopathy and myopathy
- **Horse**: Release of spasm in pharyngeal obstruction
- **Cat, dog, horse**: Colic pain
- **Rabbit**: Very effective for pain in the area of the head

▶ **Contraindications/precautions**
- Acute or chronic diseases of the gastrointestinal mucosa, ulcers
- Acute or chronic renal insufficiency (may reduce renal perfusion)
- Damage to the haematopoietic system
- Do not use in **cats** (says one manufacturer, but can be and has been used clinically)
- Caution in bronchial asthma, may increase bronchospasm
- Caution in hypotensive patients!

▶ **Adverse effects**
In general, there are a variety of undesirable effects. The most important are:
- Rarely haemorrhagic gastroenteropathy
- Damage to blood cells: leucocyte depression, agranulocytosis after multiple administration of high doses, so far only reported in people
- Bronchospasm (especially in asthmatic patients), may cause allergic reactions
- Salivation

▶ **Miscellaneous**
- May cause tissue damage if injected SC
- Fatal shock may occur with fast IV injection, therefore **inject IV slowly and diluted**
- May (rarely) cause organ damage, e.g. renal failure, if administered chronically
- Should not be administered simultaneously with other NSAIDs or steroids in cats (24 h interval), but in general a combination is possible and works clinically very well

▶ **Dosages**
- Dosages are listed in ▶ Table 4.27
- Administer **slowly (!) IV**
- Tablets are available and useful
- Older literature only gives doses per animal, not per kg
- In **cats**, the highest dose should be given initially and then the following doses reduced

Table 4.27 Dosages for metamizole (mg/kg, if not stated otherwise)

Species	IM/SC/PO	IV slowly
Dog	20–50, q4	20–50, q4
Cat	20–50, q6	10–30 (50), q6
Rabbit	20–50, q4	20–50, q4
Guinea pig	80, q4–6 (3 drops PO)	–
Ferret	20–50, q4–6	–
Small rodents	100–200, q6 (4–8 drops PO)	–
Horse	10–30 g/animal	20–50, q8
Cattle	10–20 g/animal	–
Sheep/goat	1–4 g/animal	20–50
South American camelids	40	–
Pig	5–10 g/animal	20–50

IV intravenous, IM intramuscular, SC subcutaneous, PO orally, q4 every 4 h, q6 every 6 h, q8 every 8 h

4.28 Methadone

- Opioid, pure μ agonist
- Analgesic
- **Scheduled drug** – comply with legal regulations!

Clinical relevance

Levomethadone in L-Polamivet

L-Polamivet is a compounded drug used in some European countries. It is a strong analgesic approved for dogs and horses, to which the anticholinergic fenpipramide is added to combat the bradycardia caused by levomethadone. Levomethadone is the levorotatory S-enantiomer of the racemate methadone (the dextrorotatory is dextromethadone). It has a much higher affinity for the μ opioid receptor and therefore acts more specifically and longer. It is twice as potent, which means that about half the dose is needed compared to racemic methadone. The desired effect, namely analgesia, is equivalent.

Especially in awake animals or when alpha2 agonists are administered simultaneously, it is doubtful whether the added fenpipramide is beneficial or rather would not be indicated.

▶ **Pharmacokinetics**
- Pure μ receptor agonist, but also shows an affinity to the NMDA receptor (like ketamine)
- Can be fully antagonised by naloxone (should only be used in emergencies); partial antagonisation may be possible with buprenorphine
- **Onset of effect:** Fast, IV 1–3 min, IM/SC 5–15 min
- **Duration of effect:** 2–4 h

▶ **Effects**
- Analgesia, very effective
- Sedation, very little effect in healthy patients

▶ **Indications**
- Preoperative analgesia, premedication
- Peri- and postoperative analgesia
- Analgesia in emergency and trauma patients

▶ **Contraindications/precautions**
- Pregnant animals for Caesarean section (causes prolonged respiratory depression in the pups)
- **Caution** in patients with **increased intracranial pressure**: Hypoventilation should be addressed by positive pressure ventilation
- Patients with **upper airway problems**: When used as a monotherapeutic in the awake dog with no or little pain, **panting** induced by methadone can become severe and actually causes hypothermia

▶ **Adverse effects**
- Vagally mediated bradycardia (in the anaesthetised animal)
- Respiratory depression (in the anaesthetised animal)
- Heavy panting (in the awake dog)
- Gastrointestinal motility is reduced
- Hyperacusis (particularly sensitive to metallic sounds)

▶ **Miscellaneous**
- Drugs of choice to control vagally mediated bradycardia: atropin (p. 72) and glycopyrrolat (p. 99)
- Mydriasis (**cat**), miosis (**dog**)

▶ **Dosages**
- Dosages are listed in ▶ Table 4.28
- When using levomethadone (L-Polamivet), the recommended dose should be halved

Table 4.28 Dosages for methadone (mg/kg)

Species	IV	IM/SC	Epidurally
Dog	0.1–0.5; 1	0.2–1	0.1–0.2
Cat	0.1–0.4; 0.8	0.1–0.6	0.1–0.2
Ferret	–	0.1–0.5	–
Horse	0.1–0.2	–	–

IV intravenous, IM intramuscular, SC subcutaneous

- As a mixture with lidocaine and ketamine (MLK) or only ketamine (MK) very suitable for peri- and postoperative analgesic **continuous rate infusion**; mixing is described in the chapter on peri- and postoperative pain (p. 404)
- Excellent for **epidural administration** (quite rapid onset of action), no urinary problems as described for morphine; use formulation without preservatives

4.29 Midazolam

- **Benzodiazepine**
- **Central muscle relaxant**

▶ Pharmacokinetics
- Enhances the effect of the inhibitory neurotransmitter GABA at its receptor
- Antagonisable with flumazenil
- **Onset of effect:** IV within 2 min, IM/SC about 10 min
- **Duration of effect: Dog** about 45 min to 2 h, **cat** can take a little longer

▶ Effects
- Dose-dependent
  - ○ Appetite stimulant (especially **cat**, but also **dog, horse**)
  - ○ Anxiolytic
  - ○ Sedative (midazolam seems to be more effective than diazepam, very much depending on species, age, temperament and state of health); no sedation is young and healthy animals
  - ○ Good sedation in
    - **Neonatal**, **geriatric** or **very sick dogs** and **cats** best in combination with butorphanol or low-dose ketamine with only minor cardiovascular or respiratory side effects
    - **Foals** up to 4 weeks

- ○ Muscle relaxation (central)
- ○ Anticonvulsive
- ○ Anterograde amnestic (**human, animal?**)

▶ Indications
- Sedation and premedication before induction of anaesthesia (in combination with other sedatives or analgesics)
- Epilepsy, tetanus (use high dose)
- Appetite stimulation
- Functional urethra obstruction
- Behavioural problems (urine marking in **cat**)

▶ Contraindications/precautions
- Do **not** use in **excited animals**, may cause paradoxical states of excitement
- **Caution** in animals **with liver and/or kidney disease**! Duration of action may be greatly prolonged
- **Caution** in animals in the **first trimester of pregnancy**! Malformations may occur

▶ Adverse effects
- In particular, there are side effects when midazolam is administered alone; the side effects disappear when it is administered in combination with other more sedating drugs (e.g. alpha2 agonists or ketamine)
- Healthy **dogs**, **cats**, **horses** that are not neonatal or geriatric: agitation, paradoxical states of arousal, possibly aggression and excitation
- **Horse**: Severe ataxia, muscle relaxation when used alone may lead to **panic states**
- In recovery, potentially agitation, dysphoria and vocalisation in **dogs** and **cats**

▶ Miscellaneous
- No **analgesic effect**
- Since midazolam is water-soluble, it is completely absorbed when administered IM in contrast to diazepam

▶ Dosages
- Dosages are listed in ▶ Table 4.29
- With increasing doses: Appetite stimulation (0.05 mg/kg) < anxiolysis < muscle relaxation, sedation < termination of status epilepticus (up to 1 mg/kg)
- Pigs seem to require very high doses; sedation for **piglets** 0.1–0.5 mg/kg IM

Table 4.29 Dosages for midazolam (mg/kg)

Species	IV	IM/SC
Dog	0.1–0.5	0.1–0.5
Cat	0.1–1	0.1–1
Rabbit	0.5–2	0.5–2
Guinea pig	–	0.5–2
Ferret	0.2–1	1–2
Small rodents	–	1–5
Horse	0.05–0.2	–
Cattle	0.2–0.5	–
Sheep/goat	0.2–0.5	–
South American camelids	0.1–0.2	0.2–0.3
Pig	1–2	1–2 (up to 5)

IV intravenous, IM intramuscular, SC subcutaneous

4.30 Morphine

- **Opioid, pure μ agonist**
- **Analgesic**
- **Scheduled drug** – comply with legal regulations!

▶ Pharmacokinetics
- Pure μ receptor agonist
- Can be fully antagonised by naloxone (should only be used in emergencies); partial antagonisation may be possible with buprenorphine
- **Onset of effect:** Rather fast, IV 1–3 min, IM/SC 10–30 min
- **Duration of effect:** 2–6 h

▶ Effects
- Analgesia, very effective
- Sedation, more than with any other pure μ receptor agonist

▶ Indications
- Preoperative analgesia, premedication
- Peri- and postoperative analgesia (**small animals**, **horse**)
- Local analgesia (epidural, intraarticular)

▶ **Contraindications/precautions**
- Pregnant animals for Caesarean section (causes prolonged respiratory depression in the pups)
- **Caution** in patients with **increased intracranial pressure**! Hypoventilation should be addressed by positive pressure ventilation

▶ **Adverse effects**
- Vagally mediated bradycardia (in the anaesthetised animal)
- Respiratory depression (in the anaesthetised animal)
- Panting (in the awake dog)
- Gastrointestinal motility is decreased
- **Horse**: Risk of ileus, especially after repeated administration; relaxes anal sphincter (defecation)
- **Cat, small rodent, horse**: May cause excitement, excitation and convulsions at very high doses and when used alone
- Rapid IV administration may cause histamine release (with vasodilation and hypotension), so **give IV slowly**
- Nausea and vomiting in **dogs** and **cats** are more common than with other pure μ agonists (can be used deliberately)
- With epidural administration:
  ○ Possibly urinary retention due to relaxation of the detrusor vesicae muscle, regular bladder control for 24 h recommended
  ○ Pruritus

▶ **Miscellaneous**
- Drugs of choice to control vagally mediated bradycardia: atropine (p. 72) and glycopyrrolate (p. 99)
- Mydriasis (**cat**), miosis (**dog**)

▶ **Dosages**
- Dosages are listed in ▶ Table 4.30
- Can be used as continuous rate infusion postoperatively (but causes more sedation and nausea compared to methadone): Dosage 0.05–0.2 mg/kg/h
- Epidural administration very effective (slow onset of action but long duration of action, up to 24 h), note side effects: see "Small animals" (p. 417), "Horse" (p. 442)!
- Very good intraarticular analgesic due to the presence of local μ receptors

Table 4.30 Dosages for morphine (mg/kg)

Species	IV slowly	IM/SC
Dog	0.1–0.5	0.2–1
Cat	0.1–0.4	0.1–0.6
Rabbit	0.1–0.4	2
Guinea pig	0.1–0.4	2–5
Ferret	–	0.1–0.6
Small rodents	–	2.5–5
Horse	0.1–0.2	–

IV intravenous, IM intramuscular, SC subcutaneous

4.31 Naloxone

- **Pure opioid antagonist**

▶ Pharmacokinetics
- Acts as a competitive **antagonist** at all opioid receptors (μ, κ and δ receptors); antagonises the effect of endogenous (endorphins, enkephalins) and exogenous opioids
- **Onset of effect:** After IV administration a few minutes (1.5–3 min)
- **Duration of effect:** Dose-dependent 15–45 min, sometimes shorter

▶ Effects
- Reversal of all opioid effects (analgesia) and side effects (primarily respiratory depression and bradycardia)

▶ Indications
- **Emergency medication only!**
- Antidote in case of opioid overdose
- Antagonist after termination of anaesthesia to shorten the recovery phase: **only in special cases**; caution after painful operations; **only if indicated and alternative pain management is provided**
- Endogenously or exogenously induced respiratory depression in puppies after birth

▶ Contraindications/precautions
- Caution in animals with cardiovascular insufficiency!

▶ **Adverse effects**
- Excitation, tremor
- Panting
- Vomiting
- Hypertension, tachycardia

▶ **Miscellaneous**
- Sometimes it makes sense to administer the dose partly IV and partly IM to prolong the duration of action

▶ **Dosages**
- Dosages are listed in ▶ Table 4.31
- Due to the extremely low dosages, the drug should be diluted before application in order to be able to apply the correct dose

Careful!

Caution with naloxone after painful operations!
Naloxone should only be administered in an emergency situation, as the abrupt recurrence of pain can cause **severe shock and even sudden death** – always start with a **low dose, dilute and administer slowly**!

Careful!

Rebound effect!
When the effect of the (short-acting) naloxone wears off, the effect of the initially administered opioid reappears! The antagonisation therefore wears off again.

Table 4.31 Dosages for naloxone (mg/kg)

Species	IV	IM/SC
Dog	0.002–0.02 titrate	0.02
Cat	0.005–0.01	0.01
Rabbit	–	0.03
Guinea pig	–	0.03
Ferret	–	0.001
Small rodents	–	0.12 (rat)–1.2 (mouse)
Horse	0.01–0.02	–
IV intravenous, IM intramuscular, SC subcutaneous		

4.32 Pentobarbital

- **Barbiturate, long-acting**
- **Hypnotic**

▶ Pharmacokinetics
- Barbiturates are GABA-mimetic and interact with the GABA receptor, resulting in membrane hyperpolarisation and thus reduced nerve excitability
- **Onset of effect:** After IV application several minutes
- **Duration of effect:** Very highly dose-dependent, a few minutes to hours or (with high doses) euthanasia

▶ Effects
- Effect is highly dependent on dosage, mode of application and animal species, as well as age and condition of the individual patient
- Hypnosis
- Little muscle relaxation; should always be combined with muscle relaxant
- Reduces intracranial pressure

▶ Indications
- In laboratory animal science in **small mammals** and occasionally in **dogs**, **cats** and **small ruminants**, partly as a hypnotic or anaesthetic
- Euthanasia (p. 480) of **large and small animals**
- Secondary epilepsy

▶ Contraindications/precautions
- **Anaesthesia:**
  ○ Pregnant animals (except for euthanasia)
  ○ Patients with impaired respiratory function

▶ Adverse effects
- **Extremely tissue irritatıng** (pH value approx. 11), should therefore only be administered IV! If IV is not possible use intraperitoneal (IP) administration (**small mammals**)
- Pain on injection, may cause thrombophlebitis
- Muscle twitching, excitation, defensive movements, restlessness on induction
- **As anaesthetic:**
  ○ Dose-dependent severe respiratory depression
  ○ Hypotension due to vasodilation, often concomitant (reflex) tachycardia
  ○ Arrhythmogenic

- Duration of action is determined by redistribution into fat; re-dosing leads to accumulation with very long recovery times
  - Excitation in recovery phase
  - Hypothermia
  - Dilates the spleen (complicates abdominal surgery)
- **For euthanasia:**
  - Gasping after cardiac arrest
  - Delayed death

▶ Miscellaneous

- Pentobarbital is **not recommended as sole anaesthetic** (for painful procedures) because the **lack of analgesic effect** means that it must be dosed so high that severe respiratory and cardiovascular depression leads to high mortality rates
- Before euthanasia (p. 480), the animal should first be sedated, then deeply anaesthetised and only then euthanised; the process is then calm, free of excitation and gasping for breath and "appealing" to the owner

▶ Dosages

- Dosages are listed in ▶ Table 4.32
- Should not be administered strictly according to dosage, but **according to effect**
- Mode of application is **slow IV**, other modes of application are not recommended; in exceptional cases, IP administration is also feasible for euthanasia (e.g. **small mammals**)

Table 4.32 Dosages for pentobarbital (mg/kg)

Species	IV – sedation	IV – hypnosis	IV – euthanasia
Dog	2–4	10–30	50–60, 90–150*
Cat	2–4	20–30	50–60, 120–180*
Rabbit	–	20–45	50–150, 150–300*
Guinea pig	–	15–45	50–60, 90–150*
Ferret	–	25–35	–
Small rodents	–	30–90	50–800
Horse	3–15	15–18	50–60, 90*
Cattle	–	–	50–60, 30–150*
Sheep/goat	–	20–30 (up to 50)*	50–60
Pig	–	10–30	50–60
IV intravenous; *different dose recommendations depending on the product			

- Depending on the commercial preparation, there are very different dose recommendations for euthanasia; as always, death after euthanasia should be confirmed beyond doubt

Careful!

Caution with
- **Paravascular administration:** Due to the very basic pH value (approx. 11), pentobarbital can lead to severe tissue necrosis
- **Hypovolaemic and anaemic animals:** Hypotension can occur due to vasodilation. At the same time, (reflex) tachycardia often occurs

4.33 Pethidine (= Meperidine)

- **Fully synthetic opioid, pure μ agonist**
- **Analgesic**
- **Scheduled drug** – comply with legal regulations!

▶ Pharmacokinetics
- Pure μ receptor agonist
- Similar effects and side effects as morphine
- During metabolism, the active metabolite norpethidine is formed, which can accumulate and trigger seizures; more suitable for acute pain therapy or in the context of premedication, less suitable for long-term therapy
- Antagonisable with naloxone
- **Onset of effect:** Fast, IV within a few minutes, IM/SC after up to 5 min
- **Duration of effect:** IV bolus 45–60 min, max. up to 2 h in the **dog**, **cat** potentially up to 3 h, **horse** rather short, up to 20 min

▶ Effects
- Analgesia (not really proven in the **cat**)
- Sedation (in **dogs** and **cats**)
- Spasmolysis

▶ Indications
- Used rarely overall in veterinary anaesthesia, not licenced for animals
- **Horse:** Control of colic pain (spasm colic, urinary colic) or prepartum labour
- **Cattle:** Intestinal spasms, prepartum labour, urinary colic, additional therapy for severe diarrhoea

- **Dog** and **cat**: For premedication before induction of anaesthesia or (less frequently because of the short duration of action) for postoperative pain and spasms of the gastrointestinal tract

▶ **Contraindications/precautions**
- **Caution** in case of **impaired liver or kidney function**: The duration of action may be considerably prolonged
- **Caution** in **cats**: Should not be used, as the therapeutic range is low. High dosages should be avoided!

▶ Adverse effects
- Overall, less pronounced side effects (less frequently bradycardia, panting or vomiting) than other pure μ agonists
- Has a negative inotropic effect (atypical for opioids)
- Painful on IM injection
- May cause **histamine release** (with vasodilation and hypotension as well as bronchoconstriction) **with rapid IV administration**, therefore give IM/SC or only very slow IV over several minutes

▶ Miscellaneous
- Works particularly well against postoperative tremors (shivering)
- Pethidine has a structure similar to atropine and can thus even cause tachycardia (instead of bradycardia, as opioids normally do)
- Also has some local anaesthetic efficacy

▶ Dosages
- Dosages are listed in ▶ Table 4.33
- Can also be administered as an **antitussive drug in dogs**; the dose is then around 4 mg/kg every 3 to 6 h PO (tablets are available)

Table 4.33 Dosages for pethidine (mg/kg)

Species	IV slowly	IM/SC
Dog	2–6	2–6 (up to 10)
Cat	2–4	2–4
Guinea pig	–	10–20
Small rodents	–	10–20
Horse	1–2 (up to 5)	–
Cattle	1–2	–
IV intravenous, IM intramuscular, SC subcutaneous		

▶ Literature

[1] Golder FJ, Wilson J, Larenza MP, Fink OT. Suspected acute meperidine toxicity in a dog. Vet Anaesth Analg 2010; 37: 471–7

[2] Vettorato E, Bacco S. A comparison of the sedative and analgesic properties of pethidine (meperidine) and butorphanol in dogs. J Small Anim Pract 2011; 52: 426–32

4.34 Propofol

- **Phenol derivative**
- **Hypnotic (short-acting)**

Milky-white emulsion with soy and egg protein, therefore highly perishable: Work cleanly, opened propofol should be stored in the refrigerator for max. 24 h and then discarded. Only effective after IV administration.

▶ Pharmacokinetics
- Propofol enhances the effect of GABA at the receptor
- **Onset of effect:** After IV administration 1–2 min
- **Duration of effect:** About 10 min

▶ Effects
- Hypnosis
- Reduces intracranial and intraocular pressure
- Appetite stimulant
- Antiemetic
- Antioxidant effect, free radical scavenger
- Both proconvulsant (especially during induction without adequate premedication) and anticonvulsant (third choice antiepileptic) effects

▶ Indications
- Anaesthesia induction/short anaesthesia
- Maintenance of anaesthesia
- Sedation (for painless procedures)
- Permanent sedation (**caution in cats!**)

▶ Contraindications/precautions

Careful!

Caution with
- **Cats:** Do not use as a continuous rate infusion or more than once on consecutive days. There is a risk of formation of Heinz bodies (p. 183), a visible clumping of haemoglobin in erythrocytes due to oxidative denaturation!
- **Anaemic cats:** Propofol may further reduce oxygen-carrying capacity due to Heinz body formation!
- **Hypovolaemic patients:** Propofol-induced vasodilatation can cause hypotension!

▶ Adverse effects
- **Respiratory depression** and temporary apnoea with rapid injection or high dose; therefore, always inject slowly, wait for effect, preoxygenate and be prepared for intubation and positive pressure ventilation
- **Hypotension** due to vasodilation and reduction of the contractility of the heart (negative inotropy)
- Occasional spontaneous movements, opisthotonos, vocalisation and seizures during induction; especially if there has been little/no premedication or if the environment is noisy
- Occasional vomiting, excitations (**dog**) or retching, licking of paws or face (**cats**)

▶ Miscellaneous
- **No analgesic effect!**
- Can be used in **patients with liver or kidney failure**
- Good for **pregnant small animals** for Caesarean section surgery
- If animal does not fall asleep during induction with propofol: Check IV catheter! Non-tissue irritant if accidentally administered paravenously, but has no or delayed effect
- There is a formulation that contains preservatives (20 mg/ml benzyl alcohol), making it stable for up to 28 d. Serious side effects ("gasping syndrome") have been described when used in neonates and children; this formulation (Propovet) should therefore not be used in puppies or similar as a precautionary measure

Table 4.34 Dosages for propofol (mg/kg), CRI (mg/kg/min)

Species	IV – with premedication	IV – without premedication	CRI
Dog	2–4	5–9	0.1–0.5
Cat	2–4	6–8	0.1–0.5
Rabbit	–	5–15	–
Guinea pig	5–20	–	–
Ferret	2–6	4–10	–
Small rodents	7–10	–	0.6
Horse	2–6	–	0.1–0.3
Cattle	4–6	–	–
Sheep/goat	2–4	4–7	0.3–0.6
South American camelids	2	–	0.4
Pig	2–6	Up to 10	–

IV intravenous, CRI continuous rate infusion

▶ Dosages
- Dosages are listed in ▶ Table 4.34
- Propofol should always be **titrated slowly IV** based on effect
- Induction should be fractionated (e.g. inject ¼ of the calculated dose first, wait, then inject another ¼, and so on)

4.35 Remifentanil

- **Opioid, pure μ agonist**
- **Analgesic**
- **Scheduled drug** – comply with legal regulations!

▶ Pharmacokinetics
- Pure μ receptor agonist, **ultra-short** acting
- Metabolised by plasma esterases, is independent of liver metabolism, does not accumulate
- Fully antagonisable by naloxone; is rarely necessary as remifentanil has a very short duration of action
- **Onset of effect:** Very fast, within 1 min after IV administration
- **Duration of effect:** After IV bolus about **5 min**, after that, the effect is completely gone!

▶ Effects
• Analgesia, very effective

▶ Indications
• Peri- and postoperative analgesia
• In multimorbid patients, can also be used as part of the induction of anaesthesia (e.g. in combination with midazolam) if a CRI is then immediately started as well

▶ Contraindications/precautions
• Caution in patients with **increased intracranial pressure**: Hypoventilation should be counteracted by positive pressure ventilation!

▶ Adverse effects
• Vagally mediated bradycardia, hypotension
• Respiratory depression
• Vomiting
• Muscle rigidity

▶ Miscellaneous
• **Ultra-short-acting**, pay attention to the rapid loss of effect after the end of use
• **Use other analgesics in a timely manner** so that their maximum effect has already been reached when the effect of remifentanil wears off
• Be prepared to ventilate the patient after bolus administration or with high CRI doses

▶ Dosages
• Dosages are listed in ▶ Table 4.35
• The dry substance (powder) can be **dissolved in aqua** ad injectionem, 5% dextrose, 0.9% NaCl or 0.45% NaCl
• CRI is actually the only sensible method of application, as the duration of action is extremely short

Table 4.35 Dosages for remifentanil

Species	IV bolus (µg/kg)	CRI (µg/kg/h)
Dog	1–10	12–36
Cat	1–5	6–30
Ferret	–	6–30

IV intravenous, CRI continuous rate infusion

4.36 Romifidine

- **Alpha2 agonist, imidazole derivative**
- **Sedative**
- **Analgesic**

▶ Pharmacokinetics
- Stimulates the central alpha2 receptors, thereby inhibiting nerve impulses in the CNS
- Duration and intensity strongly dose-dependent
- Alpha1 to alpha2 ratio is 1:340
- Partially antagonisable by atipamezole (not quite specific, as more alpha1 involvement than e.g. medetomidine)
- **Onset of effect: Dog, cat:** IV 2–10 min, IM/SC delayed onset of action after 10–15 min (max. effect after approx. 50 min); horse: IV within 2 min (max. effect after 10 min)
- **Duration of effect:** Sedative effect dose and species dependent:
  Dog 60–120 min, **cat** about 60 min, **horse** 40–80 min

▶ Effects
- Sedation and analgesia (stimulation of the central alpha2 receptors)
- Muscle relaxation (inhibition of impulse conduction in the spinal cord)
- Anxiolysis (through reduced release of stress hormones)

▶ Indications
- **Used predominantly in horses**, only very rarely in small animals
- Sedation to facilitate clinical examinations and treatments
- Premedication before induction of anaesthesia
- Anaesthesia when used in combination with e.g. opioids and ketamine
- Postoperative sedation and analgesia
- Perioperative MAC reduction (= one needs less inhalation anaesthetic)

▶ Contraindications/precautions
- Cardiovascular disease, cardiomyopathy, heart failure
- Diabetes mellitus (p. 333)
- Shock
- **Caution** in animals with respiratory problems
- **Caution** in animals with renal insufficiency
- **Caution** in pregnant animals (it is not known whether romifidine has an influence)

▶ Adverse effects

- Biphasic effect on blood pressure: Initially severe **vasoconstriction** (pale mucous membranes) leads to **hypertension**; then the baroreceptor reflex causes **bradycardia** with return to normotension, possibly hypotension
- Bradycardia can become severe, 1st and 2nd degree **AV blocks** are possible
- Cardiac output is drastically reduced
- Diuresis, increased urine volume (due to inhibition of antidiuretic hormone, ADH)
- Hyperglycaemia (due to inhibition of insulin synthesis), glucosuria
- Reduction of intestinal motility
- Ataxia, staggering, falling over (dose-dependent, especially after IV injection)
- Increased sensitivity to touch, may lead to sudden violent lashing out in **horses**
- Vomiting in **dogs** and **cats** (but rarely used in small animal medicine)

▶ Miscellaneous

- Combination with atropine not recommended, serious cardiac arrhythmias, increase in blood pressure and heart rate occur
- In **horses**, it seems to cause less ataxia than other alpha2 agonists and horses do not hold their heads as low during sedation

▶ Dosages

- Dosages are listed in ▶ Table 4.36
- Dose equivalence IM: 0.04 mg/kg romifidine is equivalent to 1 mg/kg xylazine or 0.02 mg/kg medetomidine

Table 4.36 Dosages for romifidine (mg/kg)

Species	IV	IM/SC
Dog	0.04–0.12	0.04–0.12
Cat	0.04–0.2	0.04–0.2
Horse	0.04–0.08	0.08–0.1
Sheep/goat	0.05	–
Pig	0.12	0.12
IM intravenous, IM intramuscular, SC subcutaneous		

4.37 Ropivacaine

I

- **Local anaesthetic (amide type)**
- **Analgesic**

▶ Pharmacokinetics
- Local anaesthetic derived from bupivacaine
- Not a racemate, but the pure S-enantiomer (= lower systemic toxicity)
- Blocks Na channels in the nerve cell membrane and thus prevents the action potential from being transmitted
- **Onset of effect:** Delayed, different data from 5 up to 20 min
- **Duration of effect:** Long, in tissue up to 6–8 h (longer than bupivacaine), epidural in **dogs** 2–3 h (shorter than bupivacaine)

▶ Effects
- Local analgesia, dose- and concentration-dependent sensory and (in low doses) **less motor blockade**

▶ Indications
- Surface, infiltration, peripheral nerve block, epidural and spinal anaesthesia, intraarticular application
- Very well suited for neuroaxial (e.g. epidural anaesthesia) and peripheral nerve block for limbs, since at lower concentrations (around 0.2–0.5 mg/kg) analgesia (= sensory blockade) is still well maintained with largely preserved motor function (**differential blockade**)

▶ Contraindications/precautions
- **Never give IV!**
- Do not use in case of local infection at the site of local anaesthesia
- Do not use in case of systemic inflammation or sepsis

▶ Adverse effects
- Lower potential for neuro- and cardiotoxicity compared to bupivacaine
- In case of overdose, initially central nervous symptoms such as:
  ○ Dizziness, headache
  ○ Nausea, vomiting
- Rarely cardiovascular symptoms such as arrhythmias

▶ Miscellaneous
- With subcutaneous infiltration, equivalent vasoconstriction in the skin as with adrenalin (therefore also longer duration of action) in contrast to lidocaine and bupivacaine, which have a vasodilatory effect

Table 4.37 Dosages for ropivacaine (mg/kg)

Species	Tissue	Epidurally
Dog	1–2	(0.2) 0.5–1
Cat	1–1.5	0.5–1

- Mixing with other local anaesthetics is possible but makes little sense
- Possibly less chondrotoxic than bupivacaine (evidence in cell culture)

▶ Dosages
- Dosages are listed in ▶ Table 4.37
- Differential blockade when using low concentrations or dosage

▶ Literature

[1] Breu A, Rosenmeier K, Kujat R, Angele P, Zink W. The cytotoxicity of bupivacaine, ropivacaine, and mepivacaine on human chondrocytes and cartilage. Anesth Analg 2013; 117: 514–22

[2] Brown DL, Carpenter RL, Thompson GE. Comparison of 0.5% ropivacaine and 0.5% bupivacaine for epidural anesthesia in patients undergoing lower-extremity surgery. Anesthesiology 1990; 72: 633–6

[3] Duke T, Caulkett NA, Ball, SD, Remedios AM. Comparative analgesic and cardiopulmonary effects of bupivacaine and ropivacaine in the epidural space of the conscious dog. Vet Anaesth Analg 2000; 27: 13–21

[4] Kim JH, Seok SH, Park TY, Kim HJ, Kim JM, Lee SW, Lee HC, Yeon SC. Analgesic effect of intra-articular ropivacaine injection after arthroscopic surgery on the shoulder joint in dogs. Veterinarni Medicina 2018; 63: 513–521

[5] Kushnir Y, Toledano N, Cohen L, Bdolah-Abram T, Shilo-Benjamini Y. Intratesticular and incisional line infiltration with ropivacaine for castration in medetomidine-butorphanol-midazolam sedated dogs. Vet Anaesth Analg 2017; 44: 346–55

4.38 Sevoflurane

- **Hypnotic**
- **Inhalation anaesthetic**

▶ Pharmacokinetics
- Halogenated volatile anaesthetic agent, the mode of action is only partially understood
- Depresses the CNS
- Should be administered by inhalation using a precision vaporiser
- **Onset of effect:** Depending on the dose, rapidly, within seconds to a few minutes

- **Duration of effect:** After discontinuation, rapid recovery phase within a few minutes, less soluble in the blood than isoflurane, therefore theoretically faster onset and recovery phase; however, this is hardly recognisable clinically

▶ Effects
- Hypnosis, unconsciousness
- Muscle relaxation
- Anticonvulsant

▶ Indications
- **Maintenance** of general anaesthesia
- Very suitable for mask induction (and maintenance) of **neonatal** or **very young puppies** and **kittens** for short, painless procedures (e.g. audiometry) or for **small mammals** for induction in a box

▶ Contraindications/precautions
- Can trigger malignant hyperthermia – careful in predisposed animals
- Should not be used alone in patients with increased intracranial pressure
- Should not be used alone for painful procedures because there is **no analgesic effect** and in higher doses a pronounced circulatory depressant effect
- Be careful when using sevoflurane without premedication in **small mammals** (e.g. in **guinea pigs**) – they may react with severe respiratory problems

▶ Adverse effects
- Dose-dependent cardiovascular depression (less overall than with isoflurane)
  - Myocardial depressant, negative inotropic effect
  - Strong vasodilation
- Dose-dependent respiratory depression (CO_2 tolerance is increased)
- Hypothermia
- Nausea, vomiting
- Degradation product of sevoflurane (compound A), which is formed under certain conditions, can have a nephrotoxic effect in **rats** at high doses; however, this does not play a role clinically

▶ Miscellaneous
- Little metabolisation via the liver (3%)
- More pleasant or less pungent odour than isoflurane, can be used for mask or box induction
- Dramatically promotes the greenhouse effect (p. 105) in the environment

139

Table 4.38 MAC values for sevoflurane (%)

Species	MAC value
Dog	2.1–2.4
Cat	2.4–2.7
Rabbit	3.7
Ferret	2.25
Small rodents	2.4–3.0
Horse	2.21–2.84
Sheep/goat	1.9–2.3
South American camelids	2.3
Pig	1.97–2.66
MAC minimum alveolar concentration	

▶ Dosages
- Dosages are listed in ▶ Table 4.38
- Definition of MAC value can be found in the chapter on "Isofluran" (p. 102)
- Although the odour is perceived as less pungent than that of isoflurane, animals react with strong defensive movements during mask induction, premedication is therefore recommended

▶ Literature

[1] Grubb TL, Schlipf JW, Riebold TW, Cebra CK, Poland L, Zawadzkas X, Mailhot N. Minimum alveolar concentration of sevoflurane in spontaneously breathing llamas and alpacas. J Am Vet Med Assoc 2003; 223: 1167–1169
[2] Mutoh T, Nishimura R, Kim HY, Matsunaga S, Sasaki N. Cardiopulmonary effects of sevoflurane, compared with halothane, enflurane, and isoflurane, in dogs. Am J Vet Res 1997; 38: 885–90

4.39 Thiopental

- **Barbiturate**
- **Hypnotic**

Powder must be dissolved in distilled water (40 ml plus 1 g powder, results in a 2.5% solution = 25 mg/ml). Loses effectiveness over a few days.

▶ Pharmacokinetics
- Thiopental inhibits the uptake of GABA, aspartate and glutamate, resulting in reduced nerve excitability (if more GABA is available, there is greater inhibition)

- Very fast and ultra-short effect
- **Onset of effect:** Within 1 min after IV administration (15–30 s)
- **Duration of effect:** About 5–10 min after IV bolus

▶ Effects
- The effect is dose-dependent: Sedation at low dose, hypnosis at higher dose
- Little muscle relaxation (should always be combined with muscle relaxant)
- Reduces intracranial pressure

▶ Indications
- Induction of anaesthesia for evaluation of laryngeal activity (retained better than e.g. with a combination of ketamine and diazepam)
- Short interventions with bolus and CRI
- Control of epilepsy
- Short-term deepening of anaesthesia in horses

▶ Contraindications/precautions
- Severe cardiovascular disease and/or cardiac arrhythmias
- Pregnancy (easily crosses the placental barrier)
- Sighthounds (p. 168)
- Obese animals: May cause relative overdose through accumulation with repeated administration
- Liver insufficiency (may prolong duration of action)

▶ Adverse effects
- **Strong tissue irritant** (pH approx. 11), should therefore only be administered **strictly IV**, i. e. an **intravenous catheter** must be available
- Pain on injection, may cause oedema, redness and thrombophlebitis
- Muscle twitching, excitation, defensive movements, restlessness on induction
- Dose-dependent severe respiratory depression
- Hypotension due to vasodilation, often simultaneous (reflex) tachycardia
- Causes transient arrhythmias, almost always **ventricular bigemini**, by sensitising the myocardium to catecholamines
- Duration of action is determined by **redistribution into fat** tissue; redosing leads to accumulation with very long recovery times
- Excitation in recovery phase
- Hypothermia

Table 4.39 Dosages for thiopental (mg/kg)

Species	IV
Dog	10–15 (titrate)
Cat	5–10 (titrate)
Horse	6–10 (up to 15 without premedication)
IV intravenous	

▶ Miscellaneous
- To reduce side effects, it is recommended to premedicate with sedatives/ opioids before induction of anaesthesia
- During the induction of anaesthesia, **horses** may rear and fall over backwards, which can be prevented by good fixation of the head with a halter

▶ Dosages
- Dosages are listed in ▶ Table 4.39
- Should not be administered strictly according to dosage, but according to effect
- Mode of application is **slow IV**, other modes of application are not recommended

▶ Literature
[1] Gross ME, Dodam JR, Pope ER, Jones BD. A comparison of thiopental, propofol, and diazepam-ketamine anesthesia for evaluation of laryngeal function in dogs premedicated with butorphanol-glycopyrrolate. J Am Anim Hosp Assoc 2002; 38: 503–506

4.40 Tramadol

- **Opioid, μ agonist**
- **Analgesic**

▶ Pharmacokinetics
- Acts like opioids agonistically at the μ receptors and additionally inhibits the reuptake of serotonin and noradrenalin; therefore similar effect as antidepressants and alpha2 agonists
- Tramadol itself has only a low affinity for the μ receptor; the first metabolite (M1), which is only formed through metabolisation, has a much greater affinity and effect but still less than pure μ agonists like methadone

- **Onset of effect:** PO about 60–80 min, IV 5–15 min (high variability), SC a little later
- **Duration of effect: Dog** up to 6 h, **cat** up to 12 h

▶ Effects
- Central analgesia
- Sedation, sleepiness
- Antitussive

▶ Indications
- All types of mild, moderate or severe pain (acute or chronic):
  - Acute postoperative pain
  - Long-term therapy of chronic pain due to the low side effects
  - Neuropathic pain
  - Orthopaedic pain e.g. osteoarthritis (accumulates in joint fluid and reduces joint inflammation)
  - Trauma
  - Abdominal colic
  - Pain patients with gastric ulcer (use of NSAIDs not indicated)

▶ Contraindications/precautions
- Caution in animals with a history of seizures, may lower the seizure threshold

▶ Adverse effects
- Tiredness, sedation
- CNS stimulation: Euphoria, dysphoria (**cat**), tremor, excitations (**dog**), sensitivity to sound, trembling, head shaking, ataxia (**horse**)
- Nausea and vomiting
- Anticholinergic effect: Reduction of gastric acid secretion, dry mouth
- More pronounced side effects in the **cat** (severe salivation, fatigue) compared to the **dog**
- **High variability in efficacy** (if the owner says the animal is still in pain, it probably is!)
- Constipation (**dog**)

▶ Miscellaneous
- No clinically relevant effects on respiratory and cardiovascular systems or renal function
- Appears to have local anaesthetic effect

Table 4.40 Dosages for tramadol (mg/kg)

Species	IV slowly	PO
Dog	1–4	1–5 TID
Cat	2	1–4 TID
Rabbit	–	10 SID
Small rodents	–	5
Horse	1–2 BID	5 BID*
Pig	–	5

IV intravenous, PO orally, SID 1 × daily, BID 2 × daily, TID 3 × daily, * i.e. for chronic laminitis

- Combines very well with NSAIDs
- Oral formulation tastes bitter and is reluctantly eaten (especially by **cats**)
- Efficacy in **small mammals** and **horses** is controversial (little metabolisation to the first metabolite, short half-life)
- Duration of action in **dogs** appears to be shorter than previously thought

▶ Dosages
- Dosages are listed in ▶ Table 4.40
- **Retard tablets** do not seem to be really effective in **dogs** because very little of the active metabolite M1 is formed, but if **dogs** chew the retard tablet, very high plasma levels can occur quickly
- Give **slowly** with **IV** application!

Practice tip

Fill oral formulation into capsules
The oral formulation tastes particularly bitter, so that acceptance by **dogs** and especially **cats** is relatively poor. However, it is possible to fill the required amount into tasteless capsules and administer it this way. This significantly increases the acceptance.

4.41 Xylazine

- **Alpha2 agonist, imidazole derivative**
- **Sedative**
- **Analgesic**

Alpha1 to alpha2 ratio is 1:160, i.e. it is not very specific for the alpha2 receptor mediating the desired effects. It also binds to the alpha1 receptor to a large extent.

"Old generation" alpha2 agonists, still used in large animals, is largely replaced by more specific alpha2 agonists in small animal anaesthesia!

▶ Pharmacokinetics
- Stimulates the central alpha2 receptors, thereby inhibiting the nerve impulses in the CNS, duration and intensity strongly dose-dependent
- Only partially antagonisable by atipamezole (due to very high binding fraction also to alpha1 receptors, which are not antagonised)
- Partially antagonisable by yohimbine or tolazoline
- **Onset of effect:** IV 3–5 min, IM 10–15 min
- **Duration of effect:** Sedative effect dose- and species-dependent up to 1–6 h, analgesic effect only about 15–30 min

▶ Effects
- Sedation and analgesia (stimulation of the central alpha2 receptors)
- Muscle relaxation (inhibition of conduction in the spinal cord)
- Anxiolytic (through reduced release of stress hormones)

▶ Indications
- Used predominantly in **large animals**, for small animals there are more modern and specifically antagonisable alpha2 agonists available
- Sedation to facilitate clinical examinations and treatments
- Premedication before induction of anaesthesia
- Anaesthesia, when used in combination with e.g. opioid and ketamine
- Postoperative sedation and analgesia
- Perioperative MAC reduction (= less inhalation anaesthetic is needed)

▶ Contraindications/precautions
- Shock
- **Puppies** < 6 months, **kittens** < 5 months
- Pregnant animals
- Animals with diabetes mellitus (p. 333)

- Obstruction within the urinary tract (if it is not certain whether the obstruction can be solved)
- **Careful** in animals with cardiovascular diseases, in particular dogs with dilated cardiomyopathy (p. 279) and/or mitral valve insufficiency (p. 285)

▶ Adverse effects

- Biphasic effect on blood pressure: Initial severe **vasoconstriction** (pale mucous membranes) causes **hypertension**; then the baroreceptor reflex causes **bradycardia** with return to **normotension**, possibly hypotension
- Bradycardia can become severe, 1st and 2nd degree **AV blocks** are possible
- **Cardiac output is drastically reduced**
- IV catheterisation may become difficult due to vasoconstriction
- Decrease in respiratory rate without change in blood gas levels; increases respiratory depressant effects of other anaesthetics
- **Sheep** may be sensitive especially after IV administration: More pronounced cardiovascular and respiratory side effects, which may lead to severe hypoxaemia
- Diuresis, increased urine output (due to inhibition of antidiuretic hormone, ADH)
- Hyperglycaemia (due to inhibition of insulin synthesis)
- Vomiting (**cat**, but also **dog**)
- Reduction of intestinal motility
- **Horse**: Small intestinal peristalsis is maintained, large intestinal peristalsis is decreased
- Ataxia, staggering (dose-dependent, especially after IV injection)
- Hypothermia (e.g. **horses** can sweat profusely and therefore lose a lot of heat)
- Increased uterine contractility in pregnant animals
- Temporary increase, followed by decrease in intraocular pressure
- Can increase sensitivity of the myocardium to catecholamines and lead to cardiac arrhythmias

▶ Miscellaneous

- **Essential disadvantage** compared to dex-/medetomidine is that **no specific antagonist** is available!
- Can be combined well with ketamine
- **Combination with atropine not recommended**, serious cardiac arrhythmias, increase in blood pressure and heart rate occur
- **Cattle**: Diarrhoea or premature birth (clenbuterol approved for tocolysis)

Table 4.41 Dosages for xylazine (mg/kg)

Species	IV	IM/SC
Dog	0.25–0.5–1–3	0.5–1–3
Cat	0.25–0.5–1–3	0.5–1–2–4
Rabbit	–	1–6
Guinea pig	–	3–5
Ferret	–	0.5–2
Small rodents	–	5–10
Horse	0.6–1	–
Cattle	0.02–0.1	0.05–0.3
Sheep	0.05–0.1	0.05–0.2
Goat	0.05–0.1	0.05–0.1
South American camelids	0.1–0.6	0.2–0.8
Pig	1–2	1–2

IV intravenous, IM intramuscular, SC subcutaneous

▶ **Dosages**
- Dosages are listed in ▶ Table 4.41
- **Sensitivity strongly species-dependent**: **Cattle** are extremely sensitive to xylazine and need about $^1/_{10}$ of the dose of **horses** to get the same effect, **South American camelids** are about between cattle and horses, **small ruminants** about between cattle and South American camelids; thus cattle > goat/ sheep > South American camelids > horse (> = is more sensitive)
- Depending on the desired effect (sedation or anaesthesia), the dose must be chosen accordingly

▶ **Literature**

[1] Kästner SB. A2-agonists in sheep: a review. Vet Anaesth Analg 2006; 33: 79–96

Part II
Anaesthesia practice

5 Species-specific anaesthesia

For the anaesthesia of each patient, one should think in advance about a (preferably) safe and suitable anaesthesia protocol as well as the ideal perioperative management. Management includes comfortable positioning, airway and temperature management, appropriate infusion management, possible antibiotic treatment, eye protection and, in case of prolonged procedures, emptying of the urinary bladder.

This chapter discusses the pre- and perioperative management of anaesthesia patients. As this is largely valid across species, it will not be discussed again for the individual species. However, this should in no way diminish the importance of these management techniques!

5.1 Preanaesthetic examination, categorisation according to ASA classification

Anamnesis and preanaesthetic examination help the anaesthetist to assess the patient's physical condition, evaluate the individual risk and formulate a tailored plan for anaesthesia.

▶ Table 5.1 lists the factors to be evaluated for the categorisation of patients according to the American Society of Anesthesiologists (ASA) classification system.

Table 5.1 ASA classification for the categorisation of patients before anaesthesia

ASA classification	Description	Example
ASA 1	Normal, healthy animals, no known diseases	Young, healthy animal for castration
ASA 2	Animals with mild systemic disease, compensated	Animal with severe obesity or e.g. dog with cruciate ligament rupture and signs of inflammation
ASA 3	Animals with moderate to severe systemic disease	Anaemia, moderate dehydration, fever, heart disease (moderate)
ASA 4	Animals with severe systemic disease associated with constant threat to life	Severe dehydration, shock, uraemia, high fever, non-compensated heart disease
ASA 5	Multimorbid animals likely to die without intervention	Severe cardiac, hepatic, renal failure or endocrine disease, severe trauma or shock

ASA American Society of Anesthesiologists

▶ **Anamnesis**
- Reactions to previous anaesthesia?
- Known diseases?
- Is the patient receiving any medication?
- Fasted?

▶ **Clinical examination**

Special attention to:
- Physical condition: Obesity, cachexia, pregnancy, temperature
- Hydration status
- Heart murmur, arrhythmia
- Lung sounds
- Further examinations like blood work, radiographs, ultrasound necessary/available?

▶ **Age**
- Young or old age is not a disease, but one must pay special attention to physiological characteristics or concomitant disease symptoms, because compensatory mechanisms may be limited. For more details see chapter on "Physiology and pathophysiology" (p. 262).

▶ **Breed**
- Some breeds show specifics in relation to different anaesthetics or breed-associated diseases. See chapters on preanaesthetic considerations in the "Dog" (p. 168) and "Cat" (p. 178) for more details.

▶ **Temperament**
- In a highly aggressive or wild animal, preanaesthetic examination may be limited and one will usually induce deep sedation or anaesthesia with an IM injection in order to be able to perform further treatment
- Conversely, in very anxious animals, it may be helpful to work with only calming, anxiolytic sedatives
- Very calm, very young, sick or old animals can be premedicated with low-dose, gentle, only mildly sedating drugs or analgesics

▶ **Intervention**
- Invasiveness?
- Painful?
- Risk of haemorrhage?
- Duration?
- Is **anaesthesia** needed or is **deep sedation** sufficient? This depends on the procedure and how much monitoring is needed for a safe procedure

► Other factors
- Experience and qualification of surgeon and anaesthetist
- Equipment available

For each patient, individual consideration should be given to the possible complications that may be encountered. These are explained in the chapter "Anaesthetic incidents and complications" (p. 350). You can **sort your thoughts** by dividing anticipated complications into:

1. **Complications associated with this species** in general, with this breed, **with this individual animal** (e.g. brachycephalic dog: respiratory problems in the recovery phase)
2. **Complications associated with anaesthesia** itself (e.g. hypoventilation, hypotension)
3. **Complications associated with the planned procedure** (e.g. pain, haemorrhage, but also inadequate access to the head in the case of e.g. eye surgery)

5.2 Perioperative management

Of course, **non-apparatus and apparatus monitoring** play a major role in perioperative management. Basic monitoring (p. 39) of vital parameters must be done in any anaesthesia; the extent to which additional apparatus monitoring is used must be decided individually on a case-by-case basis and depending on the monitoring equipment available.

Clinical relevance

Positioning the patient

In general, patients should be positioned comfortably, warm and dry: Do not overstretch or position limbs in a non-physiological way, but place them parallel and free of stretching and tension. Bony protrusions should be padded underneath. Choose a soft pad for longer operations. Mouth gags, especially those with a spring, should be removed to relieve pressure on the temporomandibular joint and avoid occlusion of vessels. In lateral positioning, the lower leg should be pulled slightly forward. These measures prevent nerve damage/overstretching and other injuries (permanent lameness or similar), cooling, pain and discomfort of the patient. The tongue should lie in a physiological position and not be squeezed off by the endotracheal tube. Appropriate positioning is important in any animal species but especially important in large animal species!

5.2.1 Airway management

Airway management includes a set of manoeuvres and medical procedures performed to prevent and relieve airway obstruction. This ensures an open pathway for gas exchange between a patient´s lungs and the atmosphere. In general, anaesthetised patients should always be offered oxygen-enriched air or pure oxygen. There are various ways to implement this in practice. Often a volatile anaesthetic (e.g. isoflurane or sevoflurane) is also administered for the maintenance of general anaesthesia.

Intubation with the endotracheal tube

Intubation ensures a secure airway through which oxygen, air and inhalation anaesthetics can be administered. Positive pressure ventilation is most reliably achieved via an endotracheal tube (ETT). Aspiration of regurgitated or vomited gastric contents or infectious material after dental cleaning can be partially prevented by an appropriately cuffed ETT. The cuff should be tested for leakage before each use. To do this, inflate it completely and leave it for a few minutes to detect even small (slow) leaks. If after a few minutes the cuff is still inflated, it is leak-proof.

  Risks associated with (incorrect) intubation can be:
- Laryngeal spasm
- Laryngeal oedema
- Vagal reflex
- Irritation of the trachea, even necrosis caused by ischaemia
- Perforation or rupture of the tracheal mucosa or trachea itself

These risks seem to influence perioperative mortality, especially in the **cat**, but they are negligible when intubation is performed correctly and do not outweigh the benefits of a secured airway.

What types of ETT are there?

As shown in ▶ Fig. 5.1, there are ETTs made of three different materials and additionally armoured tubes.

▶ PVC tubes. These tubes are manufactured for single use in human medicine but can be used many times for veterinary patients with proper cleaning, disinfection and care. They are available in sizes from 2 to 16 mm internal diameter (ID) in 0.5 mm increments, so can only be used for small animals or small ruminants, South American camelids and small pigs. The cuff usually has a large volume and applies less traumatic pressure on the tracheal mucosa (high volume, low pressure cuff).

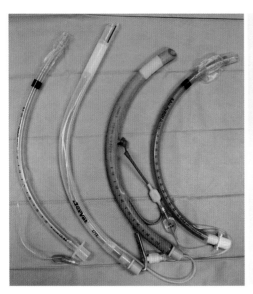

Fig. 5.1 Endotracheal tubes made of different materials; from left to right: PVC, silicone (with inserted stylet) and red rubber as well as an armoured tube.

▶ **Advantages.** Inexpensive, robust, transparent, pre-curved in physiological curve, relatively stiff, but thermoplastic, i.e. at 37 °C the material becomes soft. Intubation is relatively easy. Radiographic strip that makes the ETT visible on radiographs.

▶ **Disadvantages.** Not autoclavable; the cuff may not be sealing for liquids due to folds even when inflated correctly. These folds can be largely sealed by applying a tracheal gel onto the cuff before intubation.

▶ **Silicone tubes.** These tubes are made for repeated use for veterinary medicine. They usually come in sizes 10 to 35 mm ID. They are straight, softer and more pliable than PVC tubes, which can make intubation difficult because you do not have the angle you need for intubation. For this reason, these tubes are usually used with a stylet up to about size 12 to 16 mm ID. The cuff contains a small volume and exerts high localised pressure on the tracheal mucosa (low volume, high pressure cuff).

▶ **Advantages.** Robust, transparent, soft, autoclavable, can be used often; the cuff seals very well.

▶ **Disadvantages.** The straight form can make intubation difficult because the required angle cannot be reached, e.g. in large dogs (use a stylet!). The cuff can cause damage to the tracheal mucosa due to high pressure.

▶ **Tubes made of red rubber.** This "old generation" of tubes is disappearing more and more from veterinary practice since tubes made of the above-mentioned modern materials have become available at a lower price. They are available in all sizes from 2 to 35 mm ID.

▶ **Advantages.** Very robust, autoclavable, can be used often; the cuff seals very well (low volume, high pressure cuff).

▶ **Disadvantages.** Hard, non-transparent, expensive, becomes porous over time and cuff becomes asymmetrical and bulges; material takes up disinfectant which can damage the tracheal mucosa.

▶ **Armoured tubes.** The tube reinforced with a wire spiral is usually made of silicone and is suitable for procedures in which the tube is moved a lot and kinking is to be prevented (dental or eye procedures, operations on the cervical spine or similar). The outer diameter (OD) is often quite large compared to the inner diameter. These tubes cannot be shortened.

▶ **Very small tubes without cuff.** These have a maximum size of 5 mm ID and are very suitable for intubating rabbits (or other very small animals). Often the larynx is the narrowest part of the airway and even a thin-walled cuff is too much resistance to intubate without damaging the larynx.

▶ **Tracheostomy tubes.** They are needed to ensure a safe airway after a tracheostomy. They come in different sizes and materials, with or without cuff and with or without an inner tube.

Practice tip

Cleaning and disinfection of ETT
Some endotracheal tubes are intended for multiple use and must be cleaned appropriately after use:
- First, tubes are thoroughly cleaned inside and out under running water with bottle brushes of an appropriate size.
- After cleaning with water, the tube is soaked in a suitable disinfectant for approx. 1 hour.

- Then each tube is rinsed individually inside and out very well under running water.
- Overnight, all tubes are placed in fresh clear water and hung up to dry in the morning.
- Important: The cuff should be inflated for cleaning (especially in the case of PVC tubes with high volume, low pressure cuffs) so that mucus/blood or similar cannot get caught in folds.

Which endotracheal tube size do I use for which animal

Usually, the size of the ETT is given as the inner diameter (= the abbreviation ID found on the tube) in millimetres (mm) or French (Fr). One French corresponds to ⅓ mm. The outer diameter (OD) is often several millimetres larger.

In most cases, ETT diameter should be chosen as large as possible to minimise resistance to breathing. Which sizes are recommended for which animal species can be found in the chapter on "Species-specific anaesthesia" (p. 150) for the animal species dog, cat, rabbit, guinea pig, ferret, small rodent, horse, cattle, small ruminant, South American camelid and pig. Some animal species are so heterogeneous that no general recommendation can be made, e.g. in case of dogs. The breed can be decisive: Brachycephalic dogs often need smaller tubes, very athletic breeds, e.g. sighthounds, often need surprisingly large tubes compared to their size.

Practice tip

Shorten endotracheal tubes to reduce dead space
PVC tubes can be shortened with scissors from the distal end to just before the exit of the cuff balloon, which can significantly reduce dead space and thus CO_2 rebreathing. To do this, remove the adapter from the tube and cut off the tube. In the case of small animal tubes, you can dilate the new end of the tube with a pen or similar to make it easier to put the adapter back on. Shortening of the ETT is recommended especially for brachycephalic dogs or cats.

What equipment do I need for intubation?

▶ **For intubation I need**
- Choice of **endotracheal tubes**:
  - The size you think is right, one size smaller and one size larger
- **Laryngoscope** with light source:
  - The newer devices have LED lights that are very bright and do not get hot. When intubating blind (e.g. rabbit or horse) or with palpation (bovine), you do not need a laryngoscope
  - If animals with very long, narrow oral cavities are to be intubated (e.g. pigs, South American camelids), a very long blade is needed on the laryngoscope
- **Lidocaine** as spray, gel or solution:
  - Particularly important in animals prone to laryngospasm, such as cats, rabbits or pigs
- Something to **tie** the ETT:
  - A cotton or plastic cord is sufficient for small animals. For small ruminants, a Heidelberg extension line has proven to be effective, it does not soften when the animal salivates heavily. In large animals, no tying is necessary
- Sterile **lubricant** for the ETT:
  - Often not necessary for small animals, helpful for large animals
  - Lubricant seals the small folds in high volume, low pressure cuffs and therefore creates a better seal for liquids
- **Cuff syringe** of appropriate size or **manometer** to inflate the cuff
- **Mouth gag** if you do not have a second person to hold the mouth open. Helpful in small ruminants and large animals. It should be removed after intubation

> ## Careful!
>
> **Work cleanly during intubation!**
> - Keep the intubation equipment clean!
> - Do not place it on dirty surfaces or in the fur! Risk of infection!

What to consider when intubating?

- **Cuff** tested and **without leak**?
- ETT prepared in the **right size**? Too big it can cause injuries – too small it increases resistance to breathing exponentially
- Is the ETT **really in the trachea** and not in the oesophagus? Only if the ETT is in the trachea …

- it disappears into the depths between the arytenoid cartilages when visualised with the laryngoscope. The oesophagus lies to the right and above it when looking into the animal's oral cavity in sternal recumbency
- breath sounds in the lungs during ventilation can be auscultated
- does the tube inside fog up rhythmically with breathing (caution, can be deceptive)
- air flows out of the tube during expiration (caution, can be deceptive)
- CO_2 curves can be seen on the **capnograph**

- ETT in the **correct position**? Especially in small or brachycephalic animals, ETTs are often inadvertently pushed in too deep (one-lung ventilation). This can lead to hypoxaemia and hypercapnia. The end of the tube should be just cranial to the thoracic inlet (*apertura thoracis*). PVC tubes have centimetre markings from the tip of the tube to the distal end. Measure and determine the depth before induction of anaesthesia. To test this in the already intubated animal, a second tube of similar size is placed on the outside of the animal (▶ Fig. 5.2), the centimetres of the correctly positioned outside tube are compared with the intubated tube and the position of the tube is corrected if necessary after deflating the cuff

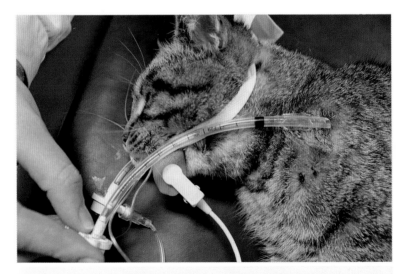

Fig. 5.2 Measuring the correct position of the endotracheal tube.

- ETT **cuffed**? In general, there is little to be said against cuffing (p. 159) and much to be said **for** it. Especially in cats, but of course also in all other animals, the tube should always be disconnected from the anaesthesia machine **before** repositioning the patient to prevent complications. To do this, turn the vaporiser off, turn the flowmeter to zero, disconnect the patient from the breathing system and then reposition slowly. After reconnecting the breathing system to the ETT, do not forget to turn on the oxygen flow and the vaporiser again! The seal of the cuff should always be checked after repositioning. A complication in cats, especially after dental treatment, is tracheal rupture, which can be caused by turning the cuff in the trachea (if not disconnected). In rabbits, it may be helpful to use a tube without a cuff, as the larynx is exceptionally small and the cuff may cause problems while intubating

Clinical relevance

Correct inflation of the cuff on the endotracheal tube

For example in patients with gastric torsion, it is particularly important that the cuff on the endotracheal tube is inflated to such an extent that the trachea is mostly sealed against stomach contents that have entered the oral cavity (aspiration protection). However, the pressure in the cuff must not completely squeeze the capillaries in the tracheal mucosa. Unfortunately, there is not yet a single technique that reliably achieves the goal (cuff is sealed, but tracheal mucosa is undamaged) for the different types of cuffs. One option without extra equipment is: As soon as the patient is intubated and connected to the breathing system of the anaesthesia machine, the APL valve is closed and positive pressure ventilation up to 15 cmH$_2$O (small animal) or 20–30 cmH$_2$O (large animal) is performed. During inspiration, listen for the passing of air between the cuff and the trachea. The cuff is inflated during inspiration until the hissing sound is just not heard anymore, which is the point where the cuff seals the trachea. Unfortunately, this method is unreliable. The cuff should be checked after each change of position. And in some animals the larynx is so tight or so much tissue is present that a hissing sound can never be heard.

In general, and especially for endotracheal tubes made of PVC with a high volume, low pressure cuff, a manometer should be used to inflate the cuff. There are even those on which colour markings (green/green shaded or yellow/red) indicate when the tube is "perfectly" inflated (▶ Fig. 5.3). There are also cuff syringes that give you a digital reading of the pressure in the cuff. However, the cuff should only be inflated to a maximum pressure of about 30–35 mmHg to avoid damage to the tracheal mucosa. If all these options are not available, the cuff must be inflated rather unreliable "by feel" to try to ensure a seal.

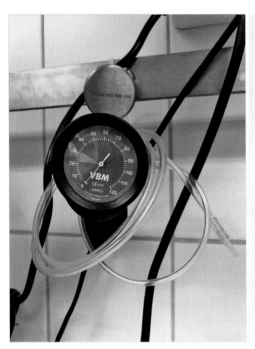

Fig. 5.3 Manometer with colour marking to check the pressure in the cuff.

Placing a laryngeal mask airway

There are only a few indications and a few suitable animal species for the placement of a laryngeal mask airway: dog, cat, rabbit and pig.

It may be useful for:

• short, light anaesthesia without change of position (e.g. radiation therapy),
• airway management during bronchoscopy in the larger dog,
• airway management in rabbits when intubation with ETT seems too difficult; or
• postoperative airway management in brachycephalic dog breeds.

Many of the laryngeal masks made for humans are too short for dogs' noses. Suitable animal patients must therefore be carefully selected. Again, a selection of different sizes (there are sizes 1 to 6) is helpful (▸ Fig. 5.4). Most human laryngeal masks have a cuff which, when inflated, wraps around the upper airway and largely seals it. Displacement of the laryngeal mask during cuffing is common, so the correct fit should be checked after inflation of the cuff. For rabbits,

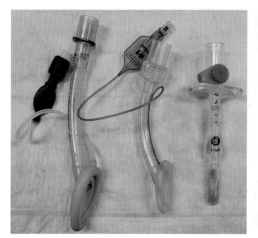

Fig. 5.4 Laryngeal mask airways for small dogs, cats and rabbits (from left to right).

cats and recently for dogs there is a special laryngeal mask airway without cuff (V-gel) available, which could be an alternative to intubation using an ETT (▶ Fig. 5.4).

▶ Advantages. Can be placed blindly and relatively easily, the distal tip blocks the upper oesophagus, large tube diameter, no laryngeal spasm or irritation of the tracheal mucosa, autoclavable

▶ Disadvantages. No protection against aspiration (therefore contraindicated in non-fasted animals, exception rabbits), possibly no positive pressure ventilation achievable, if high pressures are needed it may slip. Should only be used under capnography control!

Preoxygenation: Flow-by with mask

The tighter the mask and the higher the O_2 flow, the higher the F_iO_2, i.e. the fraction of inspiratory oxygen. The O_2 flow should be 3–5 l/min to dilute/eliminate air and CO_2. Masks should be made of transparent hard or soft plastic and ideally seal well with the help of a soft membrane (▶ Fig. 5.5). The less the mask seals, the lower the F_iO_2 will be.

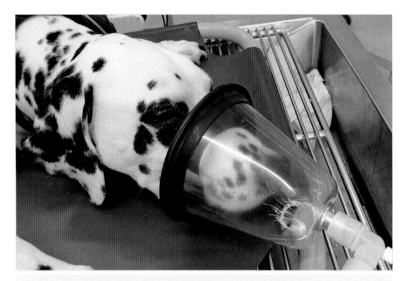

Fig. 5.5 Preoxygenation before induction of general anaesthesia with a well-fitting mask in a sedated dog.

Careful!

Caution with
- Animals with **protruding eyes**, e.g. in brachycephalic breeds, rabbits or other small mammals! Injuries to the cornea can occur if the mask is pressed on carelessly!

Especially in patients who can easily get into an oxygen deficiency situation (e.g. lung pathology, pregnancy, induction of anaesthesia), O_2 should always be administered. However, the advantages of oxygen administration should be weighed against the stress that the mask may cause the animal, so that the additional O_2 administration is practically "cancelled out". For this reason, it can often be helpful to sedate patients beforehand.

▶ **Advantages.** Easy to use, O_2 supplementation is easily possible.

▶ **Disadvantages.** No airway protection, no protection against aspiration after regurgitation or vomiting, it is hardly possible to perform positive pressure ventilation (possible in individual cases, e.g. with a tight-fitting mask in small mammals).

The mask should be cleaned after each use.

Literature

[1] Ambros B, Carrozzo MV, Jones T. Desaturation times between dogs via face mask or flow-by technique before induction of anesthesia. Vet Anaesth Analg 2018; 45:452–458

[2] Mitchell SL, McCarthy R, Rudloff E, Pernell RT. Tracheal rupture associated with intubation in cats: 20 cases (1996–1998). J Am Vet Med Assoc 2000; 216:1592–5

5.2.2 Perioperative infusion therapy

The purpose and goal of infusion therapy is to correct dehydration, maintain fluid balance and physiological electrolyte concentrations, and replace fluid losses. Each patient should be treated individually.

Evaluation of hydration balance

Prior to any sedation or anaesthesia, the degree of dehydration and volaemic status should be assessed for several reasons. Clinical signs for dehydration are found in ▶ Table 5.2. Ideally, deviations from physiologic conditions should be corrected before induction of anaesthesia. One can almost assume that patients who present fasted for anaesthesia/surgery are up to 5% dehydrated (due to excitement, panting, not eating, sometimes not drinking).

Crystalloid solutions

Perioperatively, but also for shock treatment or resuscitation, a crystalloid solution, if possible, a **balanced isotonic full electrolyte solution** (Sterofundin

Table 5.2 Clinical signs in dehydrated patients

% Dehydration	Clinical signs
< 5	No recognisable signs
5–8	Reduced skin elasticity, dry mucous membranes
8–10	Reduced skin elasticity, dry mucous membranes, possibly sunken eyeballs, slightly prolonged capillary refill time
10–12	Staying of the skin fold, prolonged capillary refill time, eyeballs sunken into the orbit, possibly signs of shock
12–15	All the above symptoms, plus shock, often life-threatening

ISO, Elomel OP, Ringer's lactate solution), should be administered. These solutions contain the important electrolytes in almost physiological concentrations and are therefore best suited to cover the fluid requirement.

NaCl 0.9% should rather be used to dilute or flush drugs than as perioperative infusion solution. Only the electrolytes sodium and chloride are added and these are present in higher concentrations than in the plasma. The solution also has an acidifying effect, shifting the pH of the blood towards acidosis.

Glucose 5% is rather unsuitable to cover the fluid requirement. The glucose is immediately metabolised and free water without electrolytes remains, which can disturb the acid-base and electrolyte balance after a short time and lead to oedema.

Clinical relevance

When to use Ringer's lactate solution?

Many patients hypoventilate under anaesthesia (hypercapnia leading to respiratory acidosis) and may also suffer from reduced perfusion due to hypovolaemia/dehydration. Accumulation of metabolic products in the tissues leads to a decrease in blood pH (metabolic acidosis). In these patients, it is useful to restore physiological fluid balance with a full electrolyte solution to which lactate has been added, e.g. Ringer's lactate solution. Lactate is metabolised in the liver to bicarbonate and then has an alkalising effect.

Infusion rates

Infusion rates are based on how much fluid loss can be expected directly and indirectly during anaesthesia/surgery:

- Fasting, no water intake pre-, peri- and immediately postoperatively
- Agitation, panting, increased urine output
- Evaporation from open surgical area

There is a generally applicable guideline in which, in healthy, normovolaemic patients, infusion rates of **up to 10 ml/kg/h balanced full electrolyte solution IV** are recommended perioperatively in dogs and cats. Especially for long procedures (> 60 min) without additional blood or other fluid losses, the infusion rate can be continuously reduced towards the simple maintenance rate. A typical recommendation may be, for example, a 25% reduction every hour until the maintenance requirement is reached. This of course is based on the assumption of a stable circulatory situation.

II

Good to know

Maintenance fluid requirement
- **Cat**: 2–3 ml/kg BW/h
- **Dog**: 2–6 ml/kg BW/h
- **Horse**: 2–3 ml/kg BW/h

BW = body weight, h = hour

Cats generally require lower infusion rates than dogs because they have a smaller blood volume.

Colloid solutions

If infusion with crystalloid solutions alone is not sufficient to normalise the volume status, colloid solutions can be infused **in addition**. They should **not be used as the sole infusion solution**.

Of the multitude of products available, one has proven very useful in practice. This colloid solution contains hydroxyethyl starch (HES) as a macromolecule (Voluven 250 and 500 ml), which cannot penetrate the vessel wall but can hold fluid in the vessel or even draw it into it due to its colloid osmotic pressure. The effect lasts until most of the HES is metabolised (6–12 h). In contrast, crystalloid solutions only remain in the vascular system for approx. 30 min and then redistribute. HES can be stored unopened for up to 3 years. It is therefore worthwhile to have a few bags in stock for emergencies.

Contraindications for the administration of colloid solutions are:
- Hyperhydration states (e.g. pulmonary oedema, congestive heart failure)
- Renal failure with oligo- or anuria
- Sepsis (increased morbidity and mortality demonstrated after administration of HES)
- Coagulopathies (increased risk of bleeding)
- Intracranial haemorrhage

Infusion rates

An initial administration to support blood pressure may be **2–5 ml/kg IV over a few minutes**, followed by further boluses as needed or continuous drip infusion. A **maximum administration of 30 ml/kg/24 h** should not be exceeded, as then the side effects increase noticeably. This applies to large and small animals.

Literature

[1] Boller E, Boller M. Assessment of fluid balance and the approach to fluid therapy in the perioperative patient. Vet Clin North Am Small Anim Pract 2015; 45:895–915

[2] Chan DL. Colloids: Current recommedations. Vet Clin Small Anim 2008; 38:587–593

[3] Davis H, Jensen T, Johnson A, Knowles P, Meyer R, Rucinsky R, Shafford H. 2013 AAHA/AAFP Fluid therapy guidelines for dogs and cats. J Am Anim Hosp Assoc 2013; 49:149–159

[4] Guidet B, Martinet O, Boulain T, Philippart F, Poussel JF, Maizel J, Forceville X, Feissel M, Hasselmann M, Heininger A, Van Aken H. Assessment of hemodynamic efficacy and safety of 6% hydroxyethyl-starch 130/0.4 vs. 0.9% NaCl fluid replacement in patients with severe sepsis: The CRYSTMAS study. Crit Care 2012; 16: R94

5.2.3 Use of antibiotics

The prophylactic use of antibiotics has been proven to be useful for certain indications. However, antibiotic prophylaxis in no way replaces clean handling, disinfection and sterilisation.

Preoperative prophylactic antibiotics should only be administered **slowly** intravenously and no longer than 30 min prior to skin incision. Intraoperative administration takes place every 1.5–2 h depending on the duration of the operation. Antibiotic administration ends at the end of surgery or within the following 24 h. Examples of surgical interventions for which prophylactic antibiotic administration is appropriate:

- Duration of the procedure > 90 min
- Existing prostheses or prostheses to be implanted
- Heavily contaminated and traumatised wounds
- Orthopaedic surgery
  - Hip surgery
  - Open fractures
  - Extensive fracture repair
  - Other elective surgery
- Gastrointestinal surgery
  - Colon, rectal or anal surgery
  - Strangulation or obstruction
  - Pancreatic abscess
  - Oesophageal surgery
- Urogenital surgery
  - Operations on genital organs (e.g. pyometra), kidney, ureter, bladder and urethra with infected urine

If at all and which antibiotic and in what dose is administered to which species should be decided individually. There are great differences from country to country as to which indications and to what extent antibiotics are used.

Literature

[1] Fossum TW. Small Animal Surgery, 4. Edition, Elsevier, chapter 9, Surgical infections and antibiotic selection, Willard MD and Schulz, KS p. 84–94

[2] Masterton RG. Antibiotic de-escalation. Crit Care Clin. 2011; 27: 149–162

[3] Weese JS, Giguère S, Guardabassi L, Morley PS, Papich M, Ricciuto DR, Sykes JE. ACVIM consensus statement on therapeutic antimicrobial use in animals and antimicrobial resistance. J Vet Intern Med. 2015; 29: 487–498

5.2.4 Protection of the cornea

In animals under general anaesthesia, the palpebral reflex is (largely) disabled and tear production is reduced. Therefore, eye ointment (without additives) should always be applied to every anaesthetised animal as protection for the cornea. The only exceptions are patients who are having surgery on the eyes themselves.

If necessary, the eye ointment should be applied repeatedly, regular checks are especially important:

- After the administration of ketamine, because the eyes often protrude and the eyelids remain open
- In small mammals (such as rabbits) or brachycephalic breeds (e.g. Persian cats or pugs); in these patients the eyes are very exposed and can be easily injured
- For any manipulation near the eyes, e.g. dental patients (small animals) where it is often necessary to hold the head and reach over the eyes
- For large animals in lateral position; a ring pad placed underneath is useful to protect the ventral eye
- When using a warm air blowing device for temperature management; warm air should not blow directly onto the unprotected cornea

Even in premedicated animals or animals that have just recovered from anaesthesia, uncontrolled movement in the cage or stall can cause injury to the eyes. A suitable environment and supervision should be provided to minimise the risk of injury. Tear production may be limited even days after anaesthesia. Drying of the cornea should be counteracted with water-based eye drops.

5.2.5 Emptying the urinary bladder

A full bladder presents a strong sympathetic and painful stimulus.

After longer procedures and/or the administration of alpha2 agonists (dexmedetomidine (p. 86), medetomidin (p. 145), xylazin (p. 145), detomidin (p. 84), romifidin (p. 135) – all induce diuresis) or opioids, the urinary bladder should be emptied before the recovery phase. This can be done by placing a urinary catheter (easy in male small animals or horses) or carefully **massaging out the bladder** (usually easy in female small animals or small mammals). This makes the recovery phase more relaxed and probably less dangerous in horses, as the animals do not feel any pressure on or pain from the bladder.

In small animal patients who have received epidural anaesthesia with morphine (p. 123), the filling of the urinary bladder should be checked regularly for at least 24 hours afterwards, as it relaxes the detrusor muscle of the bladder which may result in urinary retention.

Literature

[1] Baldini G, Bagry H, Aprikian A, Carli F. Postoperative urinary retention – Anesthetic and perioperative considerations. Anesthesiol 2009; 110: 1139–57

[2] Drenger B, Magora F, Evron S, Caine M. The action of intrathecal morphine and methadone on the lower urinary tract in the dog. J Urol. 1986; 135: 852–855

5.3 Dog

An ASA classification should be determined for each patient before anaesthesia is started (▶ Table 5.1). The perioperative management (p. 152) should be planned and prepared accordingly. If additional or different measures are recommended for individual species, these are listed under the respective species under "Preanaesthetic considerations".

5.3.1 Preanaesthetic considerations

In dogs, breeds vary in size and special characteristics more than in any other animal species.

Perioperative management depends largely on **age**, **size** and **sex** of the animal. **Breed-specific** anaesthetic **hypersensitivities** must be considered when selecting anaesthetics. Whether to sedate IM prior to catheterisation and induction of anaesthesia depends on general manageability (aggression, defensive movement, anxiety).

Classic **complications** to expect: **Hypothermia** (small dogs, dogs with little or no fur), **hyperthermia** (animals with thick, long fur and lots of undercoat, high ambient temperature), **hypotension** (often due to vasodilation), **bradycardia** and/or **negative inotropic effect** of anaesthetics, **tachycardia**, respiratory depression/**hypoventilation** with **hypercapnia** and **hypoxaemia**, problems with **intubation** (in very small or brachycephalic breeds), problems with **IV catheter placement** (i. e. in very small breeds or after high doses of alpha2 agonists).

Table 5.3 Normal values dog

Parameter (unit)	Normal values
Core body temperature (°C)	38.0–39.0
Heart rate (/min)	80–120
Respiratory rate (/min)	10–40
Haematocrit (%)	37–55
Total protein (g/dl)	6.0–7.5
Creatinine (mg/dl)	0.4–1.2

General considerations

Fasting: 8 to max. 12 h (when feeding wet food only approx. 6 h) feed deprivation before induction, no water deprivation. Do not fast suckling puppies. Some basic normal values can be found in ▶ Table 5.3.

Blood volume is about 80–90 ml/kg body weight.

Anatomical and physiological features

The "average" dog does not have any real anaesthesia-relevant special features; it is rather the different purebred dogs that require attention to special aspects. This will be discussed in the section on specific considerations (p. 170).

IV access

▶ **Cephalic vein** (*v. cephalica antebrachii*). Clearly visible. Interestingly, the small distal, medial branch is often easier to catheterise (especially in cardiovascular compromised dogs).

▶ **Lateral saphenous vein** (*v. saphena lateralis*). Well visible, but likes to "roll away". In small dogs it may not be possible to advance the catheter around the turnover point of the vein to the medial aspect of the leg.

▶ **Jugular vein** (*v. jugularis*). Very large vessel, clearly visible. Care must be taken that the catheter is long enough, otherwise it will slip out of the vessel at the first movement. Catheter should be well taped or sutured in place.

Intubation

- Endotracheal tube size is chosen from 3 to 14 mm inner diameter (ID) depending on the breed. An exception are the brachycephalic breeds. Here, a smaller tube than anticipated for the size of the animal must often be used
- As a beginner, it is easiest to intubate in sternal position with the head extended. However, this requires a helper. In lateral position, it is possible to intubate without assistance. Intubation in dorsal recumbency, which is common in human medicine, is not advantageous in dogs (it actually decreases gas exchange in that critical situation)
- The upper airways are usually easy to see, ideally with the help of a laryngoscope with a light source
- Most endotracheal tubes from human medicine are too long in small dogs, as already explained under "Airway management" (p. 153), and should be shortened. Optimal length: from the tip of the nose to the thoracic inlet (*apertura thoracis*). For more information on tube length, see "Which tube size do I use for which animal" (p. 156)
- Ideally, the epiglottis should not be touched with the laryngoscope blade, if it is necessary (and in some dogs it is!), then with care!
- Tying the tube with cotton cord, old extension lines or other can be done over the upper jaw (caution: swelling of the muzzle), over the lower jaw (caution: slipping off) or best behind the ears
- Mouth gags (especially those with springs) should be taken out

Specific considerations

It seems that more and more breed-specific characteristics or breed-associated diseases are being discovered. In the following, only the most important specific characteristics will be discussed. Whenever an unknown breed is to be anaesthetised, it is worth taking a look at a textbook or a search engine.

Many breeds of dogs are associated with cardiac diseases (p. 278), they are among others:

- **Dilated cardiomyopathy** (p. 279) and **consecutive mitral valve insufficiency**: Doberman (also Von Willebrand factor deficit), Boxer, Cocker Spaniel, Airdale Terrier and giant breeds such as Irish Wolfhound and Newfoundland dog
- **Mitral valve insufficiency** (p. 285): Dachshund, Cavalier King Charles Spaniel, Miniature Poodle, Chihuahua, Yorkshire Terrier and other small dog breeds
- **Sick sinus syndrome**: Miniature Schnauzer, Pomeranian, Dachshund, Pug and other small breeds

- **Persistent ductus arteriosus**: Poodle, Pomeranian, German Shepherd, Collie and Sheltie
- **Pulmonic stenosis**: English Bulldog, Scottish Terrier, Miniature Schnauzer, West Highland White Terrier, Chihuahua, Samoyed, Mastiff, Cocker Spaniel, Boxer and Beagle

Acepromazine sensitivity of the Boxer

▶ **Affected breed.** Some Boxer lines (coming from the UK? especially white Boxers?) or other brachycephalic breeds. However, many Boxers or other brachycephalic breeds do not show any particular symptoms after acepromazine administration.

▶ **What happens?** Affected animals react to normal doses of acepromazine with cardiovascular complications: Severe vasodilation and bradycardia, hypotension, cardiovascular collapse, shock symptoms, respiratory depression to apnoea.

▶ **Cause.** Unknown

▶ **Conclusion.** To avoid complications, the use of acepromazine in Boxers is not recommended. However, it is likely that this caution is unjustified.

Brachycephalic obstructive airway syndrome (BOAS)

▶ **Affected breeds.** Pug, English and French Bulldog, Boston Terrier, Pekinese, Shih Tsu and other brachycephalic breeds. The incidence and extent of BOAS is not uniform between or within breeds.

▶ **What happens?** Animals have increased work of breathing (active inspiration and active expiration) due to stenotic airways caused by constricted nostrils, elongated soft palate, everted laryngeal sacs, large tongue, laryngeal collapse and +/− collapsing trachea. Constant risk of hypoxaemia. Temperature management is impaired, animals are often hyperthermic. Frequent gastrointestinal problems – severity directly correlated with the degree of upper airway obstruction.

▶ **Cause.** Breeding related.

▶ **Conclusion.** Good airway management is extremely important. Continuous O_2 administration. Sedate in recovery and be ready to reintubate or perform a tracheostomy in severe cases. Administration of antiemetics and H2 blockers recommended.

Example of gastrointestinal treatment prior to anaesthesia:

- **Omeprazole** 1 mg/kg before surgery orally, then every 12 h IV – proton pump inhibitor, inhibits gastric acid production, increases pH, fewer lung problems after accidental aspiration
- +/– **Maropitant** 1–2 mg/kg at least 2 h before surgery SC or PO, better over several days, against nausea and vomiting
- +/– **Metoclopramide** 0.2 mg/kg every 8 h as prokinetic support

Thiopental sensitivity of sighthound breeds

▶ **Affected breeds.** Greyhound, Whippet, Saluki, Barsoi, Afghan Hound and other sighthound breeds.

▶ **What happens?** Thiobarbiturates have a significantly prolonged duration of action, the animals sleep for hours/days after administration, which can lead to additional secondary complications (hypotension, hypothermia, and more).

▶ **Cause.** Atypical liver metabolism especially of the cytochrome P450 enzyme system, low body fat, low volume of distribution.

▶ **Conclusion.** Thiobarbiturates (e.g. thiopental) are contraindicated in sighthound breeds and should not be used. Pentobarbital and phenobarbital can be used without restrictions.

MDR1-gene mutation (-/-) in herding dogs

▶ **Affected breeds.** Collie, Bobtail, Australian and English Shepherds, Long-haired Whippets, McNabs, Old English Sheepdogs, Shetland Sheepdogs, Silken Windhounds, Border Collie, White Shepherd Dog and German Shepherd Dog (a constantly updated list and much more information can be found on the website of the Institute of Pharmacology and Toxicology at the Justus Liebig University of Giessen, Germany, see references – unfortunately so far only in German).

▶ **What happens?** After administration of certain drugs (e.g. acepromazine, opioids), homozygous affected animals react with a prolonged recovery phase and mydriasis, loss of visual sense, ataxia, hypersalivation, disorientation and convulsions, comatose states with secondary problems (gastrointestinal motility) and death.

▶ **Cause.** A homozygous mutation of the MDR-1 gene (-/-) causes the blood-brain barrier to become more permeable, resulting in increased drug crossover into the central nervous system. Heterozygous affected animals (-/+) do not seem to show any clinical effects.

▶ **Conclusion.** Before elective surgery, it is helpful to perform an MDR-1 genetic test to detect any homozygous mutation. Drugs, not only anaesthetics, are classified in a red, yellow or green list depending on their potential to cause harm. Drugs listed in red should be avoided in affected breeds. Drugs listed in yellow, such as butorphanol, can also be used in homozygous affected animals, according to recent findings, if the dose is reduced by 25–50%.

Breeds with a thick, insulating coat

Also noteworthy are dog breeds with thick, insulating fur coat. While the majority of patients suffer from hypothermia under anaesthesia, these patients are at risk of hyperthermia (p. 384) (especially in the warm season). Rectal temperature should be taken regularly and, if necessary, the dog should be actively cooled.

5.3.2 Anaesthesia protocols

Protocols described are examples and should be understood as options. Depending on personal preferences, the availability of drugs and the individual patient, the anaesthesia protocol should be adapted.

Depending on the country and the school of thought, a combination of ketamine and dex-/medetomidine or xylazine as well as a high-dose combination of acepromazine and opioids, which are re-dosed as needed, are relatively often used in practice. These protocols are certainly old and proven, but in the meantime very controllable and less circulatory detrimental drugs and combinations are available. The following examples should serve as a suggestion and inspire to reconsider one's own protocols, especially in critically ill patients.

Of course, every patient must be checked before sedation and induction of anaesthesia as part of the preanaesthetic examinations (p. 150). The results of this clinical examination and the evaluation of laboratory parameters serve as the basis for classification into an ASA group. Perioperative management (p. 152) including airway management, infusion therapy, administration of antibiotics, protection of the cornea and emptying of the urinary bladder has already been described in detail. Monitoring (p. 39) has also been discussed in detail and is therefore not covered in repetition for the individual species.

Sedation

Below are five examples of drug combinations for sedation in dogs. The exact desired effects and side effects of the individual drugs as well as the duration of action can be found in the chapter on "Drugs" (p. 63).

Dosage

- **Acepromazine** 0.01–0.03 mg/kg AND
- **Methadone** 0.1–0.3 mg/kg mixed in one syringe IM or IV

Gentle "allrounder" sedation for healthy and slightly impaired dogs (ASA 1–3) that are nervous and also benefit from light sedation in the recovery phase (e.g. brachycephalic breeds). Slightly sedating (up to approx. 6 h, but animals are able to walk) but very good analgesic (up to approx. 4 h). One should wait up to 20–30 min after administration to obtain the desired effect. Do not use in hypovolaemic patients, be careful in dehydrated patients.

Side effects: Possibly tachycardia and hypotension due to vasodilation. Good infusion management!

Dosage

- **Medetomidine** 0.005–0.01 mg/kg IV resp. 0.01–0.02 mg/kg IM OR
  Dexmedetomidine 0.003–0.005 mg/kg IV resp. 0.005–0.01 mg/kg IM AND
- **Butorphanol** 0.2 mg/kg mixed in one syringe IM or IV

Fast and good sedation with only moderate circulatory impact for ASA 1–2 patients who are defensive or mildly aggressive. Sedation is obtained 10 min after IM injection, perfect for stress-free IV catheter placement. Mildly analgesic, short-acting (approx. 90 min to 2 h) or antagonisable (dex-/medetomidine with atipamezole).

Side effects: Vasoconstriction, resulting in reduced tissue perfusion. Bradycardia and arrhythmia. Do not use in dogs with DCM or mitral valve insufficiency!

This sedation can be enhanced by the **addition of ketamine 0.5–2 mg/kg** IM or IV. The combination of all three drugs drawn up in a mixed syringe and administered IM is very well suited to deeply sedate dogs. Depending on the individual patient and the desired effect, the dose can be increased. Addition of ketamine also stabilizes heart rate and rhythm. Intramuscular administration of ketamine is mildly painful for a short period of time – expect a response by the animal.

Dosage

- **Butorphanol** 0.2–0.4 mg/kg AND
- **Midazolam** 0.2 mg/kg mixed in one syringe IM, IV OR **Diazepam** 0.2 mg/kg IV, do not mix

This mild sedation, which is very easy on the cardiovascular system, only works well in very old and/or sick animals. All others are not sedated but rather dysphoric. Sedation occurs a few minutes after IV administration. The effect of butorphanol is mildly analgesic and short-acting, with midazolam or diazepam you get anxiolysis, relaxation and amnesia (in humans, in dogs possibly also).

Dosage

- **Methadone** 0.1–0.3 mg/kg AND
- **Midazolam** 0.2 mg/kg mixed in one syringe IM, IV OR **Diazepam** 0.2 mg/kg IV, do not mix

This combination mildly sedates very sick and painful dogs well and gently. It works very well for dogs with gastric torsion (p. 326), for example. The combination is not suitable for young or healthy animals, they pant and become rather dysphoric and agitated, but not sedated.

Dosage

- **Ketamine** 1–3 mg/kg AND
- **Medetomidine** 0.01–0.03 mg/kg OR **Dexmedetomidine** 0.005–0.015 mg/kg mixed in one syringe IM or IV

This combination produces deep sedation, in higher doses general anaesthesia. It is well suited for aggressive animals that need reliable sedation and are cardiovascularly stable. In the higher dose, short, less painful procedures can be performed. Should not be used in old and/or sick animals.

Side effects: This combination is usually well tolerated, but vasoconstriction and cardiovascular compromise occur in a dose-dependent manner.

Xylazine 0.25–1, up to 3 mg/kg SC, IM, IV is less specific than medetomidine or dexmedetomidine and cannot be fully antagonised. Therefore, dex-/medetomidine should be given preference. Dosages above 0.03 mg/kg of medetomidine or 0.015 mg/kg of dexmedetomidine only serve to prolong the duration of action (with increased side effects) and not to deepen sedation or anaesthesia!

Induction

For short procedures, the same drugs can be used for sedation, anaesthesia induction and maintenance, a classic example being the combination of ketamine and dex-/medetomidine in higher doses than mentioned for sedation (p. 175). For procedures up to about 30 min this is a good, practical approach. For longer or very painful procedures or in compromised patients, anaesthesia is usually **induced with injectable anaesthetics** and **maintained with volatile anaesthetics** (isoflurane or sevoflurane). This of course requires an anaesthetic machine (p. 20).

Propofol 2–8 mg/kg IV: With good premedication and a calm environment, 2–4 mg/kg IV is usually sufficient for an anaesthetic depth suitable for intubation. The less sedated the animal prior to induction, the higher the dosage and the more severe the side effects: Hypotension due to vasodilation and negative inotropy as well as respiratory depression and apnoea. It should always be injected slowly: Wait for the effect and preoxygenate! It is worth getting to know this drug. With good preanaesthetic sedation, practically any dog can be anaesthetised comparatively safely. For painful procedures or to induce cardiovascularly unstable patients more gently, **ketamine 0.5–1–2 mg/kg** can be added, as described for gastric torsion (p. 326).

The following drugs are also available for induction of anaesthesia:

Ketamine 2–5 mg/kg IV: Can be used for anaesthesia induction after premedication. However, it should never be given alone so that the side effects (muscle rigidity/catalepsy, salivation, bad dreams) do not get out of hand. It should only be given in high doses before long operations (about > 45 min), because otherwise the recovery phase can become restless and uncontrolled.

Thiopental 10–15 mg/kg strictly IV: However, should only be used in healthy animals and under ECG control. It causes a very rapid induction of anaesthesia.

Etomidate 1–3 mg/kg IV: Has no cardiovascular or respiratory side effects, but induction is often more agitated compared to propofol. It suppresses endogenous cortisol synthesis for 6 h after bolus injection. Etomidate dissolved in fat can be used like propofol, but it should be left at a single bolus.

Alfaxalone 2–4 mg/kg IV: Has minimal side effects, but induction seems a little rougher, intubation a little more difficult compared to propofol. Restless recoveries and vocalisations must be expected if a benzodiazepine, for example, is not co-administered. Expensive for large dogs.

In neonatal pups it may be useful to induce unconsciousness with a **mask and isoflurane or sevoflurane in O$_2$**. This is particularly indicated for short painless/low pain procedures such as audiometry. In all other dogs, mask induction is associated with too many disadvantages (inhalation anaesthetics in the room air, a lot of stress and anxiety for the patient, long induction time, no securing of the airway), is therefore not recommended and should only be reserved for exceptions.

Maintenance phase

After injection anaesthesia, the maintenance phase may be sufficient in depth and duration of effect to perform short procedures. Often anaesthesia is maintained after intubation with **isoflurane** (MAC value about 1.3%, ▶ Table 4.22) or **sevoflurane** (MAC value about 2.3%, ▶ Table 4.38). It should be borne in mind that neither isoflurane nor sevoflurane are analgesic and for this reason analgesia by other means always need to be covered if a painful procedure is performed. Well suited for analgesia is **fentanyl** continuous rate infusion or **methadone** boluses every 4 h. For visceral procedures, administration of **butorphanol** every 30–60 min is possible. **Buprenorphine** is suitable for analgesic treatment of less painful procedures. For very painful procedures, especially when skin, muscle and bone are involved, **ketamine** can additionally be used as a bolus and CRI in the dosages listed in ▶ Table 4.23. Do not forget a simultaneous use of **non-steroidal anti-inflammatory drugs**, which can also be used alone for less painful procedures.

Recovery phase

The following should be observed for the recovery phase: It should be calm and without pain, therefore – if necessary – sedation and analgesia should be provided in good time.
- Uncuffing and extubation should be done when the dog shows a swallowing reflex
- Measure core body temperature and actively warm or cool accordingly
- Continue infusion if indicated (e.g. blood loss during surgery)
- Make sure that the urinary bladder is empty

5.3.3 Literature

[1] Bednarski R, Grimm K, Harvey R, Lukasik VM, Penn WS, Sargent B, Spelts K. AAHA anesthesia guidelines for dogs and cats. J Am Anim Hosp Assoc 2011; 47: 377–385

[2] Court MH. Anesthesia of the sighthound. Clin Tech Small Anim Pract 1999; 14: 38–43

[3] Gough A, Thomas A. Breed predispositions to disease in dogs and cats. Oxford: Wiley-Blackwell 2010

[4] Neff MW, Robertson KR, Wong A, Safra N, Broman KW, Slatkin M, Mealey KL, Pedersen NC. Breed distribution and history of canine MDR1-1Δ, a pharmacogenetic mutation that marks the emergence of breeds of the Collie lineage. PNAS 2004; 101: 11725–30

[5] Sams RA, Muir WW. Effects of phenobarbital on thiopental pharmacokinetics in Greyhounds. Am J Vet Res 1988; 49: 245–9

[6] Website of the Institute of Pharmacology and Toxicology at the Justus Liebig University of Giessen, Germany: https://mdr1-defekt.transmit.de

5.4 Cat

Cats are not small dogs and must therefore be cared for differently. In the meantime, there is also a large selection of breeds of cats, some of which also have anaesthesia-relevant special considerations.

5.4.1 Preanaesthetic considerations

Preoperative **handling** but also perioperative management can be difficult as cats are comparatively small and can be so aggressive (pain? fear?) that injection or fixation for catheter placement is almost impossible without endangering yourself (and the cat). Breed-specific anaesthetic hypersensitivities (p.181) must be considered when choosing anaesthetics.

Classic complications to be expected: Fast **hypothermia** (due to large surface area compared to the small mass), **hyperthermia** (rather rare, possibly after ketamine or opioid administration in recovery phase due to excitement), **hypotension** (often due to vasodilation), **bradycardia** and/or negative inotropic effect of anaesthetics, **tachycardia**, **respiratory depression/hypoventilation** with **hypercapnia** and **hypoxaemia**, problems with **intubation** (laryngeal spasm), problems with **IV catheter placement** (in small animals or after high doses of alpha2 agonists).

General considerations

Fasting: About 8 h (when feeding wet food only approx. 6 h) feed deprivation before induction, no water deprivation. Do not fast suckling kittens. Some basic normal values can be found in ▶ Table 5.4.

Blood volume in the cat is comparatively low at 43–67 ml/kg body weight.

Table 5.4 Normal values cat

Parameter (unit)	Normal values
Core body temperature (°C)	38.0–39.3
Heart rate (/min)	108–132
Respiratory rate (/min)	20–30
Haematocrit (%)	27–47
Total protein (g/dl)	6.0–7.5
Creatinine (mg/dl)	0–1.9

Anatomical and physiological features

- Cats **metabolise drugs differently** than almost all other pets, which is an adaptation to an extremely carnivorous diet:
  - Lower cytochrome P450 enzyme activity compared to other mammals (phase 1 of liver metabolism)
  - Lower glucuronyl transferase, which is one of the most important enzymes for conjugation in other mammals (phase 2 of liver metabolism)
  - Instead, conjugation occurs with sulphate, but this biotransformation step is **slower** than glucuronidation
  - Therefore, drugs that are metabolised via the liver (e.g. ketamine, diazepam and other) accumulate
- They are **particularly sensitive** to the depressant effects of **inhalational anaesthetics** on the cardiovascular system, especially in the absence of a stimulus. This means that a balanced anaesthetic protocol should always be used
- Cats are more likely to respond to **opioid** administration alone with (happy) excitement and, depending on the dose, some dysphoria due to additional stimulation of dopaminergic receptors. They show mydriasis. Despite these particular side effects, pure µ agonists are very good analgesics: An aggressive, painful cat suddenly becomes friendly purring and happily pain-free!
- Administration of **benzodiazepines** in healthy cats (midazolam, diazepam) is followed by (friendly) excitement and not sedation, on the contrary!
- In an unbalanced anaesthetic protocol, cats like to move or "wake up" during surgery. They show fluctuating physiological parameters (heart and respiratory rate, blood pressure) depending on the degree of stimulation

IV access

▶ **Cephalic vein** (*v. cephalica antebrachii*). Clearly visible. Is well suited for routine placement of the IV catheter. Catheter is easy to fix with tape.

▶ **Lateral saphenous vein** (*v. saphena lateralis*). Well visible, but likes to "roll away". It may not be possible to advance the catheter around the turnover point of the vein to the medial aspect of the leg.

▶ **Medial saphenous vein** (*v. saphena medialis*). Larger than the lateral saphenous vein, does not roll away easily. Catheter is more difficult to fix, however. Relatively cranial on the inner side of the distal thigh. Often this vein is the last chance if one has not been successful with the smaller vessels.

▶ **Jugular vein** (*v. jugularis*). Well suited for puncture for blood collection and placement of larger catheters.

Intubation

- Endotracheal tube size is chosen from 2.5–5 mm ID depending on size of the cat, the average cat can be intubated with size 3.5–4.0 mm ID
- The upper airway is relatively small and delicate, but usually easy to see using a laryngoscope with a light source
- Cats have pronounced laryngeal protective reflexes, therefore before intubation 1. the **depth of anaesthesia** should be **sufficient** and 2. **lidocaine** should be sprayed/dripped on **topically to avoid laryngeal spasm**
- It should always be intubated into the open larynx (at expiration), which sometimes requires some patience
- Ideally, the epiglottis should not be touched with the laryngoscope blade, if it is absolutely necessary to safely intubate, then with a lot of care!
- Most endotracheal tubes used in human medicine are too long and should be shortened, as already explained under "Airway management" (p. 153) and "Which tube size do I use for which animal" (p. 156). Ideal length: From the incisors to the thoracic inlet (*apertura thoracis*) (▶ Fig. 5.2)
- Secure with a cord or an infusion line behind the ears
- If the cuff is overinflated or the cat is repositioned often without disconnecting the ETT from the breathing system of the anaesthesia machine, tracheal rupture may occur. This can also occur in cats that are "suspended" for neutering due to traction on the breathing tubes. First signs are subcutaneous emphysema, coughing, retching, dyspnoea and fever

- Due to the small internal diameter, the ETT can obstruct more quickly with secretion or similar. Monitoring of the free airway should be continuous (ideally with capnography)
- A laryngeal mask airway for the cat is available (e.g. V-Gel)

Breed-specific considerations

There are some cat breeds with which anaesthesia-related diseases are (or seem to be) associated.

▶ **Devon Rex.** Hypertrophic cardiomyopathy, myopathy/spasticity, hairlessness (also patellar luxation, hip dysplasia).

▶ **Maine Coon cat.** Hypertrophic cardiomyopathy, polycystic kidney disease, very large-framed cat, not fully grown until about 3–4 years of age (also hip joint and elbow dysplasia, spinal muscular atrophy).

▶ **Persian cat.** Brachycephalic syndrome, see also "Preanaesthetic considerations" (p.178), brain damage due to skull deformation, polycystic kidney disease (also entropion).

Other cat breeds (e.g. such as the Burmese cat) are also said to be particularly sensitive to anaesthetics. These statements are mostly general, emotional, not scientifically proven and sometimes simply wrong. It is true and correct that anaesthetics, regardless of whether they are used on an expensive pedigree cat or a random street cat, have a cardiovascular and respiratory depressive effect and, in the worst case, can lead to the death of the animal! This risk exists in particular when too much is administered too quickly, without careful clinical examination and without modern monitoring and equipment. In this case, the anaesthetic itself or the breed cannot be held responsible for the incident! Every purebred cat can be anaesthetised fairly safely – even with associated diseases – if the appropriate requirements (including clinical examination, patient-specific choice of anaesthetic protocol, perioperative management, continuous monitoring) are met.

In the section below, the most important anaesthesia-relevant diseases are discussed in more detail.

Hypertrophic cardiomyopathy

▶ **Affected breeds.** Maine Coon, Persian, Ragdoll, Devon Rex, American and British Shorthair and mixed offspring of these breeds, also European Shorthair cat.

▶ **What happens?** Concentric cardiac hypertrophy especially of the left ventricle.

▶ **Cause.** Primary (inherited) or secondary (due to pressure overload or hormonal stimulation) disease.

▶ **Conclusion.** Perioperative management must be adapted, see also "Hypertrophic cardiomyopathy in the cat" (p. 290).

Myopathy/spasticity of the Devon Rex cat

▶ **Affected breeds.** Devon Rex, Cornish Rex and possibly Sphynx cat.

▶ **What happens?** It seems that especially after anaesthesia with ketamine (dose??), convulsions, severe agitation with rapid hyperglycaemia, hypothermia, and death may occur during the recovery phase (acute phase) or progressive intense muscle pain, increase in blood creatinine kinase levels, hypothermia, hypoglycaemia and uraemia (subacute phase) about 24–48 h after anaesthesia.

▶ **Cause.** Unknown

▶ **Conclusion.** To avoid complications, the use of ketamine in high doses is probably not recommended in these breeds. If used, it should be done cautiously, at a low dose and in combination with a muscle relaxant (e.g. midazolam).

Polycystic kidney disease

▶ **Affected breeds.** Persian, Maine Coon, British Shorthair, Carthusian, Norwegian Forest Cat, Persian Mix.

▶ **What happens?** Cyst formation in the kidney (but also in the liver and pancreas) leads to progressive renal insufficiency at a young age due to displacement of kidney tissue.

▶ Cause. Autosomal dominant hereditary disease.

▶ Conclusion. Good assessment of kidney function. Ensure a strict renal food diet before elective surgery.

Feline orofacial pain syndrome (FOPS)

▶ Affected breeds. Mainly Burmese cat, also Siamese cat.

▶ What happens? Intermittent attacks of severe pain, usually in one side of the face. Cats show exaggerated licking, conspicuous chewing movements, smacking and automutilation by pawing at the mouth.

▶ Cause. Not fully understood. Neuropathic disease with a genetic component, stress as a trigger, but also oropathological changes such as tooth root debris or resorptive lesions are suspected.

▶ Conclusion. Thorough examination and exclusion of other triggers. Very good multimodal pain management.

Other specific considerations

Heinz body formation after multiple propofol administrations

Heinz bodies are clumps of haemoglobin in erythrocytes due to oxidative denaturation. The aggregates attach themselves to the inner cell membrane. Normally, these damaged erythrocytes are broken down by the spleen. However, the cat is apparently only partially able to do this. They also occur in healthy cats, on the one hand by increased formation and on the other hand by reduced elimination compared to other species. If there is increased oxidative damage, a clinically relevant haemolytic anaemia can occur.

Possible causes are:
- Drugs: Propofol, acetaminophen (paracetamol)
- Onions
- Propylene glycol (as a preservative in some anaesthetics e.g. diazepam)
- Other: Zinc, copper, L-methionine, vitamin K3 and more

For this reason, propofol should not be used in cats as a continuous rate infusion for a prolonged period of time, nor should it be used as an anaesthetic for several days in a row.

5.4.2 Anaesthesia protocols

Again, the suggested protocols are to be understood as examples and options. They should be selected and adapted in the individual situation.

Injection anaesthesia based on a mixture of ketamine and alpha2 agonists is also frequently used in the cat. For longer procedures, general anaesthesia is continued with isoflurane or sevoflurane.

The following examples are intended to serve as a suggestion and inspire to question one's own protocols and to use new drugs and their combinations if necessary.

Examination of the patient and ASA classification: see chapter "Preanaesthetic examination" (p. 150); "Perioperative management" (p. 152) incl. airway management, infusion therapy, administration of antibiotics, protection of the cornea and emptying of the urinary bladder; "Monitoring" (p. 39).

Sedation

The choice of premedication depends on the ASA status of the patient, the respective comorbidities, the temperament (from very friendly to highly aggressive), the duration and level of pain of the procedure. In general, IM sedation followed by calm placement of the IV catheter is always preferable to struggling with unsuccessful catheter placement attempts. Particularly stressed or aggressive cats can possibly already be "pre-treated" very successfully with gabapentin (p. 97) by the owner.

In case of a healthy, friendly but nervous animal, e.g.:

Dosage

- **Acepromazine** 0.02–0.05 mg/kg AND
- **Methadone** 0.2–0.3 mg/kg mixed in one syringe IM or IV

Onset of action is somewhat delayed, the animal should be given 20–30 minutes to calm down. Mild sedation with good analgesia. Nervous animals benefit from the mild sedation and anxiolysis provided by acepromazine, even in the recovery phase. It is better to use the lower dosages, the high dosage is suitable for healthy but very agitated cats.

The "**favourite**" among cat sedations, especially for patients which are difficult to handle:

Dosage

- **Butorphanol** 0.2 mg/kg IM/IV AND
- **Medetomidine** 0.005–0.01 mg/kg IV or 0.01–0.03 mg/kg IM mixed in one syringe OR **Dexmedetomidine** 0.003–0.006 mg/kg one after the other slowly IV or 0.005–0.015 mg/kg IM mixed in one syringe

Adding **ketamine 1–3 mg/kg** to the syringe deepens the IM sedation, reliably calming even aggressive animals while reducing or even preventing severe bradyarrhythmia. Ketamine in high doses should not be used in cats with hypertrophic cardiomyopathy (HCM). In aggressive ASA 3 patients, the combination can be used if medetomidine is dosed low (e.g. 0.005 mg/kg). Xylazine 0.25–1, up to 4 mg/kg SC, IM, IV is less specific than medetomidine or dexmedetomidine and cannot be fully antagonised. Therefore, preference should be given to the more specific alpha2 agonists.

For deep sedation or general anaesthesia for a short surgical procedure, **ketamine**, **dex-/medetomidine** + /– **butorphanol** can be administered at the higher end of the IM or IV dose spectrum.

If the cat is friendly with ASA status 3–4, the following combination can be used:

Dosage

- **Butorphanol** 0.2 mg/kg AND
- **Midazolam** 0.2 mg/kg mixed in one syringe IM, IV OR **Diazepam** 0.2 mg/kg IV, do not mix

This mild sedation is rather shallow and works best when the animals are very old, calm and/or really sick. It is very gentle on the circulation and can be antagonised if necessary. Here, too, the sedative and analgesic effect can be enhanced with low-dose **ketamine** (0.5–2 mg/kg) or, alternatively, the hypnotic component can be enhanced with **alfaxalone** (1–2 mg/kg). Again, ketamine in high doses should not be used in cats with HCM.

If the cat with ASA status 3–4 is not manageable or aggressive, this combination can be used:

Dosage

- **Alfaxalone** 1–5 mg/kg IM (volume is usually the limiting factor), IV AND
- **Midazolam** 0.2 mg/kg mixed in one syringe IM, IV OR **Diazepam** 0.2 mg/kg IV, do not mix + /–
- **Opioid**, e.g. **Butorphanol** 0.2 mg/kg IM, IV OR **Methadone** 0.2 mg/kg IM, IV

This combination in a mixed syringe IM causes deep sedation, but is gentle on the circulation. If butorphanol is used instead of methadone, the sedation may be slightly deeper but the analgesic effect less. If alfaxalone is not available, it can be replaced by **ketamine** 1–2 mg/kg IM, IV if there is no potential contra-indication such as HCM.

Induction

As in dogs, for short procedures (up to 20–30 min) it is practical to use the same drugs for sedation/anaesthesia induction and maintenance.

A classic example is the combination of **ketamine** and **dex-/medetomidine** + /– **butorphanol** in higher dosages as mentioned above (e.g. **butorphanol** 0.2 mg/kg, **medetomidine** 0.03 mg/kg or **dexmedetomidine** 0.015 mg/kg and **ketamine** 3–5 mg/kg IM or IV).

For prolonged (more than 20–30 min) or very painful procedures, general anaesthesia is usually induced with injectable anaesthetics and maintained with **volatile anaesthetics**.

Propofol 2–8 mg/kg slowly IV: With good premedication and a calm environment, 2–4 mg/kg IV is usually sufficient for an adequate depth of anaesthesia for intubation. Effects and side effects are identical to those in dogs (p. 176). Preoxygenation should always be performed! For painful procedures or to induce cardiovascularly unstable patients more gently (= less propofol), **ketamine** 0.5–1 or even 2 mg/kg and/or midazolam 0.2 mg/kg can be added (procedure as for gastric torsion (p. 326) in dogs). As described under specific considerations (p. 183), propofol should not be used on several consecutive days in the cat!

Ketamine 2–5 (up to 10) mg/kg IV: Can also be used for anaesthetic induction, but it has a stronger and longer lasting effect due to the unique metabolism in cats. Always use in combination with a muscle relaxant and sedative anaesthetic! It should only be given in high doses before long procedures, because otherwise side effects (especially hallucinations and catalepsy) may become apparent in the recovery phase.

Etomidate 1–3 mg/kg IV: Can be used identically as for dogs (p. 176).

Alfaxalone 2–5 mg/kg IV: Has minimal side effects, but a somewhat more restless phase of induction with a more mobile larynx during intubation and vocalisations during the recovery phase must be expected. To minimise these side effects, it should always be combined with another sedative or muscle relaxant drug (e.g. **midazolam** 0.2 mg/kg).

In neonatal kittens, it may be useful to induce unconsciousness with the mask and **isoflurane** or **sevoflurane** in O_2, especially if placement of IV access is impossible while awake.

Maintenance phase

The maintenance phase may be sufficient to perform short procedures after induction with injectable anaesthetics. However, it is common to provide anaesthesia after intubation using volatile anaesthetics, such as **isoflurane** (MAC value 1.7%, ▶ Table 4.22) or **sevoflurane** (MAC value 2.7%, ▶ Table 4.38). The MAC value indicates that the cat generally requires higher doses of volatile anaesthetics compared to the dog.

In a painful procedure, analgesia must be provided by other means. Well suited for analgesia is **fentanyl** continuous rate infusion or **methadone** boluses every 4 h in slightly lower doses than in dogs. For visceral procedures, **butorphanol** every 30–60 min may be used. **Buprenorphine** has a very good analgesic effect in the cat and is therefore particularly suitable for peri- and postoperative pain management. It can also be administered orally transmucosally (due to the acidic pH in the oral cavity) with high bioavailability. The dose is 0.02 mg/kg every 6 h. In very painful procedures and to keep vital parameters more stable during maintenance phase, **ketamine** can additionally be administered as CRI (dosages, Table 4.23). A concomitant treatment with **non-steroidal anti-inflammatory drugs** should not be forgotten, taking into account the generally lower dosages compared to dogs and the limited duration of treatment.

Recovery phase

It should be calm and without pain, therefore – if necessary – sedation and analgesia should be used in good time.
- The cuff should be completely deflated before extubation. Extubation should be done when the cat shows a swallowing reflex, but soon enough that it does not cough against the endotracheal tube
- Be sure to measure core body temperature and actively warm accordingly
- Continue infusion and monitoring if indicated

5.4.3 Literature

[1] Andress JL, Day TK, Day D. The effect of consecutive day propofol anaesthesia on feline red blood cells. Vet Surg 1995; 24: 277–282

[2] Bednarski R, Grimm K, Harvey R, Lukasik VM, Penn WS, Sargent B, Spelts K. AAHA anesthesia guidelines for dogs and cats. J Am Anim Hosp Assoc 2011; 47: 377–385

[3] Dhasmana KM, Dixit KS, Jaju BP, Gupta ML. Role of central dopaminergic receptors in manic response of cats to morphine. Psychopharmacologia 1972; 24: 380–3

[4] Drummond JC, Todd MM, Shapiro HM. Minimal alveolar concentrations for halothane, enflurane, and isoflurane in the cat. J Am Vet Med Assoc 1983; 15: 1099–101

[5] Mitchell SL, McCarthy R, Rudloff E, Pernell RT. Tracheal rupture associated with intubation in cats: 20 cases (1996–1998). J Am Vet Med Assoc 2000; 216: 1592–1595

[6] Rusbridge C, Heath S, Gunn-Moore DA, Knowler SP, Johnston N, McFadyen AK. Feline orofacial pain syndrome (FOPS): a retrospective study of 113 cases. J Feline Med Surg 2010; 12: 498–508

[7] Warne LN, Beths T, Whittem T, Carter JE, Bauquier SH. A review of the pharmacology and clinical application of alfaxalone in cats. Vet J 2015; 203: 141–148

5.5 Rabbit

In some countries, rabbits are food-producing animals by law and the appropriate laws apply. There are few anaesthetics and analgesics licensed for this species.

The peri- and postoperative morbidity and mortality of rabbits is significantly higher in contrast to dogs and cats (mortality within 48 h in a healthy animal 0.73%). If the general condition is additionally impaired, the risk (mortality at 1.4%) associated with anaesthesia and surgery must be discussed with the owner.

5.5.1 Preanaesthetic considerations

Preoperative **handling** but also perioperative management can be difficult as rabbits are quite **small** (be sure to weigh them, it is easy to misestimate) and **susceptible to stress**. They are prone to **excessive catecholamine secretion**, which can lead to **sudden death**. Restraint should be done carefully to prevent injury to the back by kicking out with the hind legs. **Reflex activity** is **increased** compared to the dog/cat, so reflex control to determine depth of anaesthesia can be difficult. After arrival at the clinic, some time should be given in a quiet environment to allow the rabbit to calm down (**adaptation time**).

Classic complications to be expected: Rapid **hypothermia** (due to large surface area compared to small mass), **hypotension** (often due to vasodilation), **bradycardia** and/or negative inotropic effect of anaesthetics, **tachycardia**, respiratory depression/**hypoventilation** with **hypercapnia** and **hypoxaemia**, problems with intubation or **no intubation possible**, problems with **IV access** placement (in small animals, in rabbits with small ears or after high doses of alpha2 agonists). Blood should be taken preoperatively, or at the latest when an IV catheter is placed, for basic parameters haematocrit, total protein and glucose, and if suspected also for organ screening. **Corneal injuries** of the eyes protruding during general anaesthesia can be prevented by careful positioning and generous use of eye ointment (e.g. dexpanthenol).

Chronic (**subclinical**) **respiratory diseases** are common and may affect ventilation and oxygenation during anaesthesia.

General considerations

Fasting: Rabbits should generally not be fasted, the risk of vomiting is non-existent as rabbits cannot vomit! However, it seems that you can reduce the risk of bloat by not offering high carbohydrate food such as apple, carrot or dried food some hours before induction of anaesthesia. Water can always be offered. Some basic normal values can be found in ▶ Table 5.5.

The blood volume in rabbits is 45–70 ml/kg body weight.

Anatomical and physiological features

Rabbits are flight animals and therefore easily stressed. If – as is absolutely necessary before longer and more complex procedures – an IV catheter is to be placed, prior SC or IM sedation is recommended. If the catheter has to be placed while the animal is awake and there is plenty of time, it also helps to apply a local anaesthetic cream (EMLA cream) to the clipped ear over the vein. Ideally, it should be left on for up to 30 minutes.

IV access

▶ **Lateral auricular vein** (*v. auricularis lateralis*). Relatively well visible, although quite small (▶ Fig. 5.6). It is very lateral on the ear, catheterisation (24 or 26 G catheter) of the vein at the lateral rim of the ear is recommended

Table 5.5 Normal values rabbit

Parameter (unit)	Normal values
Core body temperature (°C)	38.5–40.0
Heart rate (/min)	120–330
Respiratory rate (/min)	32–100
Haematocrit (%)	36–55
Total protein (g/dl)	4.9–7.4
Glucose (mg/dl)	70–160

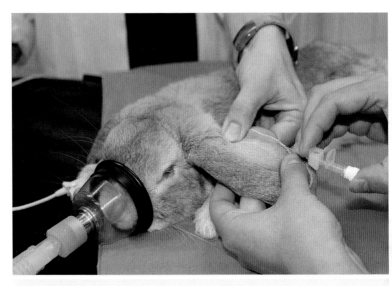

Fig. 5.6 Placement of an intravenous catheter in the lateral ear vein in the sedated rabbit.

(there is also a vein medially). In small ears, prolonged stasis and applying heat can help to make the vein more visible. For fixation, swabs can be rolled, taped together and fixed in the inner side of the ear. The catheter is then taped over this.

▶ **Cephalic vein** (*v. cephalica antebrachii*). Useful if the rabbit's ears are too small. It is small and needs a bit of practice. Sedation beforehand helps a lot. In terms of handling and placement, it "feels" like a small cat.

▶ **Lateral saphenous vein** (*v. saphena lateralis*). Also good if the rabbit has too small ears.

Intubation

Rabbits are not easy to intubate and no matter what technique you use, you should use and practise it over and over again. As the oral cavity is very long and narrow and cannot be opened wide, visualisation of the larynx is only possible in large animals. The oropharynx and airways are very small and sensitive, the larynx tends to spasm (like in the cat).

Rabbits can be intubated using several techniques, including blind, under visual control using an otoscope or laryngoscope, or using a fiberoptic endoscope.

With practice, the blind technique can be learned:

1. Anaesthetise the rabbit well and position it very straight in sternal position, a helper may administer oxygen via the nose, the animal is spontaneously breathing.
2. Hold the head with one hand and stretch it straight up.
3. Pull out the tongue and place it under the thumb of the hand holding the head.
4. With the other hand, carefully feed the tube forward until it regularly fogs up with exhalation.
5. Put one or two drops of lidocaine into the tube and let it trickle to the end of the ETT, wait briefly.
6. If intubation is attempted, the animal should not swallow; if it does, carefully deepen the level of anaesthesia.
7. Observe regular fogging of the ETT and gently advance it at the beginning of expiration.
8. If the ETT continues to fog (or if there is a capnography curve), it is in the trachea; if it stops fogging after advancement, it is in the oesophagus.
9. If it is in the trachea, tie it with a thick thread or gauze bandage behind the ears. Be careful each time you move it to avoid accidental extubation.

Do not try more than five times carefully, otherwise the risk of laryngeal injury or laryngeal spasm is too high!

There is a **laryngeal mask airway** specially designed for the rabbit that works very well and is easy to insert (V-Gel, ▶ Fig. 5.4). Even for inexperienced persons, the insertion of this laryngeal mask airway can be learned very quickly and should be available for airway management during every rabbit anaesthesia. Further information on airway management and intubation can be found under "Airway management" (p.153) and "Which tube size do I use for which animal" (p.156).

Specific considerations

About half of all rabbits (like apparently other strict herbivores) metabolise atropine very quickly through **atropine esterases**. As a result, they react less and/or shorter to atropine administration. If necessary, another parasympatholytic agent, such as glycopyrrolate (p.99), can be used. Nevertheless, it is good practice to give atropine first in an emergency, as it has a faster onset of action than glycopyrrolate.

Dwarf rabbits seem to be more sensitive to some anaesthetics. The dose should therefore be reduced slightly compared to "normal size" rabbits.

In general, all rabbits are very susceptible to stress. They should always be handled calmly and go to sleep and wake up separately from potential predators (dog, cat, ferret, …). Some breeds or colours seem to be more susceptible to stress than average (**New Zealand Whites**, possibly **tan** coloured rabbits). In these cases, special attention should be paid to calm handling and a low-stress environment.

5.5.2 Anaesthesia protocols

In rabbits, even more than in other species, it is important to think about how long the procedure will take and how painful it will be. This will largely determine the anaesthetic protocol and the doses used. The more precisely this is adapted to the needs, the safer the anaesthesia will be. This and a short duration of anaesthesia (as short as necessary) should be the goal.

Pronounced differences in the response to different anaesthetics in different strains of rabbits are known. This is especially true in laboratory animal medicine, where genetically modified animals are used.

Practice tip

SC versus IM injection of anaesthetics in small mammals

As a general rule, animals weighing less than 100 g should not be injected IM. Ketamine should not be injected IM in small mammals (even those > 100 g body weight) as it is associated with pain and muscle cell necrosis. SC injection of anaesthetic combinations with ketamine acts (almost) equally fast and causes (almost) the same depth of anaesthesia. Only the recovery time seems to be slightly delayed, but this can be compensated with the antagonisation of alpha2 agonists. SC injection also means much less stress for the animal and thus fewer defensive movements or risk of injury. For this reason, it is recommended to inject in the lateral chest wall or neck fold.

Preanaesthetic examination of the patient and ASA classification: see chapter "Preanaesthetic examination" (p. 150); "Perioperative management" (p. 152) incl. airway management, infusion therapy, administration of antibiotics, protection of the cornea and emptying of the urinary bladder; "Monitoring" (p. 39).

Sedation

Sedation before IV induction is useful in rabbits if the procedure is long and painful. In addition, sedation is useful if the procedure is short and essentially pain-free (e.g. oral cavity examination, radiography, CT scan or minor procedure under local anaesthesia) or would simply be associated with too much stress. The following protocols are suitable for these cases:

Dosage

- **Medetomidine** 0.05–0.12 mg/kg OR **Dexmedetomidine** 0.025–0.06 mg/kg AND
- **Butorphanol** 0.2–0.5 mg/kg mixed in one syringe SC or IM

Depending on the condition of the rabbit and the dosage, a moderate to deep sedation is achieved, which is well suited for more detailed examinations (e.g. oral cavity examination) or the placement of an IV access without stress. To deepen the sedation (e.g. for an ear examination or endoscopy), **ketamine 5–20 mg/kg** can be added. In that way, short, even painful procedures can be performed. If the dosages are chosen in the higher dose range of the anaesthetics, induction (p. 194) of anaesthesia is achieved.

Dosage

- **Midazolam** 0.5 mg/kg AND
- **Butorphanol** 0.5 mg/kg mixed in one syringe SC or IM

This combination is particularly useful for already sick or compromised rabbits that need to be gently sedated in order to place an IV access for induction of anaesthesia. The sedation is rather mild and is not sufficient for painful procedures.

Induction

Dosage

- **Ketamine** 10–30 mg/kg AND
- **Medetomidine** 0.05–0.12 mg/kg OR **Dexmedetomidine** 0.025–0.06 mg/kg + /–
- **Butorphanol** 0.2–0.5 mg/kg mixed in one syringe SC or IM

With this combination, one usually gets a stable anaesthesia that is sufficient (for a limited time) for castrations or painful dental treatments. Ketamine should not be used alone to avoid severe side effects such as catalepsy, salivation and hallucinations. Even when used in combination, exophthalmos occurs, especially in rabbits. The cornea must therefore be protected by generously applying ophthalmic ointment and correct positioning. Dex-/medetomidine can be antagonised with atipamezole (p. 70) (same volume) SC or IM at the earliest 30, better 40 min after injection of ketamine.

Case example

Castration of a young healthy male rabbit

This type of procedure is the perfect example of how the dose and thus the side effects of anaesthetics can be reduced with the help of 1. a balanced anaesthetic protocol and 2. local anaesthesia:

- **Ketamine** 5 mg/kg AND
- **Medetomidine** 0.05 mg/kg OR **Dexmedetomidine** 0.03 mg/kg AND
- **Butorphanol** 0.5 mg/kg mixed in one syringe IM

Wait (!) until patient is deeply sedated, then **local anaesthesia** in the **testicles** AND the **incision line** (e.g. lidocaine 2%, per testicle 0.2 ml, SC below the incision line 0.1 ml in a 1 kg rabbit). In addition, SC or IV administration of **meloxicam** 0.5 mg/kg. Wait a short time, then start castration.

These quite low dosages are usually sufficient in almost all patients and ensure great cardiovascular and respiratory safety. If the anaesthesia needs to be deepened somewhat, a small bolus of propofol slow IV (0.5–1 mg/kg) or alfaxalone IM (0.5–1 mg/kg) is a good idea.

Often you have to let the rabbit sleep for a while postoperatively (do not forget: infusion, eye lube, temperature management etc.) before antagonising with atipamezole (same volume as the dex-/medetomidine) at the earliest 30 min, better 40 min after the injection of the anaesthetics SC or IM.

Xylazin 2–4 mg/kg can also be used instead of dex-/medetomidine. However, this drug no longer meets today's standard, it is more unspecific in its effect and cannot be reliably antagonised.

Dosage

- **Propofol** 2–15 mg/kg slowly IV, titrate to effect (depending on premedication) OR **Alfaxalone** 1–5 mg/kg very slowly IV (depending on premedication) +/–
- **Ketamine** (2–10 mg/kg) very slowly IV, titrate to effect

An IV catheter is a requirement for this combination. Propofol administered slowly IV is a very good way to induce anaesthesia in rabbits but be careful with respiratory depression. If intubation is to be performed, a good premedication should be administered beforehand. The dose of **propofol** should be chosen as low as possible and **titrated slowly** to avoid periods of apnoea. Continuous O_2 administration. With the additional IV administration of **ketamine**, the dose of propofol can be reduced and the anaesthesia deepened. The duration of anaesthesia is sufficient to intubate or to perform short procedures. The maintenance phase can be prolonged with additional small boluses of propofol and ketamine.

Dosage

- **Medetomidine** 0.2 mg/kg AND
- **Midazolam** 1 mg/kg AND
- **Fentanyl** 0.02 mg/kg mixed in one syringe IM

= fully antagonisable anaesthesia

Should only be used in absolutely healthy animals! Surgical tolerance sets in very quickly, but is not as reliable as with a ketamine-based protocol. For less painful/invasive procedures (especially soft tissue surgery) this combination is sufficient. It causes **severe respiratory depression**, sometimes **apnoea**! Always add O_2. In dwarf rabbits, use only ⅔ of the indicated dose.

For antagonisation, use **atipamezole 1 mg/kg, flumazenil 0.1 mg/kg and naloxone 0.03 mg/kg mixed in one syringe SC or IM**. After painful interventions, naloxone should be not be used as it antagonises any opioid effect (also endogenous).

Dosage

- Mask induction with **Isoflurane** OR **Sevoflurane** in O_2

Mask induction is associated with a lot of stress for the animal, so it should only be done in exceptional cases. Rabbits are usually so easy to handle that induction in a box with inhalation anaesthetics should also be the exception. Sevoflurane is less irritating to the mucous membranes than isoflurane, so it should be preferred for this type of induction.

Maintenance phase

Usually, anaesthesia is continued with isoflurane or sevoflurane in O_2 for longer procedures. Intubation with an endotracheal tube or the use of a laryngeal mask airway is very helpful, but a mask can also be used. MAC values can be found in ▶ Table 4.22 and ▶ Table 4.38. Both inhalation anaesthetics depress the respiratory and circulatory system in a dose-dependent manner.

Ketamine 0.1–0.5 mg/kg can be titrated very carefully and diluted IV in this phase. If too much is given too quickly, there is a risk of respiratory arrest. If given carefully and slowly, it has a MAC-reducing effect and stabilises the maintenance phase.

If no inhalation anaesthetic is available, it is possible (when the depth of anaesthesia begins to decrease) to add about ⅓ to ½ of the initial dose of SC or IM. Problems with this approach are the poor titratability, the non-specific effect and the accumulation of the drugs.

Practice tip

"Rabbit Mix" infusion

As ideally with any other animal under anaesthesia, intravenous infusion (p. 163) should be given perioperatively. The "rabbit mix" used by the author consists of 50% colloidal solution (HES) and 50% balanced electrolyte solution (e.g. Sterofundin ISO). This is infused perioperatively using a syringe pump at 10 ml/kg/h IV, or more if perioperative losses increase.

Analgesia should be administered in a timely fashion, ideally before the painful procedure. NSAIDs such as **meloxicam** 0.4–0.6 mg/kg PO or SC 1 × /d (or up to 1 or even 1.5 mg/kg are necessary to achieve effective plasma concentrations!) or **metamizole** 20–50 mg/kg SC every 6 h and **buprenorphine** 0.01–0.05 mg/kg IM or IV every 6 h have proven effective.

The option of local anaesthesia should also be considered. It is very easy to perform, for example, when castrating male animals or, with a little practice, for dental procedures.

Recovery phase

The animal should be **monitored** for several hours at regular intervals, at least by inspection. A quiet, warm, dry environment is ideal.

It is important (especially in compromised/inappetent animals) to **start feeding** as soon as possible after the animal wakes up, ideally with high-quality powdered formula mixed with water (e.g. RODICARE instant). Feeding as soon as possible after routine surgery has also proven useful in assessing the post-operative condition of the animal.

Active **temperature management** is very important in this phase and must not be neglected. Temperature should be measured at least immediately after anaesthesia and again during the recovery phase.

As needed and available, anaesthetics should be **antagonised** to shorten the recovery period. If the animal appears weaker or sedated again after some time, re-sedation may occur as the antagonist effect wears off. It often helps to antagonise one more time.

5.5.3 Literature

[1] Aeschbacher G. Rabbit anaesthesia. Exotic Animal Medicine 2001; 17: 1003–1010

[2] Avsaroglu H, Versluis A, Hellebrekers LJ et al. Strain differences in response to propofol, ketamine and medetomidine in rabbits. Vet Rec 2003; 152: 300

[3] Brodbelt DC, Blissitt KJ, Hammond RA, Neath PJ, Young LE, Pfeiffer DU, Wood JL. The risk of death: the confidential enquiry into perioperative small animal fatalities. Vet Anaesth Analg 2008; 35: 365–373

[4] Fredholm DV, Carpenter JW, KuKanich B, Kohles M. Pharmacokinetics of meloxicam in rabbits after oral administration of single and multiple doses. Am J Vet Res 2013; 74: 636–641

[5] Longley L. Anaesthesia and analgesia in rabbits and rodents. In Practice 2008; 30: 92–97

[6] Williams AM, Wyatt JD. Comparison of subcutaneous and intramuscular ketamine-medetomidine with and without reversal by atipamezole in Dutch belted rabbits. J Am Assoc Lab Anim Sci 2007; 46: 16–20

5.6 Guinea pig

Domestic guinea pigs are usually friendly animals that are easy to handle. However, safe and well monitored anaesthesia is a major challenge: venous access is difficult to obtain (no big ears like the rabbit) and intubation is almost impossible. Common reasons for the need of anaesthesia are castration, further diagnostics (radiography, CT) or the treatment of dental diseases. Unfortunately, due to the lack of intubation options and the often missing IV access, anaesthesia incidents can only be responded to inadequately. **Chinchilla** and **degu** are not described further in the context of this book, but like guinea pigs they belong to the same infraorder "caviomorpha" and are similar in physiology and anaesthetic management.

5.6.1 Preanaesthetic considerations

Preoperative **handling** is comparatively easy, as guinea pigs are quite calm. Nevertheless, they are **susceptible to stress**. One should definitely **weigh** the animals with a digital scale, as one should not rely on an estimate, especially with emaciated animals. Fixation should be done carefully. After arrival at the clinic, the animal should spend some time in a quiet environment so that it can calm down (**adaptation time**).

Classic complications to be expected: Rapid **hypothermia** (due to large surface area compared to mass), **hypotension** (often due to vasodilation), **bradycardia** and/or negative inotropic effect of anaesthetics. **Tachycardia** with pain and too light anaesthesia.

Guinea pigs have physiologically very high respiratory rates, therefore a respiratory rate < 25 /min must already be called a respiratory emergency. **Respiratory depression/hypoventilation** will lead to **hypercapnia** and **hypoxaemia**.

Intubation is very difficult to impossible due to a mucous membrane ring (*ostium palatinum*) located rostral to the larynx. **IV access** can also be a challenge. Preoperatively, but at the latest when an IV catheter is placed, blood should be taken for measurement of the basic parameters haematocrit, total protein and glucose, and in case of prolonged inappetence also organ parameters (liver). Guinea pigs often have **food remains in their oral cavities**, there is a **risk of aspiration**. Before sedation/anaesthesia induction, the mouth should be rinsed with water if necessary. These animals also tend to **regurgitate**.

General considerations

Fasting: Like rabbits, do not fast, but avoid high carbohydrate food. No water deprivation. Some basic normal values can be found in ▶ Table 5.6.

Blood volume in the guinea pig is approx. 65–90 ml/kg body weight.

Anatomical and physiological features

Guinea pigs are small animals, IV access, intubation and monitoring are difficult. "Safe" anaesthesia is therefore a challenge. Pulse oximetry on the paws, ECG, temperature and blood-pressure measurement as well as non-apparatus monitoring are possible.

Table 5.6 Normal values guinea pig

Parameter (unit)	Normal values
Core body temperature (°C)	37.2–39.5
Heart rate (/min)	150–280
Respiratory rate (/min)	100–130
Haematocrit (%)	39–55
Total protein (g/dl)	4.4–6.6

IV access

▶ **Cephalic vein** (*v. cephalica antebrachii*). This vein is a little more lateral than you would expect. You can try to catheterise it with a 24 G catheter. With a little practice you will be quite successful, which makes the maintenance phase of long anaesthesia periods much easier.

Intubation

Intubation is **almost impossible** and is generally not recommended. This is not due to the size alone, but rather on the one hand to the *ostium palatinum*, which is characteristic of guinea pigs. It is a very well perfused mucosal ring that runs from the soft palate to the tongue and forms a ring between the oropharynx and pharynx. This tissue is easily injured and then bleeds profusely. The second reason is that guinea pigs often have **food remains in their oral cavity**, which can then be displaced into the trachea with the ETT or during dental procedures. However, these can be flushed out with 1 ml syringes with warm water without pressure (because of the risk of aspiration) until clear fluid comes out. Nevertheless, clinically the mask is really the only possible "airway".

Specific considerations

Guinea pigs seem to be particularly **sensitive to sevoflurane**, but also to **isoflurane**. Especially in higher doses, they show severe respiratory depression, asphyxia and severe bronchial secretion. It is worthwhile to **premedicate well** in order to keep the dose of inhalants low. If premedication is not possible, it may be worthwhile either to use atropine already during sedation (p. 200) or to have it within reach. In addition, inhalation anaesthetics show a dose-dependent depression of the cardiovascular system. Sevoflurane and isoflurane are therefore not suitable as monoanaesthetics in guinea pigs (just as in any other species).

5.6.2 Anaesthesia protocols

Before starting sedation/anaesthesia, similar considerations should be made as for the rabbit: How long will the procedure take? And how painful will it be? The anaesthetic protocol must then be adapted accordingly.

Examination of the patient and ASA classification: see chapter "Preanaesthetic examination" (p. 150); "Perioperative management" (p. 152) incl. airway management, infusion therapy, administration of antibiotics, protection of the cornea and emptying of the urinary bladder; "Monitoring" (p. 39).

Sedation

In the guinea pig, it may be appropriate to include **atropine** 0.04 mg/kg or **glycopyrrolate** 0.02 mg/kg in the protocol. Bronchial secretions may become very profuse, especially with the use of inhalational anaesthetics, and are reduced by the addition of parasympatholytic agents. However, it would be best to **use a balanced anaesthetic protocol**, then the addition of a parasympatholytic is usually not necessary.

Dosage

- **Medetomidine** 0.08–0.12 mg/kg AND
- **Butorphanol** 0.2–0.5 mg/kg mixed in one syringe SC or IM

Depending on the condition of the guinea pig and the dosage, a moderate to deep sedation is induced, which is well suited for more detailed examinations or the attempt to place an IV access. To deepen the sedation, **ketamine 10–20 mg/kg** can be added, so that short, even painful procedures can be performed. At higher doses, general anaesthesia is induced.

Dosage

- **Midazolam** 0.5 mg/kg AND
- **Butorphanol** 0.5 mg/kg mixed in one syringe SC or IM

This combination is particularly recommended for already sick or compromised guinea pigs that need to be carefully sedated. The sedation is rather mild and is not at all sufficient for surgical tolerance.

Induction

Sedation is often omitted in the guinea pig when the goal is general anaesthesia. The following protocols are suggestions for the "classic" guinea pig procedures such as dental treatment or castration.

Dosage

- **Ketamine** 15–40 mg/kg AND
- **Medetomidine** 0.08–0.12 mg/kg OR **Dexmedetomidine** 0.04–0.06 mg/kg + / –
- **Butorphanol** 0.2–0.5 mg/kg mixed in one syringe SC or IM

This combination usually provides stable anaesthesia sufficient for routine castrations or short painful dental procedures. **Ketamine** should not be used alone to avoid severe side effects such as catalepsy, salivation and hallucinations. At the earliest 40 min after injection, dex-/medetomidine can be antagonised with **atipamezole** (same volume) SC or IM.

Xylazine 2–4 mg/kg can also be used instead of dex-/medetomidine. However, this drug no longer meets today's standard, it is more unspecific in its effect and cannot be reliably antagonised.

Dosage

- **Medetomidine** 0.2 mg/kg OR **Dexmedetomidine** 0.1 mg/kg AND
- **Midazolam** 1 mg/kg AND
- **Fentanyl** 0.025 mg/kg mixed in one syringe SC or IM

= fully antagonisable anaesthesia

This combination should be administered IM, as apparently absorption after SC application is very irregular. Surgical tolerance occurs after about 15 min, but anaesthesia is **not as deep** as with a ketamine-based protocol. If isoflurane or sevoflurane is also administered by mask, longer and more painful procedures can be performed. This combination causes **severe respiratory depression**, one should always give O_2! For antagonisation use **atipamezole 1 mg/kg, flumazenil 0.1 mg/kg and naloxone 0.03 mg/kg mixed in one syringe SC or IM**. After painful interventions, naloxone should not be used, as it antagonises any opioid effect (including that of endogenous opioids).

Maintenance phase

Similar to rabbits, anaesthesia is continued with **isoflurane** or **sevoflurane** for longer procedures. As intubation is almost impossible, a tight-fitting face mask must be used. MAC value of isoflurane in the guinea pig is 1.15% (▶ Table 4.22) which is lower than in other small mammals and indicates that guinea pigs are more sensitive to inhalation anaesthetics (including severe bronchoconstriction); see "Specific considerations" (p. 199).

Ketamine 0.1–0.5 mg/kg can be titrated very carefully and diluted IV in this phase. If too much is given too quickly, there is a risk of respiratory arrest. If given carefully and slowly, it has a MAC-reducing effect and stabilises the maintenance phase.

Analgesia:
- NSAIDs such as **Meloxicam** 0.5–1 mg/kg SC (1 × /d) and/or
- **Metamizole** 80 mg/kg SC or PO every 4–6 h
- **Buprenorphine** 0.02–0.05 mg/kg IM or IV every 6 h

These drugs are ideally administered and effective before any painful intervention and then continued for as long as necessary.

Recovery phase

The same guidelines apply as for rabbits (p. 197). The animal should be monitored for several hours at regular intervals, at least by inspection. A quiet, warm, dry environment is ideal.

- **Start feeding** after the patient has recovered from the anaesthesia
- **Active temperature management**: Measure core body temperature several times and actively warm if necessary
- If IV access is available, **infusion** can be **continued**. Otherwise, a single SC injection of a bolus (at least 10 ml/kg, more if needed) of warm balanced electrolyte solution has proven useful
- If necessary, **antagonise** again if the animal re-sedates after some time

5.6.3 Literature

[1] Dang V, Bao S, Ault A, Murray C, McFarlane-Mills J, Chiedi C, Dillon M, Todd JP, DeTolla L, Rao S. Efficacy and safety of five injectable anesthetic regimens for chronic blood collection from the anterior vena cava of guinea pigs. J Am Assoc Lab Anim Sci 2008; 47: 56–60

[2] Heide C, Henke J, Eissner B et al. Clinical evaluation of isoflurane and sevoflurane with and without atropine premedication in guinea pigs (Cavia porcellus). Vet Anaesth Analg 2003; 30: 51–52

[3] Schwenke DO, Cragg PA. Comparison of the depressive effects of four anesthetic regimens on ventilatory and cardiovascular variables in the guinea pig. Comp Med 2004; 54: 77–85

[4] Seifen AB, Kennedy RH, Bray JP et al. Estimation of minimum alveolar concentration (MAC) for halothane, enflurane and isoflurane in spontaneously breathing guinea pigs. Lab Anim Sci 1989; 39: 579–81

5.7 Ferret

Even if you have little anaesthetic experience with this species, you do not have to be afraid of it: You can practically treat ferrets like a small cat. However, there are a few specific considerations, for example there are species-specific diseases that need to be taken into account.

5.7.1 Preanaesthetic considerations

Preoperative **handling** depends largely on whether the animal is a domestic animal accustomed to humans or more of a wild animal. Perioperative management can also be difficult as ferrets are relatively **small**. The **weight** of the animal must be determined on a digital scale as it can easily be overestimated. Wild animals can be quite **aggressive**, making injection or restraint to place the IV catheter almost impossible without endangering oneself. "Species-specific diseases" (p. 204), which are more commonly found in ferrets, should be considered in advance and the protocol should be adapted accordingly.

Classic complications to be expected: Rapid **hypothermia** (due to large surface area compared to small mass), **hypotension** (often due to vasodilation from high concentrations of isoflurane/sevoflurane), **bradycardia** and/or negative inotropic effect of anaesthetics, **tachycardia**, **respiratory depression/hypoventilation** with **hypercapnia** and **hypoxaemia**, rarely problems with **intubation** (very small but easy to see), problems with **IV access placement** (measure baseline blood parameters if possible: haematocrit, total protein and glucose). These animals can easily **vomit** or **regurgitate** and aspirate.

General considerations

Fasting: 4 to max. 6 h food deprivation before induction, no water deprivation. Ferrets have a very short digestive tract, therefore they require only relatively short fasting times. Blood glucose values should be checked regularly in insulinoma patients. Some basic normal values can be found in ▶ Table 5.7.

Blood volume is approx. 60 ml/kg body weight.

Anatomical and physiological features

Genuine anatomical and physiological features are not present.

IV access

▶ **Cephalic vein** (*v. cephalica antebrachii*). Relatively well visible. With a little practice, the IV catheter is easy to place.

Table 5.7 Normal values ferret

Parameter (unit)	Normal values
Core body temperature (°C)	37.8–40.0
Heart rate (/min)	120–260
Respiratory rate (/min)	30–60
Haematocrit (%)	42–68
Total protein (g/dl)	5.4–7.8

▶ **Lateral saphenous vein** (*v. saphena lateralis*). Clearly visible. Catheterisation is quite easy.

▶ **Jugular vein** (*v. jugularis*). Well palpable and visible vessel for blood sampling under sedation or anaesthesia.

Intubation

Intubation is similar to that of a small cat, only the jaw tone is slightly higher.
- Tube size is chosen from 2.0 to 3.5 mm ID, depending on the size of the animal.
- Upper airway is relatively small and delicate, but usually easy to visualise using a laryngoscope with a light source when the mouth is held wide open.
- Ferrets have **laryngeal protective reflexes**, so before intubation 1. the depth of anaesthesia should be sufficient and 2. lidocaine should be sprayed/dripped on topically to avoid laryngeal spasm.
- It should always be intubated into the open larynx.
- Most endotracheal tubes used in human medicine are too long and should be shortened; see "Airway Management" (p. 153); for details; optimal length: from incisors to the thoracic inlet.
- Tie with a cord behind the ears.
- Carefully inflate the cuff to seal the airway.

Species-specific diseases

Ferrets have some diseases that occur more frequently than average. These should be assessed in advance and the animal should be prepared accordingly.

Permanent oestrus

▶ **Symptoms.** Life-threatening pancytopenia, aplastic anaemia

▶ **Cause.** In the permanent oestrus of the female animal, oestrogen-induced bone marrow suppression may occur

▶ **Conclusion.** Routinely measure haematocrit before any sedation or anaesthesia. If it is below 15–20%, a conservative treatment attempt or a blood transfusion from another ferret (there are no significant blood groups) should be considered

Insulinoma

▶ **Symptoms.** Unspecific symptoms, weight loss, increased salivation, episodic fatigue and even ataxia of the hind legs, often an incidental finding

▶ **Cause.** Tumour of the β-cells of the islets of Langerhans' in the pancreas in middle-aged and old ferrets, cause not yet fully understood. Insulinoma secretes insulin independently of the pancreas

▶ **Conclusion.** In case of suspected disease, measure fasting glucose value (after 4–6 h fasting), if it is below 70 mg/dl, insulinoma is likely. In case of doubt, avoid alpha2 agonists in order not to additionally influence glucose values. Check glucose regularly and if necessary, administer it as a controlled continuous rate infusion; for more information see "Diabetes mellitus" (p. 331)

Hyperadrenocorticism

▶ **Symptoms.** Weight loss, bilateral hair loss on the trunk possibly with itching, in female animals swelling of the vulva, in male animals possibly prostate changes

▶ **Cause.** Increased production of sex hormones due to hyperplasia of the adrenal gland (90% the left adrenal gland), either adenoma or carcinoma

▶ **Conclusion.** Confirm suspected diagnosis by history, then by further diagnostics like ultrasound, fine needle biopsy, etc. If adrenalectomy is planned, organise a blood donor in case of emergency, and be sure to place an IV catheter. If the tumour has already penetrated the vena cava, allow hypothermia during anaesthesia in order to have a higher chance of survival in case of severe perioperative bleeding

Dilated cardiomyopathy (DCM)

DCM in the older ferret is very similar to that in the dog. It is much more common in the ferret than hypertrophic cardiomyopathy

▶ **Symptoms.** Weight loss, weakness, dyspnoea, tachycardia, cardiac murmur, in advanced stages also ascites, liquidothorax and pulmonary oedema

▶ **Cause.** Unknown, sometimes secondary to viral disease

▶ **Conclusion.** Diagnosis with ultrasound and ECG, adjustment of the anaesthesia protocol, details under "Dilated cardiomyopathy (DCM)" (p. 279) in dogs

5.7.2 Anaesthesia protocols

As mentioned earlier, ferrets can be anaesthetised very similarly to cats. The following protocols can be used, but must be adapted to the individual patient.

Examination of the patient and ASA classification: see chapter "Preanaesthetic examination" (p. 150); "Perioperative management" (p. 152) incl. airway management, infusion therapy, administration of antibiotics, protection of the cornea and emptying of the urinary bladder; "Monitoring" (p. 39).

Sedation

In animals that are difficult to handle, sedation may be necessary to perform an examination. It is also a good option for placing an IV catheter without stress. Whenever ketamine is included in the protocol, the mixture should not be injected IM in small animals.

Dosage
• **Acepromazine** 0.1–0.3 mg/kg IM or IV

Should only be administered in young, healthy animals, never in hypovolaemia, anaemia or shock. Mild to moderate sedation is achieved, which lasts for a long time.

Dosage

- **Butorphanol** up to 0.5 mg/kg AND
- **Midazolam** up to 0.5 mg/kg mixed in one syringe SC, IM, IV OR **Diazepam** up to 0.5 mg/kg IV, do not mix

Very gentle sedation for sick animals, light to deep sedation depending on general condition and age. A small dose of **alfaxalone** may be added (1–2 mg/kg) to deepen sedation. Midazolam/diazepam is antagonisable with **flumazenil** 0.05 mg/kg SC.

Dosage

- **Butorphanol** 0.2–0.5 mg/kg AND
- **Medetomidine** 0.04–0.12 mg/kg OR **Dexmedetomidine** 0.02–0.06 mg/kg (equals **Xylazine** 1–2 mg/kg) +/–
- **Ketamine** 2–15 mg/kg mixed in one syringe SC

With this combination, aggressive animals are moderately to deeply sedated or anaesthetised depending on the dose. The usual side effects are to be expected from alpha2 agonists, so caution should be exercised in sick or very old animals, and the dose may have to be considerably reduced. This combination can also be used for induction of anaesthesia, in which case the dose must be chosen at the higher end of the range and ketamine must be used in any case.

Induction

Induction of anaesthesia in ferrets can be carried out in the same way as in other small animals and is mainly based on ketamine with a muscle relaxant and sedative additive.

Dosage

- **Ketamine** 10 mg/kg AND
- **Medetomidine** 0.02–0.04 mg/kg OR **Dexmedetomidine** 0.01–0.02 mg/kg +/–
- **Midazolam** 0.5 mg mixed in one syringe SC

This protocol is sufficient for castration of male and female animals. After 40 min at the earliest, dex-/medetomidine can be antagonised with atipamezole (0.1 mg/kg SC, equivalent to the same volume as dex-/medetomidine). If slightly more analgesia is desired, midazolam can be replaced by butorphanol.

Dosage

- **Ketamine** 10–30 mg/kg AND
- **Midazolam** 0.5–2 mg/kg mixed in one syringe SC

This is a commonly used protocol in practice for painful procedures, ideally a long-acting opioid (e.g. **buprenorphine** 0.02–0.04 mg/kg SC, IM, IV) and/or an NSAID (e.g. **meloxicam** 0.3 mg/kg SC, PO) should then be administered post-operatively depending on the level of pain. Midazolam/diazepam may be antagonised.

Dosage

- **Ketamine** 10–20 mg/kg AND
- **Medetomidine** 0.06–0.1 mg/kg OR **Dexmedetomidine** 0.03–0.05 mg/kg mixed in one syringe SC

This protocol is relatively simple, but its high dosages can be quite **respiratory and circulatory depressive**. However, a young, healthy animal will (usually) be anaesthetised without problems. Attention should be paid to O_2 administration and temperature management. **Atipamezole** can be administered for antagonisation after 40 minutes at the earliest.

Dosage

- **Propofol** 4–8 mg/kg IV

Induction is particularly calm and controlled after sedation. For painful procedures, **ketamine 1–3 mg/kg** IV can be used along with the induction. The dose of propofol is then reduced.

Maintenance phase

Because ferrets are relatively easy to intubate despite being so small, maintenance of anaesthesia for a longer duration is performed with **isoflurane** (MAC approx. 1.3–1.5%, ▶ Table 4.22) or **sevoflurane** (MAC approx. 2.3%, ▶ Table 4.38). For shorter procedures, the duration of action of the injectable anaesthetics is sufficient; if anaesthesia has to be prolonged, about ⅓ of the initial dose of injectable anaesthetics should be administered.

For very painful procedures, a continuous rate infusion of **ketamine** and/or **fentanyl** can be considered, as in dogs and cats.

Analgesia:
- NSAIDs such as **meloxicam** 0.3 mg/kg SC and/or
- **Metamizole** 50 mg/kg PO, SC and/or
- **Buprenorphine** 0.02–0.05 mg/kg IM, IV

Recovery phase

The same guidelines apply as for rabbits (p. 197). The animal should be **monitored** for several hours at regular intervals, at least by inspection. A quiet, warm, dry environment is ideal.

- **Active temperature management**: Measure core body temperature and actively warm if necessary
- If IV access is available, **infusion** can be **continued**
- **Antagonise** again if necessary if the animal re-sedates after some time

5.7.3 Literature

[1] Busch R, Henke J, Lendl C et al. Klinischer Vergleich dreier Medetomidin – Midazolam – Ketamin Narkosen auf ihre Eignung zur Kastration von Frettchen. Berl Münch Tierärztl Wschr 2008; 121: 1–10
[2] Cantwell SL, Heard B. Ferret, rabbit and rodent anesthesia. In Vet Clin North Am Exot Anim Pract 2001; 4: 169–191
[3] Chinnadurai SK, Messenger KM, Papich MG, Harms CA. Meloxicam pharmacokinetics using nonlinear mixed-effects modeling in ferrets after single subcutaneous administration. J Vet Pharmacol Ther 2014; 37: 382–387
[4] Hildebrandt N, Schneider M. Die dilatative Kardiomyopathie beim Frettchen – Symptomatik, Diagnostik und therapeutische Möglichkeiten. Tierärztl Prax (K) 2009; 2: 115–123
[5] Ko J, Kuo W, Nicklin C et al. Comparison of anaesthetic and cardiorespiratory effects of diazepam-butorphanol-ketamine, acepromazine-butorphanol- ketamine and xylazine-butorphanol-ketamine in ferrets. J Am Anim Hosp Assoc 1998; 34: 407–416

5.8 Small rodents

The term "small rodents" is used to refer to rats, mice and hamsters. Of course, these are separate animal species with individual differences. Some of them are described below insofar as they are relevant to anaesthesia.

Unfortunately, anaesthesia incidents occur more often in small rodents and can often only be responded to poorly due to the small size of the animal.

5.8.1 Preanaesthetic considerations

Preoperative **handling** strongly depends on how accustomed the animals are to humans, which species they are (mouse and rat are basically friendlier than hamster, but this may be due to the fact that hamsters usually sleep during the day and are roused from sleep by the vet) and from which strain they are (especially with mice, there are nice and easy to handle as well as rather aggressive strains). They are all prey animals and therefore **susceptible to stress**. You should definitely **weigh** the animals with an accurate digital scale. Restraint should only be used in an emergency and with care. After arrival at the clinic, some time should be given in a quiet environment to allow the animal to calm down (**adaptation time**).

Classic complications to be expected: rapid **hypothermia** (be sure to warm the animals from the beginning, they cool down within minutes!), **hypotension** (often due to vasodilation) and **bradycardia**. Bradycardia can be caused by hypothermia and is then resistant to therapy. **Tachycardia** with pain and too light anaesthesia. **Respiratory depression/hypoventilation** results in **hypercapnia** and **hypoxaemia**. There is a risk of **hypoglycaemia** due to the high metabolic rate.

Intubation is very difficult to perform in routine clinical practice, as is getting an **IV access**. Hamsters and guinea pigs can have **food debris** in their oral cavities, and there is a **risk of aspiration**. Monitoring vital signs is very difficult and consists almost exclusively of clinical monitoring (respiratory rate and depth, heart rate, temperature). Apparatus **monitoring** very quickly reaches its limits. Therefore, special high-speed devices are needed that can also measure high frequencies.

Practice tip

What to do in case of apnoea of a non-intubated small mammal?
If intubation of a small mammal is not possible, apnoea will cause an acute life-threatening condition. One way to get air in and out of the lungs is by rhythmically swaying the animal: To do this, place the animal in the sternal position in both hands and lower alternately front and back. The forward and backward movement of the abdominal organs towards the diaphragm causes a kind of respiration. Ideally, one fixes a mask with 100% oxygen over the nose and mouth at the same time. With this technique, it is possible to provide some kind of ventilation during apnoea phases.

The aim must be to have the animal wake up from anaesthesia as quickly as possible. The objective should be normothermia, sternal position and continuous O_2 supply.

General considerations

Fasting: No food withdrawal, no water withdrawal, there is a risk of hypoglycaemia and acidosis. Rats, hamsters and mice cannot vomit. Some basic normal values can be found in ▶ Table 5.8.

Blood volume in the rat is approx. 60 ml/kg body weight (i. e. 30 ml for a 500 g rat; maximum blood loss should therefore be 15%, i. e. 4.5 ml).

In mice, blood volume is about 50–60 ml/kg body weight (for a 25 g mouse, this is 1.4 ml; maximum blood loss should not exceed 0.2 ml).

Hamsters have a relatively large blood volume of 65–80 ml/kg body weight.

Table 5.8 Normal values rat, mouse, hamster

Parameter (unit)	Rat	Mouse	Hamster
Core body temperature (°C)	37.0–39.5	35.0–39.0	37.0–38.0
Heart rate (/min)	200–500	310–840	200*–500
Respiratory rate (/min)	70–150	100–160	35*–135
Haematocrit (%)	36–54	35–50	39–59
Total protein (g/dl)	5.6–7.6	3.5–7.2	4.3–7.7
Glucose (g/dl)	50–135	107–190	60–150

* during hibernation

Anatomical and physiological features

Rat

- Often subclinical infections of the respiratory tract, frequently diagnosed after anaesthesia/surgery
- The Harder's glands above the eyes produce a reddish secretion. In healthy animals, this is regularly cleaned away and cannot be seen. In sick animals, the secretion can be seen as red circles around the eyes. This can be interpreted as an indication of a poor general condition

Mouse

- Very susceptible to stress from changes in the environment (temperature, noise)
- Very high metabolic rate, therefore requires comparatively high doses per kg
- Large differences in anaesthetic sensitivity between breed, strain and sex

Hamster

- Nocturnal animals, can be very skittish and defensive during the day
- Very large cheek pouches: After induction of anaesthesia, the oral cavity should be inspected and, if necessary, cleared out to avoid aspiration. Weight should only be measured with empty cheek pouches!

Methods of application

Subcutaneous (SC) and intraperitoneal (IP) routes are suitable methods of administration in small rodents. Analgesics can also be administered orally (PO) or orally transmucosally (OTM). IM injection should not be performed in animals weighing less than 100 g. Placing an intravenous access in such small animals is only possible with good fixation/anaesthesia, practice and a bit of luck. A 24 or 26 G catheter should be used.

IV access

▶ **Cephalic vein** (*v. cephalica antebrachii*). In rats, this IV access can be placed with fixation or after sedation/anaesthesia with some practice.

▶ **Median caudal vein** (*v. caudalis mediana*). The tail vein of the rat (and mouse) is also suitable for placing a 24 or 26 G catheter. Warming the tail with warm water or heating lamp helps to dilate the vessel. Scraping off the tail scales increases visibility.

▶ **Jugular vein, jugular vein angle** (*v. jugularis*). Suitable for blood collection with fixation or after sedation/anaesthesia. The blood volume of the respective animal must be considered.

Intubation

Intubation of such small animals requires special equipment and although it is possible and routinely performed in laboratory animal settings, it is the exception in practice.

Specific considerations

Sensitivity to different anaesthetics varies greatly between different breeds and strains. In order to obtain more detailed information on specific breeds or strains (especially in laboratory animal science), the study of further literature is recommended.

5.8.2 Anaesthesia protocols

An indication of too light anaesthesia may be the vibration of the whiskers. If the anaesthesia is too deep, pronounced exophthalmos will occur. An anaesthetic depth with surgical tolerance is usually reached when the interphalangeal reflex on the forelimb is negative.

Examination of the patient and ASA classification: see chapter "Preanaesthetic examination" (p. 150); "Perioperative management" (p. 152) incl. airway management, infusion therapy, administration of antibiotics, protection of the cornea and emptying of the urinary bladder; "Monitoring" (p. 39).

Sedation

Preanaesthetic sedation is of little use in such small animals as there are few benefits. Usually, anaesthesia is induced immediately with either injection or inhalation anaesthesia. However, sedation is useful, for example, to allow a detailed examination or to perform a radiological examination (radiography, CT or MRI).

Dosage

- **Medetomidine** 0.08–0.25 mg/kg OR **Dexmedetomidine** 0.04–0.12 mg/kg AND
- **Butorphanol** 0.2–0.5 mg/kg mixed in one syringe SC

Depending on the health status and size of the animal, one chooses its dose (small and/or healthy animal = higher dose). This combination allows for deep, non-arousable sedation, which, in combination with local anaesthesia, allows even small painful procedures to be performed.

The effect of dex-/medetomidine can be antagonised at any time with **atipamezole** (same volume as the dex-/medetomidine administered) SC. The duration and effect of butorphanol is relatively short and weak, so antagonisation with naloxone makes little sense. If dex-/medetomidine is also combined with **ketamine**, it should always be antagonised not earlier than after 30 minutes.

Induction

The choice of anaesthetics depends largely on the planned procedure.

After injection of the induction drugs, it is crucial to let the animals go to sleep undisturbed in a quiet environment. The calmer this phase is, the better the anaesthetics work. During this phase, the animal should be warmed (heating mat, gloves filled with warm water, warm air blower), as heat loss already occurs.

Rat

Dosage

Protocol 1:
- **Ketamine** 30–60 mg/kg AND
- **Medetomidine** 0.15–0.2 mg/kg OR **Dexmedetomidine** 0.07–0.1 mg/kg + /–
- **Butorphanol** 0.2–0.5 mg/kg mixed in one syringe SC or IP

Dosage

Protocol 2:
- **Medetomidine** 0.15 mg/kg OR **Dexmedetomidine** 0.08 mg/kg AND
- **Midazolam** 2 mg/kg AND
- **Fentanyl** 0.005 mg/kg mixed in one syringe IM or IP

= fully antagonisable anaesthesia

Dosage

Protocol 3:
- Box induction with **Isoflurane** > 2.5–3.5% OR **Sevoflurane** > 4–6% in O$_2$

Mouse

Dosage

Protocol 1:
- **Ketamine** 30–100 mg/kg AND
- **Medetomidine** 0.15–0.2 mg/kg OR **Dexmedetomidine** 0.07–0.1 mg/kg + / –
- **Butorphanol** 0.5 mg/kg mixed in one syringe SC or IP

Dosage

Protocol 2:
- **Medetomidine** 0.5 mg/kg OR **Dexmedetomidine** 0.25 mg/kg AND
- **Midazolam** 5 mg/kg AND
- **Fentanyl** 0.05 mg/kg mixed in one syringe IM or IP

= fully antagonisable anaesthesia

Dosage

Protocol 3:
- Box induction with **Isoflurane** > 2.5–3.5% OR **Sevoflurane** > 4–6% in O$_2$

Hamster

Dosage

Protocol 1:
- **Ketamine** 30–80 mg/kg AND
- **Medetomidine** 0.15–0.2 mg/kg OR **Dexmedetomidine** 0.07–0.1 mg/kg + /–
- **Butorphanol** 0.5 mg/kg in mixed in one syringe SC or IP

Dosage

Protocol 2:
- **Medetomidine** 0.33 mg/kg OR **Dexmedetomidine** 0.16 mg/kg AND
- **Midazolam** 3.3 mg/kg AND
- **Fentanyl** 0.033 mg/kg mixed in one syringe IM or IP

= fully antagonisable anaesthesia

Dosage

Protocol 3:
- Box induction with **Isoflurane** > 2.5–3.5% OR **Sevoflurane** > 4–6% in O_2

These protocols are **quite respiratory and circulatory depressant** due to their high dosages. The dosages should therefore always be adapted to the individual condition and size of the patient. A young, healthy animal will (usually) undergo anaesthesia even with the high dosages for a short period of time without problems. Supplemental oxygen should be administered continuously and active temperature management should be performed.

▶ Protocol 1. This protocol is sufficient for castration of male and female animals as well as for other painful procedures (tumour removal, tail amputation, etc.). After 30–40 min at the earliest, dex-/medetomidine can be antagonised with **atipamezole** (same volume as dex-/medetomidine, SC).

Instead of dex-/medetomidine, the non-specific **xylazine** can also be used. However, as its effect cannot be reliably antagonised, dex-/medetomidine should be preferred. The dosage of xylazine is between 2 and 5 mg/kg.

▶ **Protocol 2.** This combination should be administered IM (in animals with > 100 g body weight), as apparently the absorption after SC application is very irregular. Surgical tolerance occurs after approx. 15 min, but anaesthesia is not as deep as with a ketamine-based protocol. For mildly painful soft tissue procedures this combination is sufficient. **Severe respiratory depression**, always administer O_2!

Antagonisation of protocol 2 is performed with the following drugs in a mixed syringe:

Dosage

Rat:
- **Atipamezole** 0.75 mg/kg AND
- **Flumazenil** 0.2 mg/kg AND
- (**Naloxone** 0.12 mg/kg SC)

Dosage

Mouse:
- **Atipamezole** 2.5 mg/kg AND
- **Flumazenil** 0.5 mg/kg AND
- (**Naloxone** 1.2 mg/kg SC)

Dosage

Hamster:
- **Atipamezole** 1.7 mg/kg AND
- **Flumazenil** 0.33 mg/kg AND
- (**Naloxone** 0.8 mg/kg SC)

Naloxone should be avoided after painful interventions, as it antagonises any opioid effect (also that of endogenous opioids).

▶ **Protocol 3.** Box induction can take longer depending on the concentration of the inhalation anaesthetic and is associated with stress for the animal. Therefore, it should only be used in exceptional cases in an already sedated animal or when there is no alternative. Compared to isoflurane, sevoflurane is less irritating to the mucous membranes and animals salivate less. The high concentrations always cause respiratory depression, so O_2 should be chosen as sole carrier gas. As soon as the anaesthesia is induced (righting reflex and interdigital pinch reflex negative), the concentration of the anaesthetic must be reduced.

Maintenance phase

Similar to other small mammals, anaesthesia is continued with **isoflurane** or **sevoflurane** via mask (or endotracheal tube) for longer procedures. MAC values of the different animal species can be found for isoflurane in ▶ Table 4.22 and for sevoflurane in ▶ Table 4.38. If the procedure is painful, an analgesic must be administered in time, as the inhalation anaesthetics per se do not have an analgesic effect.

If anaesthesia was induced with injectable anaesthetics and an anaesthesia machine is not available (O_2 should, however, always be administered!), approx. ⅓ of the initial dosage can be re-administered. This degree of deepening and prolongation of anaesthesia is relatively unspecific and not very controllable. As a result, it can be associated with severe respiratory and circulatory depression as well as a long recovery phase.

Recovery phase

The same guidelines apply as for the other small mammals. The patient should be **monitored** for several hours at regular intervals, at least by adspection. A quiet, warm, dry environment is ideal. Allotriophagia (= eating everything) can occur, especially in rats, so neither bedding nor cellulose should be nearby at the beginning of the recovery phase.

Analgesia:
- NSAIDs such as **Meloxicam** 1–5 mg/kg PO, SC (1 × /day) and/or
- **Metamizole** 100–200 mg/kg PO, SC (1 × /d) and after very painful procedures and/or
- **Buprenorphine** 0.03–0.1 mg/kg IM, IV (every 4–6 h)

These drugs are ideally administered before painful procedures and then continued for as long as necessary.
- **Feeding**: After waking up. This is not as important for rats, mice and hamsters as for rabbits and guinea pigs, but it helps to assess the condition of the animal
- **Temperature management**: Measure core body temperature and actively warm if necessary

- If IV access is available, continue **infusion**, otherwise single SC injection of a bolus (10–30 ml/kg) of warmed balanced electrolyte solution has been shown to be effective
- If necessary, **antagonise** again if the animal is not properly awake after some time

5.8.3 Literature

[1] Henke J. Analgesie und Anästhesie beim Kleinsäuger. Prakt Tierarzt 2010; 91: 294–304

[2] Kilic N, Henke J, Erhard W. Die Ketamin-Medetomidin-Anästhesie beim Hamster: Ein klinischer Vergleich zwischen subkutaner und intraperitonealer Applikation. Tierärztl Prax (K) 2004; 32: 384–8

5.9 Horse

Horses are food-producing animals and are primarily considered as animals for slaughter within the EU. Pharmacological treatments of all kinds are subject to the relevant laws in order to protect the consumer and to make it easier to control animal diseases. Whether a drug is licensed for horses for slaughter can be found in the EU Commission Regulation on pharmacologically active substances and their classification regarding maximum residue limits in foodstuffs of animal origin from 2009 (on the Internet: https://op.europa.eu/en/publication-detail/-/publication/7155d8e1-b40e-11e3-86f9-01aa75ed71a1; as of May 2023).

An exemption comes into effect if the horse has an identification document (equine passport) and it is noted in it that this animal is not intended for slaughter. In this case, drugs/anaesthetics not specifically approved for this species can be administered. In addition to the drugs also authorised for horses for slaughter, there is a so-called "positive list" containing drugs according to the EU regulation establishing a list of substances essential for the treatment of equidae. This applies to equidae, so includes horses and donkeys. If an animal is treated with substances on this list, a waiting period of 6 months applies to the meat (on the Internet. https://eur-lex.europa.eu/legal-content/EN/TXT/HTML/?uri=CELEX:32006R1950&from=DE; as of May 2023).

5.9.1 Preanaesthetic considerations

Unfortunately, general anaesthesia of horses is associated with a relatively high mortality rate (0.5–1%). The most serious problems usually occur during the recovery phase (p. 228).

On the one hand, preoperative **handling** depends on the breed, age, temperament and purpose of use of the horse. On the other hand, however, it also depends to a large extent on whether it is a pet that is used to humans or rather an animal that has little human contact. Horses can pose a **risk of injury** to humans, especially if they are not fully awake. They can **kick**, **bite** and **hit** with their **heads**. The sheer **mass** alone can be a danger, so caution is advised. It is always worth asking if there have been any abnormalities with previous anaesthesia. Some procedures are very well suited to be performed with standing sedation in combination with local anaesthesia (such as dental procedures).

A current **weight** should be determined. As the anaesthesia time should be kept as short as possible, the fur in the surgical field should already be clipped before induction (if possible). The horseshoes should be removed for safety reasons.

Due to the size of the animals, care must be taken to ensure **good positioning** during general anaesthesia, **neuropathy/nerve damage** and **myopathy** may occur. Attention should be paid to pressure points, traction on the legs should be avoided, the lower lying legs should be positioned forward, the legs should not "cross" in lateral position. **Position** during anaesthesia is a crucial factor for oxygenation and ventilation: standing or sternal recumbency is better than lateral recumbency, and lateral recumbency is better than dorsal recumbency. Positioning often causes **congestion of the nasal mucosa**.

Classic complications to be expected: Severe **respiratory depression/hypoventilation** with **hypercapnia** and **hypoxaemia** (therefore oxygen or oxygen-enriched air should always be given to the anaesthetised horse if possible!), **hypotension** or **hypertension**, **bradycardia** or **tachycardia**. Hypoxaemia is not only caused by hypoventilation, but to a large extent by **atelectasis** (collapse of the alveoli) and the resulting **ventilation-perfusion mismatch**.

A **blood sample** with the basic parameters should be taken and assessed pre-anaesthetically: Haematology plus total protein, albumin and fibrinogen. In case of illness or suspicion, also perform blood chemistry: Glucose, lactate, urea, creatinine, electrolytes, possibly liver enzymes, other parameters if further suspicion for disease.

General considerations

Fasting: 8 to max. 12 h food withdrawal before induction, no water withdrawal. If fasted for more than 18 h, metabolic acidosis may occur. Horses cannot vomit. Fasting increases the functional residual capacity of the lungs (= the volume still in the lungs after a normal expiration) by up to 30%, which is helpful for oxygenation and ventilation during anaesthesia. The oral cavity should be rinsed with water before induction of anaesthesia! Do not fast foals that are nursing. Normal values can be found in ▶ Table 5.9.

Table 5.9 Normal values horse

Parameter (unit)	Normal values
Core body temperature (°C)	37.5–38.0
Heart rate (/min)	28–40
Respiratory rate (/min)	10–14
Haematocrit (%)	32–48
Total protein (g/dl)	5.2–7.7

Blood volume in horses is approx. 70 ml/kg body weight.

Anatomical and physiological features

The anatomy and physiology of horses is that of a flight animal that seeks its salvation in getting up and running away quickly. In summary: The physiology is not designed to be placed in dorsal recumbency.

- Horses are **obligate nasal breathers** (like the South American camelids). Care should be taken to ensure that the nasal mucous membranes are decongested at the latest by the time of extubation to allow airflow through the nose
- Ideally, the **mean arterial blood pressure** should be maintained **above 75 mmHg** to ensure perfusion and supply of O_2 to all organs
- **Gas exchange** (oxygen in, carbon dioxide out) is severely **impaired** when the horse is positioned in lateral or (even more unfavourable) dorsal recumbency under general anaesthesia

IV access

▶ **Jugular vein** (*v. jugularis*). Very large vessel, clearly visible after compressing. Care must be taken that the catheter is long enough, otherwise it will slip out of the vessel at the first movement. Work cleanly/sterilely. Inject a local anaesthetic into the tissue at the puncture site beforehand. The catheter should be well sutured to the skin. Very stressed or aggressive animals should be sedated beforehand.

▶ **Lateral auricular vein** (*v. auricularis lateralis*). Not particularly large, but quite easy to catheterise in sedated animals with a 22 or 20 G catheter. This access is not suitable for infusion therapy in large animals as the flow rate is not high enough. Do not confuse with the auricular artery, which is located in the center of the ear! If sedation is not possible, it helps to apply EMLA cream (lidocaine/prilocaine mixture) to the puncture site and leave it to take effect for about 30 minutes.

Intraarterial access

In patients with ASA status 3–5, inhalation anaesthesia and prolonged surgery in particular, an intraarterial access should be placed for continuous invasive blood pressure measurement and regular blood gas analyses after the start of standing sedation or induction of general anaesthesia.

▶ **Facial artery and transverse facial artery** (*a. facialis* and *a. facialis transversalis*). Depending on the position of the horse, one or the other localisation is preferable. Work in a sterile manner, tape well to avoid traction on the catheter (▶ Fig. 5.7).

▶ **Dorsal metatarsal artery** (*a. metatarsalis dorsalis*). For procedures on the head, this localisation is more practical.

Intubation

The easiest way to intubate horses is blindly. For this, prepare the appropriate size endotracheal tube (average horse over 500 kg 26, 28 or 30 mm ID, very large horses 30 or 35 mm ID), lubricant, mouth gag and cuff syringe. Tying is not necessary. After induction of anaesthesia, the ETT coated with lubricant is inserted centrally into the oral cavity. Be careful not to damage the cuff on the teeth. As soon as you reach the arytenoid cartilage and feel resistance, pull the tube back a little, turn it a little and push it forward again carefully. This can be done several times. If the animal swallows, the anaesthesia should be deepened. As soon as the ETT has slid in without resistance, the correct fit must be checked: Press briefly on the thorax (controversially discussed) and feel the air flow coming out of the ETT. Then immediately inflate the cuff to prevent aspiration of possible reflux material.

Specific considerations
Coldblooded/draft horses

- Need **less anaesthetics** in mg/kg overall than warmblooded or average sized horses. They can be easily overdosed.
- **Myelomalacia** may occur after general anaesthesia. This is a rare neurological complication. The horses try to stand up in the recovery phase and then go into a dog sitting position. Pathophysiologically, congestion and axonal swel-

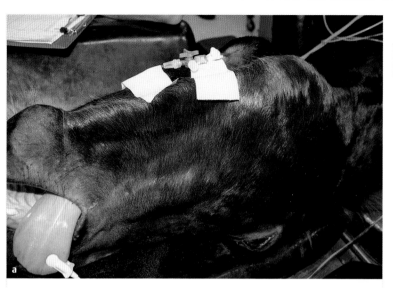

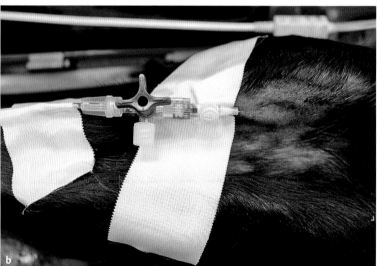

Fig. 5.7 Intraarterial access in the horse.
a Intraarterial catheter for invasive blood pressure measurement in the facial artery.
b Placed catheter with 3-way stopcock for arterial blood sampling for blood gas analysis.

ling are found in the spinal cord at the level of T16 to S1. Ischaemic neurons are found from L1 to L6.
- In case of breed predisposition, the owner should be informed of possible perianaesthetic risks.

Donkey

- Donkeys are closer to cattle than horses in terms of **behaviour**, they tend to be stoic, show pain and distress less and are more easily restrained.
- They generally seem to **metabolise drugs more quickly**, so either higher dosages or shorter application intervals must be used (e.g. ketamine).
- The **same anaesthetics** can be used as for horses.
- **Intubation** can be very difficult since the larynx has a similar angle to the trachea as in pigs. In very young animals, intubate under visualisation with a stylet.
- **Recovery phase** is usually good. Donkeys stand up in a very controlled and slow manner after remaining in sternal position for as long as necessary.

Anaesthetic-related specific reactions and features

Equine-specific effects of commonly used anaesthetics in horses (listed alphabetically). The general effects can be found in the chapter on "Drugs" (p. 63).
- **Acepromazine** (*Phenothiazine*)
  - Causes penile prolapse in rare cases, can be permanent, drug can still be used also in male horses
- **Atropine** (*Parasympatholytic agent*)
  - Should only be administered in absolutely exceptional cases, as the risk of intestinal stasis/colic increases significantly
  - Use e.g. if heart rate < 25 /min and mean arterial blood pressure < 60 mmHg and other methods/drugs have already been unsuccessful
  - One way of administration: 500 kg horse gets a total of 1 mg atropine IV slow, wait 2–3 min, if no effect another dose of 0.4 mg IV slow, again wait 2–3 min. Repeat as needed, but do not give more than 2–3 mg atropine in total
  - Do not administer at the same time as a sympathomimetic (e.g. dobutamine), the risk of arrhythmias increases
- **Butorphanol** (*Opioid, κ agonist, μ antagonist*)
  - Most commonly used opioid in horses
  - Very good sedation, especially in combination with xylazine, very good visceral analgesia

○ Only short duration of action 30–60 min, very suitable as continuous rate infusion as postoperative analgesia after colic surgery (p. 336): shorter hospital stays, lower costs

- **Diazepam** (also **Midazolam**, *benzodiazepine, central muscle relaxant*)
  ○ Administration alone causes excitement and the urge to move in the adult horse
  ○ Good for sedation of foals (< 2 weeks)
  ○ Very good as an addition to anaesthetic induction (with ketamine or thiopental) as a muscle relaxant

- **Guaifenesin 5%** (*Central muscle relaxant*)
  ○ Very nice, "soft" induction phase in combination with i. e. ketamine
  ○ Large volume, should be administered with a pressure bag IV. Relaxes the laryngeal and pharyngeal muscles, making intubation easier
  ○ Hyperosmolar solution, should not be used in a higher concentration than 5%, otherwise it causes haemolysis and vascular irritation

- **Ketamine** (*Dissociative anaesthetic*)
  ○ Should never be given alone, causes catalepsy and a dissociative state (bad dreams, hallucinations)
  ○ Good somatic analgesia, especially for muscles, skin, periosteum
  ○ Dose for induction should be considerably reduced in exhausted or very sick horses

- **Morphine** (also **Methadone**, *opioid, pure μ agonist*)
  ○ Administration alone causes excitement, urge to move and mydriasis in the adult non-painful horse
  ○ However, very good analgesic in the painful horse with hardly any side effects
  ○ Minimal effects on cardiovascular and respiratory systems
  ○ Decreases gastrointestinal motility
  ○ Tends to increase the MAC of isoflurane (i. e., you need more isoflurane to reach the same level of anaesthesia)

- **Thiopental** (*Barbiturate*)
  ○ If available, well suited for anaesthetic induction (3–6 mg/kg strictly IV) of "CNS cases" with prior good sedation
  ○ Very rapid induction, somewhat more agitated than with ketamine, only effective for a few minutes
  ○ Horses have a tendency to rear and go "over backwards" with head held high. Therefore, keep head down, support horse going down
  ○ Causes severe tissue necrosis if administered paravascularly

- **Xylazine** (also **Detomidine** or **Romifidine**, *alpha2 agonist*)
  ○ Very good sedation (analgesia also effective for a short time) before induction of anaesthesia
  ○ Horses are arousable, e.g. they can startle at loud noises. Therefore, ideally always combine with opioid

225

- Causes ataxia, in higher doses, the horse may go down
- Due to increased sweating, horses can easily become hypothermic when sedated while standing
- Decrease in gastrointestinal motility
- Diuresis (therefore place urinary catheter if necessary)
- Hyperglycaemia

5.9.2 Anaesthesia protocols

Compared to small animals, there are considerably fewer drugs and combination options available for horses. Also, adapting the protocol to certain disease states is only possible to a limited extent. Of course, the dose should always be adapted to the weight, age and condition of the patient.

Examination of the patient and ASA classification: see chapter "Preanaesthetic examination" (p. 150); "Perioperative management" (p. 152) incl. airway management, infusion therapy, administration of antibiotics, protection of the cornea and emptying of the urinary bladder; "Monitoring" (p. 39).

Sedation

Before surgical procedures in healthy horses, **acepromazine** 0.02 mg/kg IM or IV can be administered approx. 30 min beforehand to mildly relax the horse.

The actual sedation is then usually provided by IV administration of an **alpha2 agonists** in combination with an **opioid**.

Dosage

- **Xylazine** 0.4–0.6 mg/kg OR **Detomidine** 0.01 mg/kg (prolonged cardiovascular impairment) OR **Romifidine** 0.08 mg/kg IV (less ataxia) AND
- **Butorphanol** 0.01–0.02 mg/kg OR **Morphine** 0.1 mg/kg (for very painful procedures, give IV slowly) OR **Methadone** 0.1 mg/kg IV

Clinical relevance

Characteristics of deep sedation in horses
- Low hanging head with relaxed lower lip
- Half-closed eyes
- Hardly any ear movement, "drooping" ears
- Hardly any reaction to stimulus
- Wide-legged stance, partly buckling, ataxia

Induction

After the horse is well sedated, anaesthesia can be induced. As mentioned above, it should be ensured at this stage at the latest that the **mouth has been flushed out**. The protocol for induction of anaesthesia is usually based on ketamine with or without an additional muscle relaxant drug (benzodiazepine or guaifenesin).

Dosage

- **Ketamine** 2–2.2 mg/kg IV AND
- **Midazolam** 0.05–0.1 mg/kg OR **Diazepam** 0.05–0.1 mg/kg OR **Guaifenisin** 5% in a pressure bag titrated to effect (usually 30–50 mg/kg) IV

If anaesthesia needs to be deepened quickly, either **ketamine** 0.2–0.5 mg/kg or **thiopental** 0.5–1 mg/kg can be administered as bolus IV and should therefore always be available for safety reasons.

Careful!

Propofol is NOT suitable as a sole induction drug!
Propofol is not suitable for induction of anaesthesia in adult horses (and is also not licenced for horses). The induction phase is very restless and the horses literally "gallop" when they have already gone into lateral position. Another disadvantage is the large volume to be administered and the associated costs. In foals and young animals, propofol (2–8 mg/kg IV) works very well and results in a calm, controlled induction phase.

In adult horses, propofol may be used as an exception in combination with ketamine or guaifenesin for the induction of general anaesthesia after sedation.

Ideally, induction takes place in a safe environment like a padded box or a tilt table designed for this purpose.

Maintenance phase

Anaesthesia is usually maintained with an inhalation anaesthetic: **Isoflurane** MAC 1.3% (▶ Table 4.22) or **sevoflurane** MAC approximately 2.3–2.8% (▶ Table 4.38) with or without additional IV anaesthetics (e.g. ketamine or combined drips).

Only for procedures under field conditions or of short duration, a pure IV protocol is recommended.

Vienna Triple Drip
In the Vienna Anaesthesia Department, in addition to inhalation anaesthesia, a triple drip is routinely administered via an infusion pump to (cardiovascularly stable) horses. This Vienna Triple Drip consists of:
500 ml NaCl 0.9%, into which are added:
- 10 ml ketamine (100 mg/ml),
- 3 ml midazolam (5 mg/ml) and
- 12.5 ml xylazine (20 mg/ml).
Mix well and label!

Initially, **0.6 ml/kg of this mixture** are administered from the beginning using an IV infusion pump. After about 1 h, the dose can be titrated down. Physiological parameters fluctuate less, animals hypoventilate less often and are more cardiovascularly stable than with inhalation anaesthetics alone. The recovery phase appears calmer. In colic horses (p. 336), omit the xylazine from the mixture and use a **double drip**.

At the earliest 15 min after switching off the drip and inhalation anaesthesia, midazolam can be antagonised with **flumazenil** (unfortunately expensive). To do this, administer 0.01–0.02 mg/kg **very** slowly IV when the animal is already showing clear signs of recovering from anaesthesia.

Recovery phase

This phase has a higher risk for complications than average compared to other species. The lowest morbidity and mortality rate during the recovery phase seems to be observed when
- the anaesthesia time was short,
- the horse sleeps longer in the recovery box,
- the urinary bladder was emptied,
- oxygen was always given,
- minimally invasive surgery techniques were used,
- the heart rate was low during induction (good premedication?),
- the animal is not in pain, and
- the environment is quiet.

In preparation for recovery, the **congestion of the upper airways should be treated with a local vasoconstrictor**, e.g. 10–20 ml of 0.5% **phenylephrine** should be applied to each nostril. It should not be extubated until the horse swallows. Depending on the clinical routine, this can be done while the horse is still lying on its side or while it is already standing. Keeping the endotracheal tube in place until the horse is standing is also a good idea if the upper airways are blocked (e.g. gauze packs after sinus surgery). To do this, first tape the cuff balloon to the ETT and then the ETT to the lower jaw hanging out of the side of the mouth. As an alternative, **nasal tubes** can be used. At the latest when the horse starts chewing on the ETT, the cuff should be deflated and the horse extubated.

Potential complications in the recovery phase

In addition to **hypoxaemia**, **hypercapnia**, **hypotension** and **hypothermia**, the following complications may occur:

▶ **Myopathy.** Tying up syndrome. It develops when regional ischaemia due to hypotension occurs perioperatively, e.g. due to poor positioning. Signs are sweating, weakness in the hindlimbs, myoglobinuria, elevation of the laboratory values AST and CK.

▶ **Neuropathy.** Can be confused with myopathy, but is less painful. This is also caused by incorrect positioning, e.g. when bony protrusions have not been padded underneath.

▶ **Obstruction of the upper airways.** As horses are **obligate nasal breathers**, it must be ensured that the upper airways (nasal passage) are patent after extubation (by applying phenylephrine and/or placing a nasal tube). The nasal airways often become congested during anaesthesia for orthostatic reasons.

▶ **General weakness.** Preventive infusion therapy, analgesia, temperature management

▶ **Fracture.** When a fracture occurs, the tibia often seems to be affected

▶ **Other injuries.** Skin abrasions, injuries to the cornea

Field anaesthesia

In order to minimise the risk of injury to humans and animals, it must be ensured for anaesthesia under field conditions that

- the environment is safe: No fences, creeks, cars or other obstacles nearby; ideally, choose a large flat meadow,
- the staff is appropriately instructed or experienced, and
- the procedure does not take too long (ideally < 1 h).

The same conditions apply as under controlled conditions in the clinic (see above): Fasting, clinical examination, IV catheter (in lateral position in the upper jugular vein), rinsing the mouth, removing horseshoes beforehand or possibly covering them with tape and possibly administering antibiotics and analgesics preoperatively if indicated.

Protocol

Sedation (p.226) and induction (p.227) of anaesthesia are performed as under operating theatre conditions.

The difference lies in the maintenance phase of the anaesthesia. Anaesthesia is maintained exclusively with IV anaesthetics, usually **ketamine** in combination with an **alpha2 agonist** (xylazine) administered as boluses as needed or as a CRI, e.g. Vienna double drip for colic horses (p.336). The dose of the CRI must be titrated according to the depth of anaesthesia of the patient.

Management

Anaesthesia and surgical intervention in the field should be shorter than 1 h, with progression of time potential complications and problems increase.

- The horse should be secured with a halter and rope
- Work cleanly despite field conditions
- Ideally, an IV infusion should be given with a crystalloid solution of 10 ml/kg/h, which also makes it easy to flush in the anaesthetic drugs using a 3-way stopcock
- Label all syringes well to avoid confusion
- The animal should be protected from ambient temperature; a rescue blanket made of aluminium-vapourised polyester foil is very useful here (protection against cold: silver on the inside, wrap the patient up; protection against heat: silver on the outside, spread out like a sun sail)
- It is not absolutely necessary to intubate, but the option must be available. If anaesthesia time > 1 h, at least O_2 should be insufflated via the nostrils
- Monitoring is usually limited to clinical, non-apparatus monitoring; a hand-held pulse oximeter can be used

Standing sedation

For many procedures, standing sedation is a good option for the horse. Sedation avoids the disadvantages of general anaesthesia in lateral or dorsal recumbency and the risk of the horse injuring itself during recovery.

Basically, there are 3 groups of anaesthetics available:
1. Phenothiazines: Acepromazine
2. Alpha2 agonists: Xylazine, detomidine and romifidine
3. Opioids: Butorphanol (morphine, methadone – for very painful procedures)

Ketamine can be added as an additional analgesic component at a very low dose (0.4–0.8 mg/kg/h) as a continuous rate infusion. This addition seems to help particularly well in very painful procedures (e.g. burn patients).

Protocol

Dosage

- **Acepromazine** 0.02 mg/kg IV to calm down

Then after approx. 30 min beginning of the sedation:
- **Xylazine** 0.5–1 mg/kg IV (e.g. for shorter interventions) OR
  Detomidine 0.01–0.02 mg/kg IV (for longer interventions) OR
  Romifidine 0.04–0.12 mg/kg IV (apparently less ataxia)

For prolonged or painful/invasive procedures, alpha2 agonists are best combined with an opioid:

Dosage

- **Butorphanol** 0.01–0.03 mg/kg IV

With this drug combination, a stable, deep sedation is obtained that lasts 20–60 min, depending on the dose and choice of alpha2 agonist. Continuous attention should be paid to the horse's responses to stimuli and the depth of sedation/degree of ataxia and re-dosed accordingly. The dose of the repeat boluses is lower than the initial bolus.

Clinical relevance

Detomidine gel

Detomidine gel is administered sublingually and absorbed through the oral mucosa. It takes about 30 minutes for the effect to start. Depending on the dose, it causes mild to deep sedation. The duration of action is stated as 2–3 h. To continue the sedation, detomidine, xylazine or romifidine can be used.

Management

- An IV catheter should be placed before induction of prolonged sedation or painful procedures
- Ideally, an IV infusion with crystalloid solution 10 ml/kg/h should be administered
- Animals often sweat profusely and become hypothermic due to the administration of alpha2 agonists. The rectal temperature should be measured at regular intervals and passive or active temperature management should be provided (blanket, solarium, warm air blower etc.)
- The administration of alpha2 agonists leads to increased diuresis. A urinary catheter should be placed for longer procedures
- The head should be supported to prevent congestion of the nasal mucosa
- Cotton wool can be stuffed in the ears to keep acoustic stimuli low
- The oral cavity should be rinsed prior to sedation as a precaution
- Finally, it can never be ruled out that the horse may become severely ataxic, collapse and go down, despite careful titration of the sedatives. Precautions should be taken for this possible complication

5.9.3 Literature

[1] Bidwell LA, Bramlage LR, Rood WA. Equine perioperative fatalities associated with general anaesthesia at a private practice – a retrospective case series. Vet Anaesth Analg 2007; 34: 23–30

[2] Brosnan RJ, Steffey EP, Escobar A, Palazoglu M, Fiehn O. Anesthetic induction with guaifenesin and propofol in adult horses. Am J Vet Res 2011; 72: 1569–1575

[3] Goodrich LR, Clarck-Price S, Ludders J. How to attain effective and consistent sedation for standing procedures in the horse using constant rate infusion. Proceedings Am Assoc Eq Pract 2004; 50: 229–232

[4] Johnston GM, Eastment JK, Wood JLN, Taylor PM. The confidential enquiry into perioperative equine fatalities (CEPEF): mortality results of phases 1 and 2. Vet Anaesth Analg 2002; 29: 159–170

[5] Knych HK, Steffey EP, McKemie DS. Preliminary pharmacokinetics of morphine and its major metabolites following intravenous administration of four doses to horses. J Vet Pharmacol Therap 2014; 37: 374–381

[6] Matthews NS, Fielding CL, Swinebroad E. How to use a ketamine constant rate infusion in horses for analgesia. Proceedings Am Assoc Eq Pract 2004: 50: 227–228

[7] Michou J, Leece E. Sedation and analgesia in the standing horse 1. Drugs used for sedation and systemic analgesia. In Practice 2012; 34: 524–31

[8] Posner LP, Kasten JI, Kata C. Propofol with ketamine following sedation with xylazine for routine induction of general anaesthesia in horses. Vet Rec 2013; 173: 550

[9] Sellon DC, Roberts MC, Blikslager AT, Ulibarri CT. Continuous butorphanol infusion for analgesia in the postoperative colic horse. AAEP Proceedings 2002; 48: 244–246

[10] Steffey EP, Howland D Jr, Giri S et al. Enflurane, halothane, and isoflurane potency in horses. Am J Vet Res 1977; 38: 1037–9

[11] Taylor P, Coumbe K, Henson F, Scott D, Taylor A. Evaluation of standing clinical procedures in horses using detomidine combined with buprenorphine. Vet Anaesth Analg 2014; 41: 14–24

[12] Von Ritgen S, Auer U, Schramel J, Moens Y. A commercial foot pump for emergency ventilation of horses, proof-of-principle during equine field anaesthesia. Equine Vet Edu 2013; 25: 581–584

[13] Wagner AE, Mama KR, Contino EK, Ferris DJ, Kawak CE. Evaluation of sedation and analgesia in standing horses after administration of xylazine, butorphanol, and subanesthetic doses of ketamine. J Am Vet Med Assoc 2011; 238: 1629–33

5.10 Cattle

Bovines are food-producing animals and the relevant laws apply. There are few anaesthetics and analgesics approved for this species.

Many procedures are performed on this species using only local anaesthesia. Although economically indicated, this practice should be viewed critically, because although these animals are stoic and rarely show their stress, it has been repeatedly demonstrated that restraint also causes a massive stress reaction. This is relatively easy to counteract with sedation.

Cattle show very subtle signs that they are in pain and distress. It is the veterinarian's responsibility to watch for these signs very carefully so as not to miss them. Major or very painful procedures should ideally be performed under general anaesthesia. With a little knowledge of the special considerations of the "anaesthesia patient cattle", general anaesthesia can be performed without increased risk in large animal practices with appropriate anaesthetic equipment.

5.10.1 Preanaesthetic considerations

Preoperative **handling**, or the degree of difficulty in preoperative handling, depends largely on whether the animal is used to humans or is more likely to have little human contact. Cattle are generally very stoic and easy to handle. More resistant cattle can **kick in all directions**, so caution is advised. Logistics in terms of **size** and manageability need to be considered (e.g. how do I transport an anaesthetised 1000 kg bull back to its stall?). Due to their stoic behaviour, cattle are very well suited for procedures under **sedation** in combination with **local anaesthesia**.

As with all ruminants, **regurgitation** must be expected and the associated **aspiration** of stomach contents must be prevented. Complications seem to be less frequent in **right lateral position**. Bloating of the first stomach (rumen **tympany**) must be checked regularly, and a stomach tube may have to be placed after induction of anaesthesia. The animals show constant **salivation**, even during anaesthesia. The head must be positioned in such a way that saliva can flow out of the mouth (nose lower than the pharyngeal area). Due to the size of the animals, good positioning must be ensured during general anaesthesia, as **nerve damage** and **myopathy** may occur.

Clinical relevance

Perioperative rumen tympany – what should I do?
If rumen tympany is diagnosed perioperatively, 1. a stomach tube should be inserted as soon as possible and/or 2. trocarisation should be performed.

The physiological effects of the distended rumen are pain, a cranially displaced diaphragm which greatly reduces lung and respiratory volume and alters the breathing pattern. The diaphragm is mechanically impeded in its function, resulting in hypoxaemia, hypoventilation, reduced venous return to the heart and thus reduced cardiac output.

Other classical complications to be expected: Massive **respiratory depression/ hypoventilation** with **hypercapnia** and **hypoxaemia** (therefore, always give oxygen to the animal in lateral position), especially if the rumen is bulging or gassed up (due to cranial displacement of the diaphragm), **hypotension, hypertension, tachycardia**, problems with intubation (p. 236), problems with IV access (p. 235). A **blood sample** to measure basic parameters (haematology, total protein, albumin and chemistry: glucose, lactate, urea, creatinine, electrolytes, possibly liver enzymes, other parameters if suspected) should be taken and examined prior to anaesthesia.

Clinical relevance

Methane causes faulty measurements of inhalation anaesthetic concentrations
In gas analysis devices that measure absorption with low-spectrum infrared light, methane in exhaled air falsifies the values of inhalation anaesthetics (isoflurane). The values are usually displayed falsely high!

Table 5.10 Normal values cattle

Parameter (unit)	Normal values
Core body temperature (°C)	38.3–38.8
Heart rate (/min)	60–80
Respiratory rate (/min)	10–30
Haematocrit (%)	30–40
Total protein (g/dl)	6.0–8.0

General considerations

Fasting: 18–24 h food withdrawal before induction, 8–12 h water withdrawal. Do not fast any longer than this, as the animals react with severe bradycardia, sinus arrhythmia and increased cortisol levels. Do not fast nursing calves. Normal values of the most important physiologic parameters can be found in ▶ Table 5.10.

Blood volume in cattle is approx. 56 ml/kg body weight.

Anatomical and physiological features

Cattle are ruminants and therefore have a special digestive system. They have four stomachs, of which especially the rumen (up to 150 l filling volume) can have an influence on vital parameters during general anaesthesia.

IV access

For animals that are difficult to handle, it is recommended to sedate the animal for catheter placement.

▶ **Lateral auricular vein** (*v. auricularis lateralis*). Is good to catheterise with an 18 G catheter. Do not confuse with the auricular artery located centrally on the ear!

▶ **Jugular vein** (*v. jugularis*). Very large vessel, easily visible after occlusion. A local anaesthetic should be injected subcutaneously over the puncture site. The skin over the puncture site can be incised with a scalpel blade beforehand. Care must be taken to ensure that the catheter is long enough, otherwise it will slip out of the vessel with the first movement. Catheter should be well sutured to the skin.

Intubation

Adult cattle are usually intubated **blind** with **direct palpation of the larynx**. In very small or young animals, it may be possible to intubate in sternal position under visual control using a long laryngoscope blade. The technique is then similar to the procedure for intubating small ruminants (p. 241).

- Endotracheal tube size in adult animals is approximately 22–26 mm ID. Cattle have smaller tracheas than horses. Prepare lubricant, mouth gag and cuff syringe
- For intubation, there should be a depth of anaesthesia that allows manipulation in the oral cavity without defensive movement, swallowing or coughing
- Position the animal as required (preferably in sternal or right lateral recumbency) and administer O_2 at this stage if possible
- After placing the mouth gag, go deep into the oral cavity with one bare arm (no rings or watch!) and palpate the larynx. The epiglottis is pressed down. With the other hand, insert the ETT, which has been coated with lubricant, centrally into the oral cavity. Be careful not to damage the cuff on the teeth! Then use two fingers to spread the arytenoid cartilage and feed the ETT forward into the trachea
- Immediately inflate the cuff to prevent aspiration of regurgitated material
- Tying is not necessary

Respiratory function and consequently gas exchange in anaesthetised cattle is exceptionally poor. The pH and p_aO_2 decrease, while the p_aCO_2 increases. A spontaneously breathing anaesthetised bovine is generally (severely) tachypnoeic (>60 breaths/min), hypoxaemic (p_aO_2 50–60 mmHg) and hypoventilated (high p_aCO_2). For optimal management, positive pressure ventilation with 100% O_2 is almost inevitable.

  Perianaesthetic blood pressure is usually very high: MAP is around 100 mmHg, systolic arterial blood pressure is up to 170–200 mmHg. This is probably due to severe vasoconstriction. Cardiac output and tissue perfusion are reduced. For this reason, it is recommended to limit the procedure to 60–90 min if possible, but with good care and monitoring, a much longer duration of anaesthesia is certainly possible.

Specific considerations

Cattle are – depending on their temperament – **particularly sensitive to xylazine**. The dose is about ⅓ of that of horses. The dose per kg is increasing from cattle to South American camelids to horses. Whereas in other animals the administration of xylazine is initially followed by hypertension and then hypotension, in cattle hypotension occurs immediately. Aggressive (wild) cattle may require a dose similar to that of the horse. There are also breed-specific differences in sensitivity to xylazine: Brahman > Hereford > Holstein cattle (> = more sensitive than).

Thiopental may theoretically be used according to EU regulation, but there is no approved drug available. However, it is generally unsuitable in cattle as the duration of action is extremely short (< 5 min at 10 mg/kg IV). The dose would have to be increased and repeated more often, which may lead to apnoea and cardiovascular depression.

Atropine is metabolised very quickly. It is hardly useful to prevent salivation, only to reduce the water content of the saliva. Its use for this purpose is therefore discouraged.

Cattle are generally more sensitive with respect to respiratory and cardiovascular depression caused by **inhalational anaesthetics**. If possible, a balanced protocol with a decreased dose of inhalation anaesthetics should be used.

5.10.2 Anaesthesia protocols

The choice of drugs is severely limited. Any use of drugs must comply with the legally prescribed withdrawal times for milk and meat.

Examination of the patient and ASA classification: see chapter "Preanaesthetic examination" (p. 150); "Perioperative management" (p. 152) incl. airway management, infusion therapy, administration of antibiotics, protection of the cornea and emptying of the urinary bladder; "Monitoring" (p. 39).

Sedation

Sedation can be obtained with alpha2 agonists (**xylazine** or **detomidine**) or **butorphanol** or a combination of these drugs.

Xylazine has a dose-dependent effect.

Dosage

- **Xylazine** 0.02–0.05 mg/kg IM or better IV causes mild sedation, with ASA 3–4 patients rather deep sedation. Healthy animals remain standing and become manageable
- **Xylazine** 0.05–0.1 mg/kg IM or IV causes moderate to deep sedation, animal may go into sternal position

In pregnant animals, xylazine has an oxytocin-like effect. Clenbuterol can be used prophylactically for tocolysis.

When using **detomidine** instead of xylazine, a dose of 0.01 mg/kg IM or IV can be used.

To deepen the effect and add another analgesic component, **butorphanol** 0.05 mg/kg IM or IV is suitable. It should not be used without alpha2 agonists.

In wild, aggressive or painful animals, **ketamine** 0.2–1 mg/kg (as needed to deepen sedation) can also be added IM to place an IV catheter for the administration of drugs and fluids.

Induction

After good sedation, anaesthesia can be induced in sternal position. The protocol is based on ketamine. A convenient method is to connect the syringe with the induction drug to the running infusion line using a 3-way stopcock. This allows for easy titration and immediate flushing of the infusion solution into the vein.

Dosage

- **Ketamine** 2–5 mg/kg titrate until intubation is possible

The animal is preoxygenated with a mask during induction until intubation. In sternal position, intubation is performed as described above. Under field conditions for short anaesthesia without intubation, positioning should be performed as described above.

Maintenance phase

Anaesthesia is usually maintained with an **inhalation anaesthetic**.

Isoflurane MAC 1.1–1.3% (▶ Table 4.22) with or without additional IV anaesthetics (e.g. **ketamine** or **butorphanol** bolus); carrier gas should always be oxygen.

Only for procedures under field conditions or of short duration is a pure IM or IV protocol recommended. This may consist of a combination of xylazine, ketamine and butorphanol administered IM or slowly IV in a mixed syringe.

It should always be checked whether local anaesthesia (p. 413) is possible and useful. Suitable post-operative analgesics are **NSAIDs**.

> ### Careful!
>
> **No nitrous oxide in ruminants!**
> Nitrous oxide is rarely used nowadays. It is **contraindicated in all ruminants** because it diffuses very quickly into air-filled spaces (e.g. rumen) and expands them. A life-threatening rumen tympany may result.

Recovery phase

In general, the recovery phase is calm and controlled, even in large animals. While still anaesthetised, the patient should be placed in sternal recumbency and the head positioned so that saliva can drain freely. The tube should remain in place and cuffed with bite block for as long as possible. If the animal swallows, extubation can be performed with the cuff still slightly inflated to pull out saliva accumulated in the oral cavity.

5.10.3 Literature

[1] Cantalapiedra AG, Villanueva B, Pereira JL. Anaesthetic potency of isoflurane in cattle: determination of the minimum alveolar concentration. Vet Anaesth Analg 2000; 27: 22–26
[2] Klein L, Fisher N. Cardiopulmonary effects of restraint in dorsal recumbency on awake cattle. Am J Vet Res 1988; 49: 1605–1608
[3] McGuirk SM, Bednarski RM, Clayton MK. Bradycardia in cattle deprived of food. J Am Vet Med Assoc 1990; 196: 894–896
[4] Raptopoulos D. Post anaesthetic forelimb lameness in a cow. Vet Rec 1983; 112: 409
[5] Tagawa M, Okano S, Sako T, Orima H, Steffey EP. Effect of change in body position on cardiopulmonary function and plasma cortisol in cattle. J Vet Med Sci. 1994; 56: 131–134

5.11 Small ruminants: Sheep, goat

Sheep and goats (including pet animals) are food-producing animals and the relevant legislation applies. There are only a few anaesthetics and analgesics licensed for these species. In the case of sheep and goats that are anaesthetised within a laboratory setting, one does not have to limit oneself to these drugs, but can (after approval of the appropriate proposal) use any drug that one wishes. The animal remains must then be disposed of and must not enter the food chain under any circumstances.

5.11.1 Preanaesthetic considerations

Depending on the type of use of the small ruminant, the **ease of handling** varies. In general, lower dosages are sufficient in tame animals than in wild animals to obtain a comparable effect. The animal should be weighed. As in cattle, **regurgitation**, **aspiration** of stomach contents and **bloating** of the rumen (**rumen tympany**) must be expected. It may be necessary to insert a stomach tube to release gases. The animals show constant **salivation** (sheep up to 16 l in 24 h), the head should be stretched out during anaesthesia and positioned with the neck as the highest point and the tip of the mouth as the lowest point, so that saliva can flow out of the mouth easily. The administration of atropine does not reduce salivation, but only decreases the water content and thickens the saliva. To prevent **aspiration**, always intubate and cuff. Especially in lean animals with prominent bony protrusions, care should be taken to ensure soft **positioning**. The eye positioned below should be specially protected (apply **eye ointment** and close the lid).

Expected complications, especially in lateral or dorsal position, include **respiratory depression/hypoventilation** with **hypercapnia** and **hypoxaemia**, especially if the stomachs and intestines are bulging or distended. Hypoxaemia can occur simply by change of position in the awake animal. **Hypotension** (often due to vasodilation or compression of the returning vessels to the heart), **bradycardia** or **tachycardia**, **hypothermia**, major problems with intubation (p. 241), problems with IV access (p. 241). Complication rate increases with duration of anaesthesia.

Due to the way they are kept, sheep and goats often have **subclinical respiratory** or **pulmonary diseases**. It should also be remembered that they are prey animals in the wild and do not demonstrate obvious symptoms for a long time when ill. A thorough preanaesthetic examination with blood work is therefore important to detect these "hidden" pathological changes.

General considerations

Fasting: 12 to max. 18 h fasting before induction, 6–12 h water deprivation. Feed and water deprivation should (as in cattle) reduce rumen contents to reduce the risk of regurgitation, aspiration and pressure on the diaphragm. Prolonged fasting is associated with side effects. Do not fast nursing lambs and kids. Some normal values can be found in ▶ Table 5.11.

Blood volume in sheep and goats is 55–80 ml/kg body weight.

Table 5.11 Normal values sheep, goat

Parameter (unit)	Sheep	Goat
Core body temperature (°C)	38.5–39.5	38.3–39.0
Heart rate (/min)	60–80	60–80
Respiratory rate (/min)	16–30 (up to 40)	10–30 (up to 40)
Haematocrit (%)	28–39	20–38
Total protein (g/dl)	6.0–7.8	6.0–7.8

Anatomical and physiological features

Sheep and goats are ruminants with four stomachs like cattle.

In wild or resistant animals, sedation reduces stress and makes the placement of an IV catheter easier.

IV access

▶ **Lateral auricular vein** (*v. auricularis lateralis*). Not particularly large, but easy to catheterise with a 22 G catheter. Do not confuse with the auricular artery located in the centre of the ear (similar to the alpaca) (▶ Fig. 5.9)!

▶ **Jugular vein** (*v. jugularis*). Large vessel, easily visible. Use a long catheter, otherwise it will slip out of the vein at the first movement of the neck.

Intubation

- ETT size for sheep and goats is between 6–12 mm ID. However, the tube must be significantly longer than the "normal" small animal tubes
- For intubation, there should be a depth of anaesthesia that allows manipulation in the oral cavity without defensive movement or coughing
- The animal is placed in sternal position with the head extended vertically upwards; it should be continuously oxygenated
- Intubation can be very difficult due to
  - the narrow, long oral cavity that cannot be opened wide
  - the immobile tongue with the *torus linguae*, which cannot be advanced
  - the elongated soft palate, which makes it difficult to see
- There is a risk of laryngeal spasm, so lidocaine should be applied before manipulation (▶ Fig. 5.8a)
- Usually, a long flexible stylet must be used, which is first inserted into the trachea as a guide for the ETT (▶ Fig. 5.8b). The tube is then pushed over the stylet into the trachea. It is important to verify the correct fit (capnography, visual control)

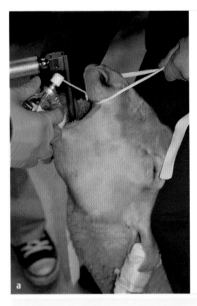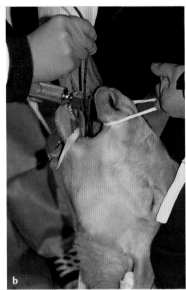

Fig. 5.8 Intubation of a sheep.
a Positioning the sheep for intubation and applying local anaesthetic.
b Insertion of a stylet into the trachea using a laryngoscope with light source.

- An infusion extension line is suitable for tying the tube behind the ears – it does not soften when the animal salivates and holds the tube securely in place
- Immediately inflate the cuff to prevent aspiration of regurgitated material

Sheep and goats prefer to breathe via the nose, i.e. spraying a locally effective vasoconstrictor into the nostrils is useful. However, they can also breathe through the mouth in case of a congested nasal passage or respiratory distress.

Specific considerations

Xylazine sensitivity in sheep

Apparently, sheep are particularly sensitive to the effects of xylazine. The typical cardiovascular (vasoconstriction, hypertension, bradycardia, 2nd degree AV block, decreased cardiac output) and respiratory side effects (initial apnoea, decrease in p_aO_2, increase in p_aCO_2) are pronounced.

Xylazine administration can lead to macrophage activation and pulmonary oedema in sheep. As in cattle, it has a similar effect to oxytocin in pregnant animals and should not be used in this case.

Goats appear to require lower doses of xylazine than sheep to obtain a comparable effect.

5.11.2 Anaesthesia protocol

Few anaesthetics are licensed for sheep and goats. Therefore, one well-established protocol is often used, regardless of the patient's ASA status.

Examination of the patient and ASA classification: see chapter "Preanaesthetic examination" (p. 150); "Perioperative management" (p. 152) incl. airway management, infusion therapy, administration of antibiotics, protection of the cornea and emptying of the urinary bladder; "Monitoring" (p. 39).

Sedation

Sedation can be induced with **alpha2 agonists** or **butorphanol** or a combination of these drugs.

Xylazine has a dose-dependent effect.

Dosage

- **Xylazine** 0.015–0.025 mg/kg IM, IV causes mild sedation. The animal remains standing and becomes manageable. Small ruminants require much lower doses than South American camelids
- **Xylazine** 0.05 mg/kg very slowly IV or 0.05–0.1 mg/kg IM (goat) or 0.1 mg/kg IV or 0.2 mg/kg IM (sheep) causes moderate to deep sedation for up to 1 h, animal goes into sternal position

To deepen the effect and add another analgesic component, **butorphanol** 0.05–0.2 mg/kg IM or IV is suitable. If used alone, sedation is weak and animals may become dysphoric.

In wild or aggressive animals, **ketamine** 0.2–1 mg/kg (as needed to deepen sedation) can also be added to place an IV catheter for permanent anaesthetic and analgesic administration after the drugs of the IM injection have taken effect.

Induction

After adequate sedation, anaesthesia can be induced in sternal position. The protocol is usually based on ketamine, but it can also be induced with propofol (be aware of legal restrictions!). A convenient method is to connect the syringe with the induction drug to the running infusion line using a 3-way stopcock. This way, it can be easily titrated and is immediately flushed into the vein with the infusion solution.

Dosage

- **Ketamine** 2–5 mg/kg OR
- **Propofol** 2–10 mg/kg, in each case titrated IV until ready for intubation

The animal is oxygenated with a mask during induction until intubation (flow-by). In sternal position, intubation is performed as described above. Under field conditions for short anaesthesia without intubation, positioning should be performed as described above.

Maintenance phase

Anaesthesia is usually maintained with an **inhalation anaesthetic**.
- **Isoflurane** MAC 1.5% (sheep) and 1.3–1.6% (goat) (▶ Table 4.22) or **sevoflurane** MAC 1.9% (sheep) and 2.3% (goat) (▶ Table 4.38) with or without
- additional IV anaesthetics (e.g. **ketamine** or **butorphanol** bolus)

Only for procedures under field conditions or of short duration is a pure IM or IV protocol recommended. This may consist of a combination of xylazine, ketamine and butorphanol administered in a mixed syringe IM or slow IV.

It should always be checked whether local anaesthesia (p.413) is possible and useful. Appropriate post-operative analgesics are **NSAIDs**.

Recovery phase

While still anaesthetised, small ruminants should be placed in sternal recumbency and the head held so that saliva can drain freely. The ETT should remain in position and cuffed for as long as possible. Make sure that the ETT is not chewed or bitten off! A bite block is recommended! The animal should not be extubated until it swallows. This reduces the risk of aspiration after active regurgitation.

5.11.3 Literature

[1] Aziz MA, Carlyle SS. Cardiovascular and respiratory effects of xylazine in sheep. Zbl Vet Med 1978; 25: 173–180

[2] Carroll GL, Hartsfield SM. General anesthetic techniques in ruminants. Vet Clin North Am Food Anim Pract 1996; 12: 627–661

[3] Coulson NM, Januszkiewicz AJ, Ripple GR. Physiological responses of sheep to two hours anaesthesia with diazepam-ketamine. Vet Rec 1991; 129: 329–332

[4] Taylor PM. Anaesthesia in sheep and goats. In Pract 1991; 13: 31–36

[5] Uggla A, Lindqvist A. Acute pulmonary oedema as an adverse reaction to the use of xylazine in sheep. Vet Rec 1983; 113: 42

5.12 South American camelids

Although South American camelids (**SAC**) are mainly kept as pets in European countries, they are food-producing animals. Legal regulations must therefore be complied with.

In the following, the anaesthesia of **llama** and **alpaca** is discussed. In general, however, these considerations also apply to other species of South American camelids.

5.12.1 Preanaesthetic considerations

Preoperative **handling** depends largely on whether the animal is a domestic animal used to humans or more likely a wild animal. Animals used to human contact tend to be stoic and easy to handle. More defensive SAC can **kick in all directions**, so caution is advised: The safest place is next to the shoulder. You should always **weigh** the animal, because the dense fur makes it easy to mis-judge the weight. As with other ruminants, **regurgitation** must be anticipated and the associated **aspiration** of stomach contents prevented. Complications are less frequent in right lateral position. It is important to check regularly for distention of the first stomach (**tympany**) and it may be necessary to insert a stomach tube. The animals show constant **salivation**, even during anaesthesia. The head must be positioned in such a way that saliva can flow out of the mouth.

Classic complications to be expected: **Respiratory depression/hypoventilation** with **hypercapnia** and **hypoxaemia**, especially if the three stomachs and bowel are distended or bloated (due to cranial displacement of the diaphragm), **hypotension** (often due to vasodilation), **bradycardia** and/or negative inotropic effect of anaesthetics, tachycardia, **hypo- or hyperthermia**, problems with intubation (p. 248), problems with IV access (p. 247) (measure baseline blood parameters if possible: Haematocrit, total protein).

During non-apparatus **monitoring**, it is interesting to note that the **palpebral reflex** is maintained even during surgical tolerance. The animals can even blink spontaneously although they are adequately anaesthetised. The mucous membranes are highly keratinised as an adaptation to a dry climate. Therefore, they often look physiologically pale and dry.

General considerations

Fasting: 12 to max. 18 h food withdrawal before induction, 6–12 h water withdrawal. Do not fast suckling young animals (Crias). Some basic normal values can be found in ▶ Table 5.12.

Blood volume in llamas and alpacas is about 65–86 ml/kg.

Anatomical and physiological features

In general, SAC are not considered ruminants, although they have three stomachs and also ruminate their food.

- SAC have very protruding, large **eyes**, which need to be protected particularly well by lots of **eye ointment** and appropriate padding so that the cornea is not injured. The palpebral reflex is maintained for a very long time
- SAC are **obligate nasal breathers**, so they need a reliable, free airway via the nasal passage. Important: After general anaesthesia, **congestion** of the **nasal airways** can easily occur; here, as in the horse, a locally vasoconstrictive drug must be given in a timely manner: Apply nasal spray, e.g. diluted phenylephrine!
- Male camels have a so-called "dulla", which is a protrusion of the trachea. This protrusion can be accidentally intubated and injured!
- The **fur** takes about 18 months to grow back. Owners should be pre-warned!

Table 5.12 Normal values llama and alpaca

Parameter (unit)	Llama	Alpaca
Core body temperature (°C)	37.5–38.9	36.4–37.8
Heart rate (/min)	60–80	60–90
Respiratory rate (/min)	10–30	10–30
Haematocrit (%)	25–45*	25–45*
Total protein (g/dl)	5.1–7.9	5.1–7.9
Glucose (mg/dl)	88–151**	88–151**

* Deviations in haematocrit give no indication of hydration status, ** about twice as high as in other ruminants

South American camelids are extremely adapted to life at high altitude. This includes the following **physiological characteristics**:

- Special shape of the **erythrocytes** (small, ellipsoid and with high haemoglobin content) and increased number
- This explains the **lower haematocrit**. However, the number of erythrocytes and the haemoglobin concentration are far higher than e.g. in horses
- High **affinity of haemoglobin** for O_2 (P50 is low), oxygen binding curve is shifted to the left
- Physiological mild to moderate **pulmonary hypertension**

IV access

▶ **Lateral auricular vein** (*v. auricularis lateralis*). Not very large, but quite easy to catheterise with a 22 G catheter. Do not confuse with the auricular artery located in the middle of the ear (▶ Fig. 5.9)! If sedation is not possible, it helps to apply EMLA cream (lidocaine/prilocaine mixture) to the puncture site and leave it to act for about 30 minutes.

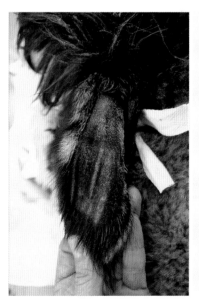

Fig. 5.9 Ear vessels in the alpaca: the vein is lateral on the ear, the artery is centrally located.

▶ **Jugular vein** (*v. jugularis*). Large vessel, but not easily visible as it lies deep next to the carotid artery. There are some **special features** to consider:

- Place the catheter in the **upper third** of the neck because otherwise the transverse processes of the vertebrae are in the way
- Place on the **right side** of the neck because the oesophagus can be accidentally punctured on the left side
- The skin is **very thick** (up to 1 cm), after local anaesthesia pre-cut with scalpel blade
- Jugular vein has **valves**, which can prevent backflow of blood when catheter is placed: If you think you are in the vein, attach syringe and aspirate!

Intubation

- Endotracheal tube size is chosen between 6–10 mm ID for alpacas and between 8–14 mm ID for llamas. The ETT should be longer than the "normal" small animal tubes
- For intubation, there should be a depth of anaesthesia that allows manipulations in the oral cavity without defensive movement or coughing
- The animal is placed in sternal position with the head extended vertically upwards, as in the sheep (▶ Fig. 5.8), the animal should be continuously pre-oxygenated
- Intubation can be very difficult due to
  - the narrow, long oral cavity that cannot be opened wide
  - the immobile tongue that cannot be pulled forward
  - the elongated soft palate that makes it difficult to see
- There is a risk of laryngeal spasm (as in the cat), so lidocaine should be applied to the arytenoid cartilages before manipulation
- It may be necessary to use a long flexible stylet. Correct positioning in the trachea should be verified (capnography, visual check)
- An infusion extension line is suitable for tying the tube behind the ears – it does not soak when the animal salivates and holds the tube securely in place
- Inflate the cuff immediately to prevent aspiration of regurgitated material

Like horses, SAC are also **obligate nasal breathers**, a free airway via the nose must always be ensured as long as the animal is not intubated.

Specific considerations

If possible, the animals should lie on their **right side** on a soft surface; the risk of regurgitation is lower then. The lower front leg should be pulled forward. The head should be positioned in a way that allows saliva to drain: Nose is the lowest point, larynx the highest, which should also be higher than the cardia.

The sensitivity of the SAC to xylazine is between that of horses and cattle, therefore, an appropriate dose is somewhere in between.

5.12.2 Anaesthesia protocols

As a rule, SAC are rewarding patients for anaesthesia, except for the difficult intubation. For short procedures IM anaesthesia can be administered, for longer procedures or in sick animals, general anaesthesia based on ketamine and inhalation anaesthetics after sedation and placement of the IV catheter is recommended.

Patient examination and ASA classification: see chapter "Preanaesthetic examination" (p. 150); "Perioperative management" (p. 152) incl. airway management, infusion therapy, administration of antibiotics, protection of the cornea and emptying of the urinary bladder; "Monitoring" (p. 39).

Sedation

Sedation can be achieved with **alpha2 agonists** or **butorphanol** or a combination of these drugs.

Xylazine or **medetomidine** IM or better IV have a dose-dependent effect.

Dosage

- **Xylazine** 0.1–0.25 mg/kg OR **Medetomidine** 0.01 mg/kg IM or IV = mild sedation, animal remains standing and becomes manageable
- **Xylazine** 0.4–0.6 mg/kg OR **Medetomidine** 0.02–0.03 mg/kg IM or IV = moderate to deep sedation, animal goes into sternal position (with support)

To deepen the effect and add another analgesic component, **butorphanol** 0.05–0.2 mg/kg IM or IV can be added. If it is used alone, the sedation is weak and the animals may become dysphoric.

In very aggressive animals, **ketamine** 0.5–2 mg/kg can also be added in order to place an IV catheter for longer procedures after the drugs of the IM injection have taken effect.

Induction

After adequate sedation, anaesthesia can be induced in sternal position. The protocol is usually based on ketamine, but it can also be induced with propofol.

Dosage

- **Ketamine** 2–5 mg/kg OR
- **Propofol** 2–10 mg/kg, in each case titrated IV until intubation is possible

The animal is preoxygenated with a mask and also supplied with oxygen through the nose during induction until intubation (flow-by). Intubation (p. 248) is performed in sternal position. Under field conditions for short anaesthesia without intubation, ideally oxygen is continuously supplied to the animal via mask.

Maintenance phase

Anaesthesia is usually maintained with an inhalation anaesthetic **isoflurane** MAC 1.1% (▶ Table 4.22) or **sevoflurane** MAC approx. 2.3% (▶ Table 4.38) with or without additional IV anaesthetics (e.g. **ketamine** or **butorphanol** bolus).

Only for procedures under field conditions or of short duration, a sole IM or IV protocol is recommended.

Practice tip

Field anaesthesia in alpacas for minor procedures

For IM or IV field anaesthesia, a combination of

- **Xylazine** 0.2–0.5 mg/kg OR **Medetomidine** 0.01–0.03 mg/kg AND
- **Ketamine** 3–8 mg/kg + / –
- **Butorphanol** 0.1–0.2 mg/kg IM or IV

is recommended.

The dose is chosen according to the temperament, size and clinical condition of the animal. IV is dosed lower than IM. Medetomidine can be antagonised with atipamezole.

It should always be checked whether local anaesthesia (p. 413) is possible and useful.

Recovery phase

In general, the recovery phase runs smoothly. While still anaesthetised, the SAC should be placed in a sternal position and the head positioned so that saliva can drain freely. The ETT should remain in position and cuffed for as long as possible. Be careful that it is not chewed or bitten off! If the animal swallows and the nasal airways have been treated with a local vasoconstrictor (phenylephrine), the animal can be extubated.

5.12.3 Literature

[1] Carroll GL, Boothe DM, Hartsfield SM, Martinez EA, Spann AC, Hernandez A. Pharmacokinetics and pharmacodynamics of butorphanol in llamas after intravenous and intramuscular administration. J Am Vet Med Assoc 2001; 219: 1263–67

[2] Fowler ME, Zinkl JG. Reference ranges for hematologic and serum biochemical values in llamas (Llama glama). Am J Vet Res 1989; 50: 2049–53

[3] Gavier D, Kittleson MD, Fowler ME, Johnson LE, Hall G, Nearenberg D. Evaluation of a combination of xylazine, ketamine, and halothane for anesthesia in llamas. Am J Vet Res 1988; 49: 2047–55

[4] Mama KR, Wagner AE, Parker DA, Hellyer PW, Gaynor JS. Determination of the minimum alveolar concentration of isoflurane in llamas. Vet Surg 1999; 28: 121–125

[5] Mama KR, Wagner AE, Steffey EP. Circulatory, respiratory and behavioral responses in isoflurane anesthetized llamas. Vet Anaesth Analg 2001; 28: 12–18

[6] Neiger-Aeschbacher G. Llamas – sedation and anesthesia. Schweiz Arch Tierheilkd 1999; 141: 307–318

[7] Reynafarje C, Faura J, Paredes A, Villavicencio D. Erythrokinetics in high-altitude-adapted animals (llama, alpaca, and vicuña). J Appl Physiol 1968; 24: 93–97

[8] Riebold TW, Kaneps AJ, Schmotzer WB. Anesthesia in the llama. Vet Surg 1989; 18: 400–404

5.13 Pig

Pigs (also pigs kept as pets, e.g. potbellied pigs) are food-producing animals and the relevant laws apply. Unfortunately, there are very few licensed anaesthetics and analgesics for this species besides various NSAIDs: in Germany and Austria, for example, only ketamine and azaperone. This and the low financial value of the individual animal severely restricts appropriate treatment.

If pigs are anaesthetised within a laboratory setting, one does not have to limit oneself to these drugs, but can (after approval of the appropriate proposal) use any drug. The deceased animals must then be disposed of and must not enter the food chain.

5.13.1 Preanaesthetic considerations

The preparations and considerations depend to a large extent on the type of use of the pig. Pigs come in **very different sizes** from the 30 kg lightweight minipig to the full-grown landrace boar weighing over 300 kg. The animal should be **weighed** if possible. The size, **use** and **behaviour/temperament** of the pig play a major role. **Manageability** and management of the animal before, during and after anaesthesia must be adapted to these factors. Piglets and small tame pigs are best taken briefly in the arm and sedated/anaesthetised intramuscularly or intravenously (lateral auricular vein). Slightly larger or less tame animals can be pressed against the wall in the pen with a board or similar. The maxillary sling works for large sows, but extreme caution should be taken with boars and wild animals – these animals can be very **dangerous**! Pigs are generally very **susceptible to stress**, a calm approach is indicated. For reasons of epidemic hygiene, pigs that are used for food production and are part of a herd may not be taken from the herd and reintroduced. It is therefore necessary to operate/**anaesthetise on site**.

Classic complications to be expected are: **Hypothermia** (no fur, large surface area, therefore measure core body temperature and warm the animal if necessary) or **malignant hyperthermia**. **Respiratory depression** with **hypercapnia** and **hypoxaemia** (therefore always give oxygen if possible and ventilate if necessary) and **hypotension**. **Intubation** can be challenging, especially in adult potbellied pigs.

For prolonged procedures, balanced electrolyte solution should be infused at about 10 ml/kg/h.

General considerations

Fasting: For 12 (there is still some food in the stomach) to 24 h (in case of gastrointestinal surgery). Edible material in the cage must be removed. Do not fast nursing piglets and do not fast older piglets for more than 3 hours. Water deprivation is not necessary, except before gastrointestinal surgery, in which case water should be removed for 4–6 h. Some normal values can be found in ▶ Table 5.13.

Blood volume in pigs is approx. 65 ml/kg.

Anatomical and physiological features

The pig is predominantly bred for food production. Anatomy and physiology are therefore not designed for physical performance. Compensatory mechanisms of the cardiovascular and respiratory systems are limited.

Table 5.13 Normal values pig

Parameter (unit)	Normal values
Core body temperature (°C)	38.3–39.0
Heart rate (/min)	70–120
Respiratory rate (/min)	20–30
Haematocrit (%)	28–47
Total protein (g/dl)	5.7–8.0

IV access

▶ **Lateral auricular vein** (*v. auricularis lateralis*). The lateral ear vein is easily accessible, even in awake, large animals. It is a relatively small vessel and not suitable for large amounts of infusion or irritating substances. Do not confuse with the central (pulsatile) auricular artery!

▶ **Cephalic vein** (*v. cephalica antebrachii*). This vein can be used for potbellied pigs that do not have "real" ears. It is difficult to see even after holding the vein off for a while. The catheter must be inserted more or less blindly. It is located cranially on the front leg, similar to the dog.

Intraarterial access

Particularly in case of long procedures (pet or experimental animal), intraarterial access for invasive blood pressure measurement is worthwhile.

▶ **Auricular artery** (*a. auricularis*). Easily accessible ear artery, it lies centrally on the ear and pulsates.

IM injection

Often the muscles of the hind legs must be spared in food-producing animals. A good access is directly behind the ears, but you have to choose a long enough cannula to get through the often relatively thick layer of fat into the muscle.

Intubation

- ETT size is usually smaller than expected and should be chosen depending on the size of the animal: Piglets up to 15 kg from 3–6 mm ID, most experimental animals at 15–25 kg about 6–7 mm ID and 10–16 mm ID for large sows or boars
- For the beginner, intubation is easiest in sternal position with a helper to hyperextend the head and hold the mouth open. In laboratory animal science, it is also popular to intubate in dorsal recumbency
- The upper airways are difficult to see because
  - the oral cavity is very narrow and tight
  - the mouth cannot be opened wide
  - the tongue is quite thick and long
  - the soft palate, which is often very long, lies in front of the epiglottis
  - pharyngeal diverticula protrude into the pharynx
  - there are two lateral ventricles into which one can accidentally intubate

- the larynx is angled downwards from the trachea and e.g. potbellied pigs and mini-pigs are often brachycephalic
- Often the long soft palate must be held up with a firm stylet to be able to see the arytenoid cartilages
- The larynx tends to spasm and tissue can be easily traumatised, be sure to spray lidocaine on the arytenoid cartilages under visualization after induction of anaesthesia (► Fig. 5.10a) and leave it to act briefly (► Fig. 5.10b)
- In small animals, the ETT can be inserted directly into the trachea after visualisation of the larynx (► Fig. 5.10c) (► Fig. 5.10d)
- In very large animals, a long soft stylet can be advanced into the trachea as a guide using the laryngoscope, the ETT is then advanced into the trachea over the stylet
- If you cannot advance the tube through the larynx, a careful rotation of the tube by up to 180° can help to overcome the angle of the larynx on its way to the trachea

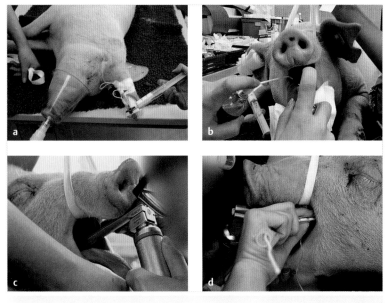

Fig. 5.10 Intubation in the pig.
a Induction of anaesthesia of an already sedated pig with oxygen administration.
b Spraying the arytenoid cartilage with lidocaine.
c Careful visualisation of the larynx.
d Advancing the endotracheal tube.

- Do not feed in too deeply, the trachea already branches relatively cranially; the tracheal bronchus is at the level of the 3rd thoracic vertebra (T3), the bifurcation is at the level of the 5th thoracic vertebra (T5)

Specific considerations

Sensitivity to anaesthetics appears to vary according to breed, e.g. potbellied pigs appear to require lower doses of some anaesthetics compared to other pig breeds. Yucatan and Yorkshire pigs seem to require higher doses.

Malignant hyperthermia

▶ **Affected breeds.** All breeds, especially those with rapid growth and large muscle mass (including Pietrain and Landrace); less affected are potbellied pigs and Duroc pigs.

▶ **What happens?** A trigger leads to continuous muscle contraction with the generation of heat. This is called hypermetabolic syndrome, in which large amounts of CO_2 and lactate are produced. If stress is already sufficient as a trigger, one speaks of **porcine stress syndrome**. Known triggers in anaesthesia are all inhalation anaesthetics (halothane, isoflurane, sevoflurane, desflurane) and non-depolarising muscle relaxants (succinylcholine). Clinical signs are hypercapnia, increase in temperature, heart and respiratory rate, as well as muscle rigidity. Animals die without treatment from severe acidosis and hyperkalaemia.

▶ **Cause.** Inherited genetic defect in the ryanidine type 1 receptor. Massive calcium release from the sarcoplasmic reticulum into the cell, resulting in prolonged muscle contraction.

▶ **Conclusion.** If trigger substances are suspected, avoid them. Possibly keep **dantrolene** on hand as a therapeutic agent (it is difficult to obtain, expensive and has a short shelf life).

Opioids

Pigs generally seem to require relatively **high doses** of opioids. Doses up to 10 times higher have been described to obtain an analgesic effect. An increase in motor activity and dysphoria can sometimes be observed. Opioids allow a dose reduction of inhalation anaesthetics (MAC reduction), but the effect seems to be rather short: e.g. morphine reduces MAC for about 60–90 min. The use of the fentanyl patch (75–100 µg/h) in potbellied pigs (50–60 kg) has been described. Mild sedation but no dysphoria was observed here.

5.13.2 Anaesthesia protocols

Unfortunately, only a few anaesthetics are approved for use in pigs as anaesthetics and various NSAIDs as analgesics.

In essence, there are three "types" of anaesthesia, depending on the use of the pig:

1. The pig as a meat producing animal as part of a herd; see "Field anaesthesia" (p. 260)
2. The hobby pig, which is treated like a pet as part of the family
3. The pig used in laboratory animal science

Examination of the patient and ASA classification: see chapter "Preanaesthetic examination" (p. 150); "Perioperative management" (p. 152) incl. airway management, infusion therapy, administration of antibiotics, protection of the cornea and emptying of the urinary bladder; "Monitoring" (p. 39).

Sedation

In unmanageable animals, sedation before induction of anaesthesia can be helpful. One option is to use lower doses of drugs than used for induction of anaesthesia. The smaller the animal, the higher the dosage should be per kg body weight; the opposite is true for large animals.

Dosage

- **Midazolam** 0.2–0.5 mg/kg IM or intranasally

In young piglets, benzodiazepines sedate quite well and very gently.

Dosage

- **Azaperone** 0.5–4 mg/kg IM

The effect of **azaperone** is very dose-dependent, at low doses (0.5–2 mg/kg) mild sedation, at higher doses more pronounced sedation with lateral recumbency (2–4 mg/kg); side effects become more likely with higher doses.

Dosage

- **Azaperone** 4 mg/kg AND
- **Midazolam** 1 mg/kg mixed in one syringe IM

Very good and gentle sedation, no analgesic effect.

Dosage

- **Ketamine** 10 mg/kg AND
- **Azaperone** 2–4 mg/kg mixed in one syringe IM

Deep sedation or light anaesthesia; when administered IV it is like a rapid induction of anaesthesia. More on this under "Field anaesthesia" (p. 260). However, there is an opinion that IV injection of azaperone is contraindicated because it can induce excitation.

Dosage

- **Ketamine** 7–10 mg/kg AND
- **Midazolam** 1 mg/kg mixed in one syringe IM, wait about 15 min

Very gentle and reliable sedation, animals are in lateral position, IV catheter and induction without resistance, stable cardiovascular parameters; especially suitable for longer procedures, otherwise possibly antagonise midazolam with **flumazenil**.

Dosage

- **Ketamine** 10 mg/kg AND
- **Medetomidine** 0.05–0.1 mg/kg mixed in one syringe IM, for further deepening of the anaesthesia
- **Butorphanol** 0.2 mg/kg can be added

Deeper sedation than the combinations above, but also more cardiovascularly challenging. Only very low doses of induction drugs are required.

Dosage

- **Tiletamine/Zolazepam** 1–3 mg/kg IM

Works well as premedication, zolazepam acts longer than tiletamine (only in pigs).

Clinical relevance

Peripheral muscle relaxants in pigs

Especially in laboratory animal science, peripheral muscle relaxants are used during general anaesthesia. In this case, it is extremely important to ensure that the animal is adequately anaesthetised and analgesics are provided, because no motor signals can indicate too light anaesthesia or pain.

Pigs seem to require higher dosages overall than other animals and these again vary from individual to individual. The duration of action appears to be shorter.

Induction

After adequate sedation, an IV catheter can be placed and anaesthesia induced.

Dosage

- **Propofol** 2–5 mg/kg IV after preoxygenation

Dosage

- **Ketamine** 2–4 mg/kg AND
- **Midazolam** 0.2 mg/kg OR **Diazepam** 0.2 mg/kg IV

Small piglets can be induced by inhalation via mask with **isoflurane** or **sevoflurane** in oxygen.

Ideally, induction is performed under controlled conditions.

Maintenance phase

Anaesthesia is usually maintained with an inhalation anaesthetic **isoflurane** MAC 1.45–1.75% (▶ Table 4.22) or **sevoflurane** MAC 1.97–2.66% (▶ Table 4.38) with or without additional IV anaesthetics (e.g. **ketamine** 0.01–0.03 mg/kg/h) or **fentanyl** (0.3–0.5 µg/kg/min).

Local blocks can be used well in pigs, e.g. incision line infiltration for Caesarean section or intravenous regional anaesthesia for claw surgery. Epidural anaesthesia is also occasionally used; the spinal cord ends at L5/L6.

Only for procedures under field conditions or of short duration is a pure IM or IV protocol used.

Clinical relevance

Characteristics of a good anaesthesia level in pigs (without the use of peripheral muscle relaxants!)
- Relaxed muscles, no jaw tone
- No reaction to triggering of the interdigital reflex
- No reaction to palpebral reflex
- Stable, normal heart and respiratory rate

Recovery phase

The most common problems in the recovery phase are **hypothermia**, **pain** and **airway management**. The animals should be placed in a warm (heat lamp), padded and dry place. If there are several animals in the herd, they should be separated so that they cannot disturb, attack or even cannibalise the recovering animal.

Analgesia should be provided before the recovery phase. For example, the following NSAIDs are available:
- **Meloxicam** 0.4 mg/kg IM every 24 h (equivalent to 2 ml for a 100 kg pig with metacam 20 mg/ml), also available as PO formulation for piglets
- **Ketoprofen** 1.5–2 mg/kg every 24 h IM, PO
- **Tramadol** can also be used in pigs: 5 mg/kg IM already before induction of anaesthesia leads to prolonged analgesia

It should be extubated as late as possible, the swallowing reflex should be present. A bite block must always be used! Sternal position facilitates ventilation and oxygenation.

Field anaesthesia

For the anaesthesia of an animal in the herd under field conditions, it must be ensured that
- the intervention does not take too long (preferably < 1 h) and
- the best possible management is performed within the scope of possibilities (in terms of space and finances)

Protocol

Often piglets up to 50 kg have to be anaesthetised because of a hernia, cryptorchidism or for diagnostic purposes (lung lavage) or adult sows for Caesarean section.

In piglets: Up to approx. 60 kg, a mixture of **ketamine** 10 mg/kg and **azaperone** 1.5 mg/kg can be injected directly IV into the lateral ear vein. This corresponds to 1 ml of ketamine (100 mg/ml) and approx. ⅓ of the volume of azaperone (40 mg/ml) per 10 kg body weight in a mixed syringe. The anaesthesia begins immediately and lasts for approx. 20–30 min. If necessary, ⅓ of the initial dose can be injected to re-dose.

For adult sows or boars: The above dose is practically **halved**. This then corresponds to approx. 5 mg/kg **ketamine** and 0.7 mg/kg **azaperone** IV.

In surgical procedures, it is essential to use local anaesthesia techniques (e.g. incision line infiltration) and to ensure postoperative analgesic care.

Management

Anaesthesia and surgery should last less than 1 h. Compensation for **hypotension**, **inadequate ventilation** and **oxygenation** gets steadily worse the longer the procedure is.
- For prolonged procedures, an IV catheter should also be placed in the lateral ear vein under field conditions and crystalloid solution infused at approx. 10 ml/kg/h (in any case in sows with Caesarean section)
- The animal should be protected from the ambient temperature, usually active warming is required
- Monitoring is usually limited to clinical, non-apparatus monitoring, a hand-held pulse oximeter can be used
- Keep the patient separated from the herd during the recovery phase

5.13.3 Literature

[1] Chum H, Pacharinsak C. Endotracheal intubation in swine. Lab Anim 2012; 41:309–311

[2] Clutton RE, Blissitt KJ, Bradley AA, Camburn MA. Comparison of three injectable anaesthetic techniques in pigs. Vet Rec 1997; 141: 140–146

[3] Lacoste L, Bouquet S, Ingrand P, Caritez JC, Carretier M, Debaene B. Intranasal midazolam in piglets: pharmacodynamics (0.2 vs 0.4 mg/kg) and pharmacokinetics (0.4 mg/kg) with bioavailability determination. Lab Anim 2000; 34: 29–35

[4] Moon PF, Smith LJ. General anesthetic techniques in swine. Vet Clin North Am Food Anim Pract 1996; 12: 663–691

[5] Pehböck D, Dietrich H, Klima G, Paal P, Lindner KH, Wenzel V. Anesthesia in swine – Optimizing a laboratory model to optimize translational research. Anaesthesist 2015; 64: 65–70

[6] Sakaguchi M, Nishimura R, Sasaki N, Ishiguro T, Tamura H, Takeuchi A. Anesthesia induced in pigs by use of a combination of medetomidine, butorphanol, and ketamine and its reversal by administration of atipamezole. Am J Vet Res 1996; 57: 529–534

6 Physiology and pathophysiology

6.1 Neonatal or paediatric patient

There is much to consider when anaesthetising the neonatal patient. The most important responsibility of the anaesthetist is to ensure that
- the oxygen supply to the tissue is maintained,
- the limited metabolism and reduced excretion of the anaesthetics are taken into account in the choice and dosage of drugs, and
- the procedure is carried out as briefly and painlessly as possible (keyword: pain memory).

Definition

Juvenile stages
The information is to be understood as a guideline, as the time specifications in the literature vary greatly in some cases.

Neonatal (newborn) animal
- Dog and cat: 0–2 weeks
- Horse: 0–7 days

Infant
- Dog and cat: 2–6 weeks
- Horse: 1–4 weeks

Adolescent animal/young animal
- Dog and cat: 6–12 weeks
- Horse: 4 weeks to 6 months

6.1.1 Physiology

The most important physiological features are summarised below:
1. **Cardiovascular system**
   - Systemic blood pressure is lower in the neonate than in the adult
   - Overall, heart rate is much higher
   - Heart can increase contractility only slightly when hypotensive, usual response is an increase in heart rate (blood pressure is heart rate dependent)
   - Body has a higher water content

- Neonatal patients respond quickly to fluid administration during hypotension, but are also less tolerant of too much infusion
- Higher vagal tone: May become severely bradycardic with vagal stimulation

2. **Respiratory system**
   - Laryngospasm is easier to induce (therefore always apply local anaesthetic, e.g. lidocaine, to the arytenoid cartilage before intubation)
   - Higher respiratory rate and higher minute ventilation
   - Reaction to hypoxia occurs in two phases: First increase in minute volume due to deeper breaths, then secondarily an increase in respiratory rate
   - Neonates are potentially able to reduce oxygen metabolism
   - Hypoxaemia and hypercapnia are weaker respiratory stimuli than in the adult animal

3. **Metabolism, excretion and more**
   - Reduced liver function – neonatal patients are generally less able to metabolise drugs, which is why anaesthetics that are metabolised via the liver (e.g. ketamine, barbiturates) have a longer duration of action
   - Very low glycogen storage! Become hypoglycaemic more quickly, especially during stress
   - Nephrogenesis is not complete until 3 weeks of age at the earliest (puppy); neonates can hardly produce concentrated urine, so fluid balance is relatively unstable
   - Thermoregulation is not yet fully developed, e.g. puppies cannot shiver to produce heat in the first days of life

6.1.2 Pharmacology

When choosing and dosing drugs, the following special considerations must be taken into account:
1. Reduced protein binding
2. Increased permeability of the blood-brain barrier
3. Higher body water content, lower fat content
4. Slower metabolism
5. Immature nervous system

6.1.3 Pre- and perioperative management

Neonates and nursing animals are generally **not fasted**, and if additional food is already being fed, they should be fasted for a maximum of a few hours. Nursing should always be allowed.

Good preparation reduces the risk of an adverse event.

- Thorough clinical examination, special attention should be paid to the cardiovascular system (dehydration? congenital heart disease?)
- Determine baseline blood values: Haematocrit, total protein, glucose
- Determine exact weight
- Correct fluid balance if necessary (infusion with balanced electrolyte solution)
- Avoid stress
- Avoid hypothermia, measure core body temperature, actively warm (possibly pre-warming)
- Place IV catheter if possible

In large animals, especially horses, the mare must be sedated (p. 226) in most cases.

6.1.4 Anaesthesia protocols

The physiological and pharmacological differences mentioned above indicate that anaesthetics have a stronger and longer effect than in the adult animal. Accordingly, the **dose must be reduced** and the dosing intervals extended.

Suitable drugs are metabolised only minimally by the liver (e.g. **inhalation anaesthetics**) or are also metabolised relatively quickly via alternative routes to the liver (e.g. **propofol**, **remifentanil**). In addition, all drugs whose effect only lasts for a relatively short time (e.g. **butorphanol**) or can be reversed by the administration of antagonists (e.g. **midazolam**) are suitable. Ideally, the drugs used also have no/very few cardiovascular or respiratory side effects.

The protocols below are examples and must be adapted to the individual patient.

Sedation

Two substance groups are used preferentially in the neonatal animal: **Opioids** and **benzodiazepines**.

Opioids, as very effective analgesics (pure and partial μ agonists such as **methadone** and **buprenorphine**) and sedatives (κ agonist/μ antagonist such as **butorphanol**), can reduce the dose of all other anaesthetics. The two main side effects, bradycardia and respiratory depression, can usually be well managed if IV access is available and the patient is intubated. The addition of **atropine** or **glycopyrrolate** can be helpful in keeping the heart rate within the normal range.

Midazolam and **diazepam** are sedative in neonates and infants, although paradoxical effects cannot be ruled out in some animals. The great advantage of benzodiazepines is that they are practically free of side effects and can be antagonised in an emergency situation.

Dosage

Premedication dog, cat, foal
- **Butorphanol** 0.2 mg/kg AND
- **Midazolam** 0.2 mg/kg mixed in one syringe IM

This combination is cardiovascularly protective and provides quite reliable sedation in the neonatal animal and infant.

Induction

If an intravenous catheter can be placed, induction of anaesthesia with **propofol**, but also **alfaxalone** or **etomidate** titrated according to effect, is possible (after premedication). If not, anaesthesia can be induced with a tight-fitting mask and inhalation anaesthetic (e.g. **sevoflurane**), but this is again associated with stress and increased morbidity/mortality for the animal and contamination of the ambient air with inhalation anaesthetic. With prior sedation, however, mask induction is again quite safe and low in stress.

The animal is preoxygenated in sternal position with a mask and also supplied with oxygen via the nose during induction until intubation.

Maintenance phase

Oxygen should be administered at all times during anaesthesia. The use of a non-rebreathing system (p. 22) helps to minimise dead space and keep breathing resistance low. **Inhalational anaesthetics** such as isoflurane (p. 102) are only minimally metabolised by the liver and are therefore particularly suitable for maintaining anaesthesia. The MAC value is lower in neonates, then higher after a few days than in adults, so it is best to dose according to effect. In order to detect and counteract complications at an early stage, extensive monitoring (p. 39) is useful.

Perioperative management largely corresponds to that of adult animals. Analgesics are often "forgotten" in young animals or only administered in insufficient doses for fear of side effects. However, because of their mild cardiovascular and respiratory side effects, the opioids **buprenorphine** and **butorphanol** in particular are well suited to control pain. The administration of **non-steroidal anti-inflammatory drugs** should be used only in slightly older juveniles when the renal and cardiovascular systems are largely mature. The perioperative use of local anaesthetics (p. 406) is always a good option. Care must be taken not to exceed the maximum dosages.

Recovery phase

A quiet, dry and warm environment is ideal. Hypothermia and stress should be avoided at all costs. A hair dryer can do a good job of warming up small young animals. Especially nursing animals should be fed again quickly to prevent hypoglycaemia.

6.1.5 Literature

[1] Mathews KA. Analgesia for the pregnant, lactating and neonatal to pediatric cat and dog. Vet Clin North Am Small Anim Pract 2008; 38: 1291–1308
[2] O'Hagan B, Pasloske K, McKinnon C, Perkins N, Whittem T. Clinical evaluation of alfaxalone as an anaesthetic agent in dogs less than 12 weeks of age. Aust Vet J 2012; 90: 346–350
[3] Milsap RL, Jusko WJ. Pharmacokinetics in the infant. Environ Health Perspect 1994; 102: 107–110
[4] Pascoe PJ, Moon PF. Peripartuent and neonatal anesthesia. Vet Clin North Am Small Anim Pract 2001; 31: 315–341
[5] Robertson SA. Sedation and general anaesthesia of the foal. Equine Vet Educ 2005; 7: 94–101
[6] Robinson EP. Anaesthesia of pediatric patients. Compend Contin Educ Pract Vet 1983; 5: 1004–1011
[7] Sokolove PE, Price DD, Okada P. The safety of etomidate for emergency rapid sequence intubation of pediatric patients. Pediatr Emerg Care 2000; 16: 18–21
[8] Tranquilli WJ, Thurmon JC. Management of anesthesia in the foal. Vet Clin North Am Equine Pract 1990; 6: 651–663

6.2 Geriatric patient

An animal that has already exceeded **more than 75% of its expected lifespan** is called geriatric. Age in and of itself is not a disease, however the number and severity of age-associated diseases are increasing. In addition, the physiology of the body changes. These characteristics must be taken into account when planning the management of anaesthesia. Mortality during anaesthesia in dogs and cats older than 12 years increases 7-fold. The risk of anaesthesia is also increased many times in geriatric horses (> 20 years old). In general, the most important goals are exactly the same as in the neonatal patient (p. 262).

6.2.1 Physiology

The most important physiological features are summarised below:

1. **Cardiovascular system**
   - Myocardium and vessel walls are less compliant, afterload is increased, which can cause hypertension
   - Catecholamine response is reduced, the system responds more slowly and to a lesser extent to hypotension
   - Increased incidence of age-related cardiovascular changes (e.g. mitral and tricuspid valve regurgitation)
   - Decreased tissue perfusion and blood flow through organs
2. **Respiratory system**
   - Increased risk of hypoxaemia and hypoventilation due to a more rigid thoracic wall and thus increased work of breathing and/or reduced lung capacity
3. **Metabolism, excretion and more**
   - Decreased metabolism of anaesthetics due to decreased liver function, possibly prolonged duration of action and increased intensity of action
   - Kidney function is reduced, therefore excretion may be delayed
   - Thermoregulation depends, among other things, on physical condition: Obese animals tend to stay warm, while anorectic animals have difficulty maintaining their own physiological body temperature

6.2.2 Pharmacology

When choosing and dosing drugs, the following considerations must be taken into account:

1. Reduced protein binding due to hypoproteinaemia (= increased free fraction of drugs and therefore increased efficacy)
2. Low body water content
3. Low or high fat content
4. Slower metabolism

6.2.3 Pre- and perioperative management

Subscribed medications should be administered according to the therapy plan (also on the morning of the anaesthesia). One exception are ACE inhibitors which should be discontinued 24 hours before anaesthesia until after recovery.

- Thorough clinical examination; special attention should be paid to the cardiovascular system

- Laboratory parameters: Complete blood count (CBC), chemistry and possibly urine analysis recommended
- Obtain accurate weight
- Correct fluid balance if necessary (infusion with balanced electrolyte solution)
- Avoid stress
- Avoid hypothermia, measure temperature, actively warm patients
- Pay particular attention to physiological positioning. Patients often suffer from chronic (orthopaedic) pain conditions
- Fasting as normal, continue to offer water

6.2.4 Anaesthesia protocols

Unfortunately, there is no "ideal" protocol for the geriatric patient. Many principles apply as with anaesthesia of the neonatal/paediatric patient (p. 262). Sedatives/anaesthetics have a stronger and longer effect in the old animal. For this reason, it is always wise to titrate drugs to effect, if possible, and to monitor the patient closely. The dose should be reduced and the dosing interval extended. It is advisable to use anaesthetics that rely little on metabolisation via the liver, whose effect is short or antagonisable and which have hardly any cardiovascular or respiratory side effects.

Often geriatric patients suffer from chronic (orthopaedic) pain conditions. This can lead to a reduction in general well-being and higher morbidity compared to the young animal. For this reason, special care must be taken to provide adequate analgesic care.

Sedation

Well-suited substance groups are **opioids** and **benzodiazepines** (midazolam, diazepam). In healthy older animals, **acepromazine**, **ketamine**, **alfaxalone** and/or **alpha2 agonists** can also be used in low doses without any problems. In large animals, the anaesthesia protocols are more or less predetermined due to the limited choice of drugs.

Midazolam and **diazepam** are generally sedating agents in geriatric or very sick small animal patients and horses. In some old dogs or cats ("who are still young in the head"), however, they have more of a dysphoria-inducing effect.

Dosage

Premedication in geriatric small animals
- **Butorphanol** 0.2 mg/kg OR **Methadone** 0.2–0.4 mg/kg (prior to painful procedures) AND
- **Midazolam** 0.2 m/kg mixed in one syringe IM or IV
- In case of bradycardia, **Atropine** 0.04 mg/kg OR **Glycopyrrolate** 0.02 mg/kg IM or very slowly and diluted IV may be given in addition

This combination is mild, cardiovascularly protective and suitable for the multimorbid patient. It reliably causes sedation in animals that are actually old or sick. If patients are not sedated with this protocol, they were not yet old or sick enough (despite old age and disease).

Induction

After placement of the IV catheter, induction of anaesthesia with **propofol** (after premedication), but also **ketamine**, **alfaxalone** or **etomidate** titrated to effect, are options. As the latter three are metabolised via the liver, a prolonged duration of action must be expected, but use in the clinically healthy patient is nevertheless acceptable. Overall, a geriatric patient requires a lower dose for anaesthetic induction compared to the young adult animal.

Ideally, the animal should be **preoxygenated** in sternal position with a mask and oxygenated during induction until intubation.

Maintenance phase

Inhalation anaesthetics are particularly suitable for maintaining anaesthesia. The **MAC value** of inhalation anaesthetics **decreases continuously with age** and is therefore best dosed according to effect: As much as necessary, as little as possible. In order to be able to recognise and counteract complications at an early stage, extensive monitoring (p. 39) is beneficial. In particular, blood pressure and temperature management as well as positioning should be performed conscientiously. Perioperative management largely corresponds to that of young adult animals.

A complete, **multimodal analgesia regime** is particularly important in chronically ill patients with painful conditions. The combination of local anaesthesia, analgesics from different substance groups in appropriate application intervals or as continuous rate infusion as well as possibly non-pharmacological pain treatments (cold, heat, physiotherapy, etc.) is ideal.

Recovery phase

Care should be taken to provide a quiet, dry, warm environment and soft bedding. Hypothermia and stress should be avoided, especially during this phase. Often geriatric patients are suffering from **dementia** and should therefore be returned to their owner and familiar environment as early as possible.

6.2.5 Literature

[1] Brodbelt DC, Blissitt KJ, Hammond RA, Neath PJ, Young LE, Pfeiffer DU, Wood JL. The risk of death: the confidential enquiry into perioperative small animal fatalities. Vet Anaesth Analg 2008; 35: 365–373

[2] Carpenter RE, Pettifer GR, Tanquilli WJ. Anesthesia for geriatric patients. Vet Clin Small Anim 2005; 35: 571–580

[3] Hosgood G, Scholl DT. Evaluation of age as a risk factor for perianesthetic morbidity and mortality in the dog. Vet Emerg Crit Care 1998; 8: 222–236

[4] Johnston GM, Eastment JK, Wood JLN, Taylor PM. The confidential enquiry into perioperative equine fatalities (CEPEF): mortality results of phases 1 and 2. Vet Anaesth Analg 2002; 29: 159–170

[5] Matthews NS. Anesthetic considerations of the older equine. Vet Clin Equine 2002; 18: 403–409

7 Case management

This chapter discusses the perianaesthetic management of patients with special needs. **Physiology** and **perioperative management** are largely **cross-species**. If not noted separately, mainly the **small animal** is discussed in detail. Often it is not so important which drugs/anaesthetics are used. However, pre- and perioperative management can be crucial and should be carried out appropriately for each condition.

7.1 Gravid patient, Caesarean section

A pregnant animal requiring a Caesarean section is (almost) always an **emergency**. If it is certain that the foetus or foetuses are already dead, management can be tailored primarily to the mother. If one or more live foetuses are still expected, management must be adapted to ensure that, if possible, both mother and offspring are safely managed through the Caesarean section. In a less urgent situation, such as an indication for a Caesarean section due to weakness in labour or exhaustion, it is worthwhile to first obtain a more comprehensive overview of the mother's condition (clinical examination including blood parameters).

7.1.1 Physiology

Some of the most important physiological **characteristics during pregnancy** and their significance in the context of anaesthesia are discussed below.

1. **Cardiovascular system**
   - Cardiac output increases by approx. 30–40%, mainly due to an increase in heart rate; avoid decreasing heart rate!
   - Especially in dorsal recumbency, compression of the gravid uterus on vessels returning to the heart can lead to massive hypotension/collapse within a very short time; in this case it is essential to change the position (of the gravid uterus)

2. **Respiratory system**
   - Increased minute ventilation with mild hyperventilation (p_aCO_2 approx. 28–32 mmHg instead of 35–45 mmHg, ▶ Table 2.3)
   - Increased work of breathing due to increased abdominal pressure. Often ventilation/oxygenation must be supported by positive pressure ventilation
   - Oxygen consumption is increased, any respiratory depression will immediately lead to hypoxaemia

3. **Gastrointestinal system**
   - Increased risk of reflux/regurgitation/vomiting due to reduced gastrointestinal motility and lower tone of the sphincter cardiae muscle; therefore intubate as soon as possible and secure the airway by inflating the cuff
4. **Blood parameter**
   - Increased plasma volume, therefore **decreased haematocrit** and lower total protein; therefore increased free fraction of drugs, which means stronger effect
   - Decreased release of fibrinolytic activators (thus inhibition of fibrinolysis)
5. **Other/anaesthesia-related**
   - Almost all anaesthetics can cross the blood-brain barrier, which means they also cross the placental barrier
   - Inhalation anaesthetics such as isoflurane are up to 40% more potent (MAC value is reduced)

Careful!

"Normal" haematocrit in pregnant animals
A pregnant animal with an apparently "normal" haematocrit is (usually) dehydrated, as haematocrit physiologically decreases during pregnancy. A venous catheter should be placed and the animal should be infused with balanced electrolyte solution.

7.1.2 Pre- and perioperative management

The most important factor in a Caesarean section is TIME!
The following applies across species:
- Work should be done quickly and (if possible) as much as possible should be prepared on the awake animal: clipping, washing and disinfecting the surgical field
- Place IV catheter and administer infusion (as required by the patient, infusion rates should be higher than in the "normal" patient, up to 30 ml/kg/h); blood pressure should be kept within the norm
- Continuous monitoring, attach equipment if possible (ECG pads or clamps, blood pressure cuff, pulse oximeter sensor, if possible)
- Administer oxygen at all times to avoid fetal hypoxia; preoxygenate (▶ Fig. 7.1)
- Ventilate perioperatively if necessary (manual or mechanical ventilation with 100% O_2)

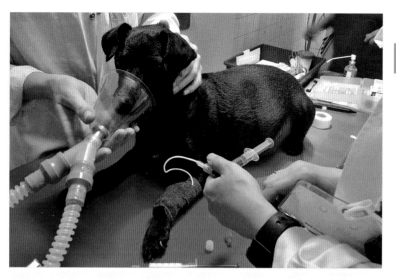

Fig. 7.1 Preoxygenation before induction of anaesthesia in the pregnant dog.

- If possible, do not allow anaesthesia to become too deep
- **Positioning**: Keep dorsal recumbency as short as possible; possibly slight lateral position or inverted Trendelenburg position (head/chest high) to avoid compression of large vessels (venous backflow) by the uterus
- Avoid hypothermia
- Continue monitoring and supportive care (especially infusion of crystalloid solutions) until full recovery from anaesthesia
- Preoperatively (if time permits) determine baseline blood parameters: Haematocrit, total protein, glucose, creatinine, electrolytes including calcium

Careful!

Avoid teat injuries!
Despite all urgency, caution is required: Teat injuries, which can easily happen especially with the cat, must be avoided!

Definition

Trendelenburg position

In the **Trendelenburg position**, the operating table is tilted so that the head, front legs and torso are positioned low and the abdomen, hips and hind legs are positioned high. This position allows viscera to fall cranially towards the diaphragm and enables a better view, especially during laparoscopic procedures.

The **reverse Trendelenburg position** relieves the diaphragm and facilitates ventilation and return of blood to the heart especially when there is increased abdominal pressure (pregnancy, gastric distention, colic, etc.).

7.1.3 Anaesthesia

In general, until the foetus(es) is/are developed, anaesthetics should be chosen that
- minimally stress the cardiovascular system and respiratory function,
- have a short duration of action,
- are antagonisable.

Once the foetus(es) is/are separated from the mother's "system", the mother can receive longer and more effective analgesic agents.

In contrast to large animals, where the "normal" protocol is usually used due to the limited choice of drugs, there are different opinions on what is the "best" anaesthetic management for a Caesarean section in **dogs** and **cats**. Among others, the protocol below has proven to work well.

Sedation

Dosage

- **Butorphanol** 0.1–0.4 mg/kg IV

- Short-acting, few cardiovascular and respiratory side effects, visceral analgesia, can be antagonised with naloxone in an emergency situation
- Do not expect true sedation
- A non-steroidal anti-inflammatory drug (NSAID) can also be administered at this time, e.g. **carprofen** 4 mg/kg IV or SC in dogs, if hydration status and blood pressure are normal

Induction

Dosage

- **Propofol** 2–8 mg/kg IV titrate to effect; as much as necessary, as little as possible

- Due to the little sedation caused by butorphanol, high doses of propofol are often necessary to induce anaesthesia
- Very short duration of effect
- Ensure a quiet environment. Always preoxygenate, intubate quickly as soon as possible and inflate cuff, positive pressure ventilation may be necessary immediately

Maintenance

- Inhalation anaesthetics (**isoflurane** or **sevoflurane**) in O_2, dose depending on depth of anaesthesia
- In addition, **local anaesthesia** of the **incision line** should be performed, e.g. with lidocaine (p. 108). Alternatively, bupivacaine (p. 76) can be used. Another option for incision line analgesia is the so-called **splash block**: The local anaesthetic is dripped onto the tissue after closure of the abdominal wall but before closure of the skin. This is to reduce the pain during the first suckling attempts and thus increase the acceptance of the puppies by the mother
- Another option is an **epidural analgesia** with e.g. lidocaine. The time lost in administering local anaesthesia must be weighed against the status of the foetus and mother and the benefit of this type of analgesia
- As soon as the foetuses are developed, a more effective analgesic should be administered to the mother e.g. **methadone** 0.2 mg/kg IV in dogs and cats

7.1.4 Postoperative management – care of the neonates

After surgery, the **mother's teats** should be cleaned with water to remove any residual soap or disinfectant. The mother should continue to be infused and warmed as needed. As the mother has often already entered surgery dehydrated, then lost a large volume (foetuses and blood loss) and will now produce milk, the **infusion volume may be increased** significantly (e.g. up to 30 ml/kg/h). A quiet, warm, soft and dry place is ideal for the mother and the puppies.

After a Caesarean section, **newborns** are often depressed and therapy is aimed at stimulating the cardiovascular and respiratory systems. The following measures have a supportive effect:

- Dry with a towel and warm so that the animals remain or become normo-thermic
- Continuous oxygenation (puppies often show bradycardia due to hypoxia, less often vagally induced, ▶ Fig. 7.2)
- Aspirate mucus from the nose and mouth
- If necessary, prepare small endotracheal tubes or large venous catheters for intubation
- Check vital signs with Doppler probe or pulse oximeter in addition to non-apparatus monitoring
- Is antagonisation possible?
- Possibly drip 50% glucose on the oral mucosa
- In case of respiratory depression despite normothermia, possibly
  - drip doxapram on the oral mucosa as a respiratory stimulant (the benefit is controversially discussed) and/or
  - stimulate the acupuncture point LG 26 in the middle between the nostrils in the philtrum

The neonates should be brought together with the mother as soon as possible under supervision and encouraged to nurse. The presence of the owner can have a calming effect.

7.1.5 Literature

[1] Bidwell LA. Anesthesia for dystocia and anesthesia of the equine neonate. Vet Clin Equine 2013; 29: 215–222
[2] Datta S, Alper MH. Anesthesia for cesarean section. Anesthesiol 1980; 53: 142–160
[3] Hay Kraus BL. Anaesthesia for cesarean section in the dog. Vet Focus 2016; 26: 24–31
[4] Kushnir Y and Epstein A. Anesthesia for the pregnant cat and dog. Isr J Vet Med 2012; 67: 19–23
[5] Palahniuk RJ, Shnider SM, Eger EI II. Pregnancy decreses the requirements of inhaled anesthetic agents. Anesthesiol 1974; 41: 82–83
[6] Shnider SM. The physiology of pregnancy. In: Annual Refresher Course Lectures. Park Ridge, IL: American Society of Anesthesiologists 1978: 1251– 1258
[7] Traas AM. Resuscitation of canine and feline neonates. Theriogenol 1980; 53: 142–160
[8] Wilson DV. Anesthesia and sedation for late-term mares. Vet Clin North Am Equine Pract 1994; 10: 219–236

II

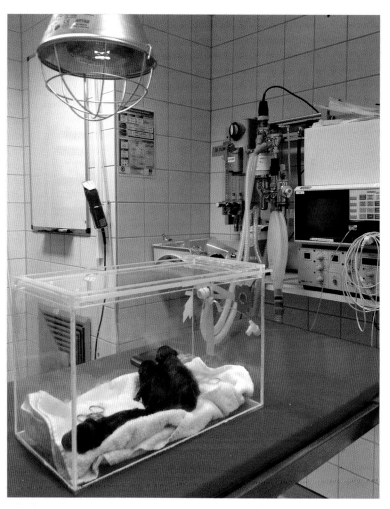

Fig. 7.2 Puppies delivered by Caesarean section shortly after birth. Until the mother wakes up, they are placed in an oxygen-enriched Plexiglas box with a heating lamp under permanent supervision.

7.2 Small animal patient with cardiac disease

Before elective surgery, an effort should be made to **stabilise** cardiac patients as much as possible. For this purpose, the diagnosis should first be established with the help of a clinical and extended cardiological examination (ECG, cardiac ultrasound), so that the appropriate supportive therapy can then be initiated. Enough time should be planned for therapeutic drugs to take effect (days to weeks, good would be at least 1–2 weeks after the start of therapy). It is of little use to start therapy today and anaesthetise the patient tomorrow. In general, before an anaesthetic, it is good to

- Reduce (congestive) oedema (diuresis)
- Maintain or improve cardiac contractility (positive inotropy)
- Reduce cardiac work (afterload reduction)
- Control cardiac arrhythmias

If the cardiac patient is well adjusted with medication, these should also be administered in the same dose on the day of the anaesthesia/surgery. The only exception are ACE inhibitors: It has been found that ACE inhibitors can make the patient severely hypotensive perioperatively. Therefore, it is recommended that ACE inhibitors be discontinued 24 h before anaesthesia and restarted postoperatively. If the oral administration in the morning only works with a treat, this is to be tolerated before anaesthesia.

The key is a balanced anaesthesia technique, administering as much as necessary and as little as possible. "Keeping everything within normal limits", good monitoring, no stress and continuous administration of oxygen are helpful. In the choice of medication there is (almost) no wrong and no right, often it is "only" a question of dose. There is no one "cardiac patient" – every patient and every disease are different and an individual regime, tailor-made for the patient, increases safety. Thinking helps!

A certain knowledge of the anatomy and physiology of the heart, circulation and lungs as well as an understanding of the terms preload and afterload is expected. The basic requirements for anaesthesia of the cardiac patient should also be met:

- IV catheter placement
- Oxygen administration
- Intubation and ventilation if needed
- Emergency drugs available
- Monitoring equipment (ECG, blood pressure, pulse oximetry, capnography, temperature)
- Knowledge of cardiopulmonary resuscitation

Definition

Vocabulary associated with the heart: What does it mean?
- **Inotropy** Influencing muscular contraction force
- **Chronotropy** Influencing heart rate
- **Dromotropy** Influencing speed of conduction
- **Bathmotropy** Influencing stimulus threshold
- **Lusitropy** Influencing relaxation (is in contrast to inotropy)
- **Preload** End diastolic wall tension, proportional to diastolic filling pressure
- **Afterload** Systolic wall tension proportional to resistance opposing systolic ejection

In any case, owners should be informed of the (increased) risk in a preanaesthetic consult, but should also be reassured that the risk will be reduced with the help of diagnostics, therapy and tailoring of the anaesthetic protocol. An overview of the cardiovascular effects of important anaesthetic agents can be found in ▶ Table 7.1.

Before any anaesthesia, the patient must be thoroughly clinically examined, with the focus on the cardiovascular (and respiratory) system.

7.2.1 Dilated cardiomyopathy (DCM) in the dog

DCM is a disease characterised by ventricular dilatation and reduced contractility. DCM is essentially idiopathic or genetic. Other diseases that can cause the same phenotype must be excluded. These include in particular congenital diseases, endogenous causes, tachycardia-induced cardiomyopathy or taurine and carnitine deficiency.

In the Doberman, a primary arrhythmogenic form of the disease has been described, which can lead to death in the course of arrhythmias before the onset of myocardial weakness.

Clinical relevance

DCM in the cat
DCM in cats used to be a relatively common disease, mainly caused by taurine deficiency. Due to the feeding of commercial diets, it has become very rare and a specific cause is usually not found. Nevertheless, the taurine level should always be measured and taurine should be substituted at a dose of 250 mg every 12 hours until the taurine level is known.

Table 7.1 Cardiovascular effects of important anaesthetic agents (in physiological doses)

Drug	Heart rate	Arrhythmia	Inotropy	Cardiac output	Vascular resistance	Arterial blood pressure
Acepromazine	↕	↕	↕	↕	↕ to ↓	↓ to ↓
Midazolam/Diazepam	↕	↕	↕	↕	↕	↕
Butorphanol	↕	↕	↕	↕	↕	↕
Buprenorphine	↕	↕	↕	↕	↕	↕
Methadone/Morphine/Fentanyl	awake ↔ anaesth ↓	↔ to ↑ (2nd degree AV-block)	↕	↕	↕	↔, with bradycardia ↓
Xylazine/Medetomidine/Dexmedetomidine	↓↓	↑	↕	↓ to ↓↓	↑ to ↑↑	first ↑ then ↔ to ↓*
Ketamine**	awake ↑ anaesth ↓	↕	↑	↑	↑	↑
Propofol	↕	↕	↓	↓	↓	↓
Thiopental	↑	↑ (bigeminy)	↓	↓	↓	↓
Alfaxalone	↑	↕	↓	↓	↓	↓
Etomidate	↕	↕	↕	↕	↕	↕
Isoflurane	↑	↕	↓	↔ to ↓	↓ to ↓↓	↓
Sevoflurane	↑	↕	↓	↔ to ↓	↓	↓

↑ = increase, ↑↑ = strong increase, ↓ = decrease, ↓↓ = strong decrease, ↔ = no or little change
* so-called biphasic effect on blood pressure
** the circulatory stimulating effect of ketamine remains mostly absent during anaesthesia

- **Systolic dysfunction** due to myocardial weakness, which is compensated by an increase in preload and therefore leads to cardiac enlargement (eccentric hypertrophy)
- **Cardiac wall** retains its thickness or becomes slightly **thinner**
- **Enlargement of the heart** leads to **secondary mitral valve regurgitation** (p. 285), which remains mild to moderate
- The disease ultimately leads to **backward** (pulmonary oedema) **or forward** (syncope) **failure**

Boxers, Doberman, Cocker Spaniels and giant breeds are predisposed, it is more likely to affect males than females and the average age is 4 to 10 years.

▶ **Anamnesis.** Weakness, weight loss, performance intolerance

▶ **Clinical symptoms.** Dyspnoea, pale mucous membranes, poor performance, loss of appetite, (congestive) lung oedema, increase in abdominal circumference, cardiac murmur

▶ **Electrocardiogram.** Ventricular and supraventricular (tachy)arrhythmias, especially atrial fibrillation

▶ **Radiography.** Cardiac enlargement, congestion symptoms

▶ **Cardiac ultrasound.** Enlargement of the left ventricle with poor systolic function, mitral valve regurgitation, left atrial enlargement

Preoperative management

As mentioned above, cardiovascular function should be stabilised in every cardiac patient before elective surgery. A general plan for anaesthesia for this condition includes:
- Improve contractility
- Reduce peripheral vascular resistance (– tendency to vasodilation)
- Keep heart rate normal to high-normal
- Treat arrhythmias
- Treat oedema/congestion

Conversely, one should therefore **avoid**:
- Drugs with a negative inotropic effect
- Vasoconstriction
- Bradycardia
- Decrease in venous return to the heart and thus stroke volume (by e.g. positive pressure ventilation or hypovolaemia)

Anaesthesia

The following protocols are examples and should be used as orientation.

Sedation

The aims of preanaesthetic sedation are stress reduction and a decrease in oxygen consumption without too much cardiovascular impairment.

For dogs that are already depressed or severely impaired by the disease (not in rather healthy animals, otherwise there will be excessive panting and thus unnecessary oxygen consumption):

Dosage

- Pure μ opioid agonist (**Morphine** OR **Methadone**) 0.2 mg/kg or higher dose IM or IV OR **Butorphanol** 0.2 mg/kg IM or IV

If animal becomes bradycardic:
- **Atropine** 0.04 mg/kg IM or slowly titrated to effect IV OR **Glycopyrrolate** 0.02 mg/kg IM or slowly titrated to effect IV

Good combination for moderately agitated animals or animals that are not yet severely affected by the disease:

Dosage

- **Butorphanol** 0.2 mg/kg AND
- **Acepromazine** 0.01–0.03 mg/kg IM or IV

Animals that would benefit from more sedation (very nervous/excited) or in aggressive/not handleable animals:

Dosage

- **Ketamine** 0.5–2 mg/kg AND
- **Midazolam** 0.2 mg/kg + /–
- **Butorphanol** 0.2 mg/kg mixed in one syringe IM

Immediately when the animal is sedated, oxygen should be administered, intravenous access established and monitoring equipment applied.

Careful!

Avoid alpha2 agonists (e.g. xylazine, medetomidine, dexmedetomidine) in dogs with DCM!
- Due to strong vasoconstriction and thus increase in afterload
- Due to drastically reduced cardiac output

Induction

In this phase, as with any sick patient, a controlled approach should be chosen with continuous monitoring and the administration of 100% oxygen. Possible protocols for induction are:

Dosage

- **Etomidate** 1.5 mg/kg or more titrated slowly IV AND
- **Midazolam** OR **Diazepam** 0.2 mg/kg IV

Dosage

- **Ketamine** 1–3 mg/kg IV, (positive ino- and chronotropy, but increases O_2 consumption; best after very good sedation at low dose) OR **Alfaxalone** 1–5 mg/kg IV AND
- **Midazolam** OR **Diazepam** 0.2 mg/kg IV

Dosage

- **Propofol** 1–3 mg/kg AND
- **Ketamine** 1–2 mg/kg + / –
- **Midazolam** OR **Diazepam** 0.2 mg/kg slowly titrated IV

> ## Careful!
>
> **Avoid in patients with DCM**
> - **Thiopental** (causes tachycardia, arrhythmias, bigeminy [p. 362])
> - **Mask induction** with **isoflurane** or **sevoflurane** (too much stress and therefore O_2 consumption)
> - **Propofol** in **high doses** (negative inotropic effect, vasodilatation causing hypotension; in low doses after good preanaesthetic sedation ok)

Maintenance

It is best to use a **balanced anaesthesia technique** with relatively high doses of opioids, as the side effects are relatively "easy" to control: careful (cardiovascularly protective) positive pressure ventilation in case of respiratory depression, administration of parasympatholytic agents (atropine/glycopyrrolate) to treat bradycardia. With fentanyl continuous rate infusion at higher doses, for example, it must be expected that a dose of atropine will have to be given every 30–45 min to control bradycardia. Inhalation anaesthetics should – if possible – only be used in low doses.

> ## Dosage
>
> - **Isoflurane** OR **Sevoflurane** low dose AND
> - **Fentanyl** CRI 0.3–0.5 µg/kg/min IV
> - For very painful procedures PLUS **Ketamine** CRI 10–30 µg/kg/min
>
> Work with **local anaesthesia** techniques if possible

Monitoring, complications and therapy

Basic monitoring should be performed continuously, with a special focus on cardiovascular parameters: ECG, pulse oximetry and blood pressure measurement, if possible, invasively. In particularly severe cases, central venous pressure measurement would be helpful to assess volume status. In general, one should check whether anaesthesia/surgery is absolutely necessary in particularly severe cases or whether stabilisation with medication is possible in terms of time.

Complications that can be **associated with DCM** are:
- **Hypotension:** Contractility and therefore stroke volume is severely limited. The myocardium has a maximum sarcomere length, which means that an increase in preload (e.g. through higher infusion rate) will only slightly increase stroke volume. Too much reduction in afterload (vasodilation) can lead to cardiovascular collapse
  - Preventive therapy can be administered by **inodilators** (pimobendan), phosphodiesterase III inhibitors (milrinone) or digoxin
  - Perioperatively, a **dobutamine continuous rate infusion** (▶ Table 8.1) can be used
  - If possible, let the patient **breathe spontaneously** (positive pressure ventilation reduces preload)
- **Arrhythmias** due to the stretching of the myocardium
  - Lidocaine to treat premature ventricular extrasystoles
  - Esmolol can reduce the ventricular rate during atrial fibrillation
- **Hypoxaemia** due to circulatory impairment and possibly congestive lung oedema
- **Cardiac failure:**
  - Furosemide (to treat pulmonary oedema)
  - ACE inhibitors
- Sudden **death**

Postoperative management

Depending on the severity of the disease, postoperative care and monitoring must be more or less intensive.

   Ideally
- **Oxygen** is administered continuously
- **Volume status** is checked and infusion rate is adjusted (at least isotonic electrolyte solution should be administered at the maintenance dose of 2–4 ml/kg/h)
- **Vital signs** such as heart rate, blood pressure and oxygenation are checked
- Continuous **ECG monitoring** is performed
- A calm and **stress-free environment** is provided

In patients with DCM, mitral valve regurgitation often occurs as well.

7.2.2 Mitral valve insufficiency in the dog

Mitral valve insufficiency is the most common cardiac disease in dogs, in which the left atrioventricular valve progressively degenerates and valve closure is no longer fully possible. This results in regurgitation into the left atrium. The dis-

285

ease can be mild, moderate or severe and in many cases leads to volume overload of the left ventricle, enlargement of the left atrium and finally pulmonary oedema. In approx. ⅓ of cases, the tricuspid valve is also affected.

The enlargement of the left atrium is caused on the one hand by the regurgitation itself, and on the other hand by a compensatory increase in preload. As a result, lung perfusion pressure increases, leading to interstitial or alveolar pulmonary oedema.

While the ventricle initially copes with the higher blood supply (Frank-Starling mechanism), chronic volume overload results in eccentric hypertrophy and a progressive deterioration of contractility (**reduced cardiac output**).

The disease is **hereditary** in Dachshunds and Cavalier King Charles Spaniels. Often small dog breeds are affected (e.g. miniature poodle, Chihuahua, Yorkshire terrier). Large breeds are less affected. In these cases, an echocardiographic differentiation from DCM is necessary. In general, older animals are affected.

▶ **Anamnesis.** Weakness, weight loss, performance intolerance, coughing

▶ **Clinical symptoms.** Shortness of breath, coughing, poor performance, loss of appetite, pulmonary oedema, (enlarged abdomen), left apical cardiac murmur, tachycardia

▶ **Electrocardiogram.** Supraventricular (tachy)arrhythmias (atrial fibrillation), ventricular arrhythmias possible

▶ **Radiography.** Enlargement of the cardiac silhouette, especially in the area of the left atrium, congestion of the pulmonary veins, interstitial or alveolar oedema, starting perihilarially

▶ **Cardiac ultrasound.** Typical thickening or prolapse of the mitral valve leaflets, insufficiency visible with colour Doppler, signs of volume overload of the ventricle and atrium. Later, clear signs of myocardial dysfunction

Preoperative management

After pharmacological stabilisation, the plan for anaesthesia is based on that of DCM (p.279). As mitral valve insufficiency has a wide range of grades of severity, it is helpful to know how far the disease has progressed and whether a (de-)compensation stage has already been reached. If decompensation has occurred, the cardiovascular system should first be appropriately decongested with afterload reduction and positive inotropy.

Anaesthesia

Sedation, induction, maintenance and postoperative management are identical to those for DCM (p. 279).

Monitoring, complications and therapy

Vital signs should be monitored continuously (already during induction).

The complications that can accompany mitral valve insufficiency are also identical to those of DCM (p. 279).

7.2.3 Persistent ductus arteriosus (PDA) in the dog

Along with pulmonary stenosis and aortic stenosis, PDA is one of the most common congenital cardiac diseases in dogs, but also occurs in cats and horses. It is a regression malformation. The foetal vitally important connection between the aorta and the pulmonary artery remains open (▶ Fig. 7.3). Usually a left-right shunt develops, i. e. blood from the systemic circulation is continuously directed into the pulmonary circulation.

Predisposed are small dog breeds like Poodle and Pomeranian, but also German Shepherd, Collie and Sheltie.

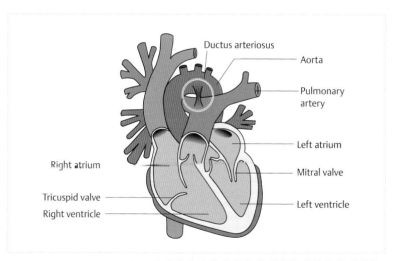

Fig. 7.3 Persistent ductus arteriosus (PDA) in a heart cross-section.

▶ **Anamnesis.** Possibly performance intolerance, often an incidental finding in young dogs. If more advanced, also pulmonary oedema and left-sided cardiac failure

▶ **Clinical symptoms.** On auscultation, a continuous loud left basal (just behind the shoulder joint) cardiac murmur (machine murmur) can be heard, chest wall buzzing

▶ **Electrocardiogram.** Often high R-wave, non-specific

▶ **Radiography.** "Over-circulation" of the lungs (pulmonary hypertension), enlargement of the cardiac silhouette, especially of the left atrium and ventricle. In the vertical image, a protrusion is often seen at 1 to 2 o'clock, which corresponds to the ductus ampulla

▶ **Cardiac ultrasound.** Depending on the haemodynamic effect, i.e. the extent of flow through the shunt vessel, the left atrium and ventricle are more or less enlarged. In the pulmonary artery, a continuous turbulent flow directed towards the transducer can be visualised. The PDA can be visualised and measured by ultrasound.

In some cases, the direction of the shunt can be reversed, i.e. a right-left shunt develops with enlargement of the right heart. This type of shunt is much more difficult to visualise and is usually treated pharmacologically (clinical signs: severe cyanosis, high haematocrit, no cardiac murmur).

Preoperative management

Therapy is the closure of the vessel under general anaesthesia either surgically via a thoracotomy or less invasively with the help of a coil or Amplatzer duct occluder, which is placed in the shunt vessel via the femoral vein or artery (*v.* or *a. femoralis*) and closes by coagulation. Often the animals are very young and compensate quite well. Therefore, special management with regard to cardiac medication prior to anaesthesia is often not necessary.

For any thoracic procedure, one must be able to ventilate the patient, preferably with a ventilator capable of positive end-expiratory pressure (PEEP). The plan for anaesthesia is

- Mild hypoventilation (controlled hypercapnia using a capnograph, target value approximately $etCO_2$ of > 45 and < 50 mmHg) causes vasoconstriction in the lungs and thereby decreases shunt fraction
- Decrease peripheral vascular resistance to avoid increasing shunt fraction

- Keep heart rate normal to high-normal (the lower the rate, the higher the outflow through the low-resistance shunt vessel); reference values (▶ Table 2.1)
- Reduce oedema/congestion

Anaesthesia

Sedation, induction, maintenance and postoperative management are identical to those used in DCM (p. 279).

Monitoring, complications and therapy

In addition to full monitoring in the cardiac patient, an attempt should be made to measure the blood pressure invasively. This will allow the typical cardiovascular signs of a PDA (low diastolic pressure) and the equally typical change in parameters after ligation (Nicoladoni-Branham sign) to be closely observed.

Definition

Nicoladoni-Branham sign

A **decrease of the heart rate** due to a sudden increase in preload and an **increase in blood pressure**, immediately after compression/occlusion of an arterio-venous fistula. In the specific case, closure of the PDA, the blood pressure increases in particular due to an increase in the extremely low diastolic pressure.

Complications that may **accompany a PDA patient** are:
- **Hypotension:** The shunt away from the systemic circulation into the pulmonary circulation creates a low diastolic pressure, which results in a low mean arterial pressure
  - Dobutamine continuous rate infusion can be used (▶ Table 8.1)
  - Before closing the PDA, the heart rate should be kept within normal or high-normal limits with atropine or glycopyrrolate
- **Hypoventilation** due to pneumothorax caused by the surgical approach: Positive pressure ventilation is necessary!
- **Hypoxaemia** due to circulatory impairment and possible congestive lung disease

Postoperative management

Depending on the patient's condition and the course of the surgery, postoperative care and monitoring must be more or less intensive. It should include

- Vital parameters such as respiratory rate, heart rate and blood pressure are checked
- Continuous ECG monitoring is performed
- Oxygen is administered, if necessary (saturation can be checked on room air with pulse oximeter)
- Infusion solutions are given
- If the patient is particularly young, it should be fed early after the procedure
- Provide good analgesia management (p. 405) (thoracotomy is severely painful)

7.2.4 Hypertrophic cardiomyopathy (HCM) in the cat

Hypertrophic cardiomyopathy (HCM) is essentially a **primary** (idiopathic, genetic) disease of the myocardium characterised by an increase in cardiac mass due to concentric hypertrophy of the left ventricle. In Ragdoll and Maine Coon cats, a mutation is known which could have an aetiological significance.

The diagnosis of HCM may only be made after ruling out diseases that can lead to **secondary** concentric hypertrophy. These include, in particular, hyperthyroidism and systemic hypertension. Acromegaly and certain cardiac tumours (lymphoma) can cause a similar phenotype, but are much less common.

Pathogenetically important factors for the progression or clinical presentation of HCM are:

- Myocardial **ischaemia** (due to hypertrophy, with subsequent fibrosis)
- Dynamic **outflow tract obstruction**
- **Diastolic dysfunction** due to ischaemia, impaired relaxation and increased stiffness of the myocardium; leading to left atrial enlargement and ultimately pulmonary oedema
- **Thromboembolism**
- **Systolic function** is regularly present in clinically ill cats, sometimes the disease ends as a so-called burnout cardiomyopathy with significant loss of contractility

Maine Coon (autosomal dominant), Norwegian Forest Cat, Persian, Ragdoll, Devon Rex and American and British Shorthair cats are predisposed. Males are more likely to be affected than females. However, most cats presented in clinics with HCM are ordinary domestic cats. In Ragdolls and Maine Coons, HCM occurs in relatively young animals.

▶ **Anamnesis.** Dyspnoea, tachypnoea, weight loss, exercise intolerance (often difficult to assess)

▶ **Clinical symptoms.** Often only noticeable at a late stage of the disease: Dyspnoea, tachypnoea, cyanosis, open mouth breathing, increased need for rest, arrhythmias, often gallop rhythm, not necessarily cardiac murmur

▶ **Electrocardiogram.** Tachycardia, ventricular or supraventricular arrhythmias (atrial fibrillation or fibrillation)

▶ **Radiography.** Enlargement of the cardiac silhouette, left atrial enlargement (less easily recognised than in dogs!). Normal radiographic findings do not exclude HCM! Pulmonary oedema, pleural effusion, dilatation of the pulmonary vessels and caudal vena cava

▶ **Cardiac ultrasound.** Concentric hypertrophy, especially of the left ventricle without dilatation, in severe cases enlargement of the left atrium. Evidence of diastolic dysfunction by Doppler, possibly dynamic left ventricular outflow tract obstruction (DLVOTO) and systolic anterior motion (SAM) of the anterior mitral valve leaflet.

Preoperative management

As mentioned above, one should cardiovascularly **stabilise** any cardiac patient before elective surgery. Plan for anaesthesia for this condition includes:
• No stress!
• Maintenance of stroke volume
• Keep contractility rather low (possibly administer β receptor blockers)
• Keep heart rate normal to low-normal
• Keep peripheral vascular resistance normal to high-normal (= tendency to vasoconstriction)
• Control arrhythmias
• Avoid (diastolic) hypotension because coronary perfusion pressure is directly dependent on it

In any case, it should be assessed whether there is an underlying primary disease. This should be treated first (e.g. by measuring blood pressure: in primary HCM there is often hypotension, in secondary HCM hypertension).

Good to know

Myocardium is perfused during diastole!
During systole, the coronary arteries are mostly compressed. During diastole, when the pressure on these vessels decreases, the heart muscle can again be supplied with oxygen and glucose and waste products can be removed. A thickened, hypercontractile myocardium requires more oxygen, has compressed coronary arteries and holds a lower volume than a physiological myocardium. Therefore, it is extremely important to allow enough time for the ventricles to fill (= diastole) and oxygen to be available. At very high heart rates, myocardial perfusion can become critically too low.

Anaesthesia

The protocols in the following are examples and serve as orientation. As a general rule, one should rather **avoid** acepromazine (vasodilation), ketamine in high doses (positive inotropy, increases the risk of outflow tract obstruction), thiopental (arrhythmias), high doses of atropine/glycopyrrolate (tachycardia), mask induction with isoflurane or sevoflurane (too much stress), and propofol without premedication (vasodilation, apnoea).

Sedation

The goals of preanaesthetic sedation are stress reduction, maintenance of (myocardial) perfusion and oxygen supply, and normotension. Good premedication, gentle handling of the animal and oxygen provided whenever possible greatly help to achieve these goals.

In cats severely compromised by the disease:

Dosage

- Pure μ opioid agonist (**Morphine** OR **Methadone**) 0.2 mg/kg or higher dose OR **Butorphanol** 0.2 mg/kg or slightly higher dose IM or IV; mild bradycardia can be allowed
- **Midazolam** 0.2 mg/kg IM or IV may be added for nervous animals

Animals that would benefit from more sedation (very nervous/excited) or in aggressive/not treatable animals:

Dosage

- **Butorphanol** 0.2 mg/kg AND
- **Medetomidine** OR **Dexmedetomidine** mixed in one syringe in lowest dosage 2– max. 10 µg/kg OR 1– max. 5 µg/kg IM, respectively (to avoid struggling with the animal when placing the catheter, costs too much oxygen)

For highly aggressive cats the following is recommended:

Dosage

- **Alfaxalone** 1–3 mg/kg AND
- **Medetomidine** 2–10 µg/kg OR **Dexmedetomidine** 1–5 µg/kg mixed in one syringe IM
- **Butorphanol** 0.2 mg/kg can be added to provide an additional sedative and analgesic component

For sick, severely compromised but aggressive cats, or cats with unknown health status, you can use this very gentle but effective protocol:

Dosage

- **Alfaxalone** 1–3 mg/kg (limiting factor is volume) AND
- **Midazolam** 0.1–0.2 mg/kg AND
- **Butorphanol** 0.1–0.2 mg/kg mixed in one syringe IM or slowly titrated IV

Immediately when the animal is sedated, oxygen should be administered, intravenous access established and monitoring equipment applied.

Induction

At this stage, as with any sick patient, vital signs should already be monitored, an IV catheter should be in place and oxygen should be administered.

Dosage

- **Etomidate** 1.5–3 mg/kg slowly titrated IV AND
- **Midazolam** OR **Diazepam** 0.2 mg/kg IV

After proper sedation:

Dosage

- **Propofol** 1–2 (up to 4 or more) mg/kg IV OR **Alfaxalone** 3–5 mg/kg IV AND
- **Midazolam** OR **Diazepam** 0.2 mg/kg IV (if not already administered as part of premedication)

Titrate everything slowly to effect.

In case of already severely depressed animals and a painful procedure is also possible:

Dosage

- **Fentanyl** 2–5 (up to 10) µg/kg AND
- **Midazolam** OR **Diazepam** 0.2 mg/kg IV
- Then immediately start the continuous rate infusion of **Fentanyl** at 0.3–0.5 µg/kg/min and (after intubation) **inhalation anaesthetics** in 100% oxygen

Maintenance

It is best to use a balanced anaesthesia technique with inhalational anaesthetics and opioids on top of good sedation. Severe bradycardia should be avoided, as should tachycardia. Inhalational anaesthetics should be used only in low doses if possible.

Dosage

- **Isoflurane** OR **Sevoflurane** low dose in O_2 AND
- **Fentanyl** continuous rate infusion 0.3–0.5 µg/kg/min IV

Work with **local anaesthesia** if possible.

If indicated, dex-/medetomidine may be partially or fully antagonised (atipamezole IM).

Monitoring, complications and therapy

Basic parameters should be monitored continuously, with particular attention to cardiovascular parameters: ECG, pulse oximetry and blood pressure measurement, invasively if possible. Cats with HCM show a particular bifid waveform on arterial blood pressure measurement: steep rise with systole, mid-systolic fall and then late systolic rise again.

Complications that can **accompany HCM** are:
- **Hypotension:** Filling of the ventricle and therefore stroke volume are severely limited
  - Perioperatively, blood pressure (heart rate normal to low-normal) should be maintained by vasoconstriction (▶ Table 8.1)
- **Arrhythmias** reduce the atrial kick, meaning the help of the atrium to fill the ventricle, which is critically important in this disease
  - Beta-blockade, e.g. with esmolol CRI
  - Calcium channel blocker, e.g. diltiazem
- **Hypoxaemia** due to circulatory impairment and possibly congested lung
  - Oxygen
  - Ventilation if indicated
  - Diuretics, e.g. furosemide if indicated
- Sudden **death**

Postoperative management

Depending on the severity of the disease, postoperative care and monitoring must be more or less intensive.

Ideally
- Oxygen is administered continuously
- Volume status is checked and adjusted
- Vital signs such as heart rate and blood pressure and oxygenation are checked
- Continuous ECG monitoring is carried out
- A calm and low-stress environment is provided
- Sufficient analgesics are administered; NSAIDs and opioids have (almost) no cardiovascularly relevant side effects in the awake animal

7.2.5 Literature

[1] Bednarski RM. Anesthetic concerns for patients with cardiomyopathy. Vet Clin North Am Small Anim Pract 1992; 22: 460–465

[2] Clutton E. Cardiovascular disease. In: BSAVA manual of canine and feline anaesthesia and analgesia. 2nd ed. Seymore C, Duke-Nowakovski T. Gloucester: BSAVA 2007; 200–219

[3] Eberspächer E, Baumgartner C, Henke J, Erhardt W. Invasive Blutdruckmessung nach intramuskulärer Verabreichung von Acepromazin als Narkoseprämedikation beim Hund. Tierärztl Prax (K) 2005; 33: 27–31

[4] Evans AT. Anesthesia for severe mitral and tricuspid regurgitation. Vet Clin North Am Small Anim Pract 1992; 47: 631–635

[5] Fayyaz S, Kerr CL, Dyson DH, Mirakhur KK. Cardio-pulmonary effects of anesthetic induction with isoflurane, ketamine-diazepam or propofol-diazepam in the hypovolemic dog. Vet Anaesth Analg 2009; 36: 110–123

[6] Fox PR, Sisson D, Moise NS. International small animal cardiac health council 1999: recommendations for diagnosis of heart disease and treatment of heart failure in small animals. In: Textbook of canine and feline cardiology. 2nd ed. Fox PR, Sisson D, Moise NS. Philadelphia: Saunders 1999; Appendix A

[7] Gelissen HP, Epema A, Henning RH, Krijnen HJ, Hennis PJ, Den Hertog A. Inotropic effects of propofol, thiopental, midazolam, etomidate, and ketamine on isolated human atrial muscle. Anesthesiol 1996; 84: 397–403

[8] Harvey RC, Ettinger SJ. Cardiovascular disease. In: Lumb and Jones' Veterinary anesthesia and analgesia. 4th ed. Tranquilli WJ, Thurmon JC, Grimm KA. Ames: Blackwell Publishing 2007; 891–898

[9] Haskins SC, Patz JD, Farver TB. Xylazine and xylazine-ketamine in dogs. Am J Vet Res 1986; 47: 636–641

[10] Ilkiw JE, Pascoe PJ, Haskins SC, Patz JD. Cardiovascular and respiratory effects of propofol administration in hypovolemic dogs. Am J Vet Res 1992; 52: 2323–2327

[11] Jones DJ, Stehling LC, Zauder HL. Cardiovascular responses to diazepam and midazolam maleate in the dog. Anesthesiol 1979; 51: 430–434

[12] Keene BW, Atkins CE, Bonagura JD, Fox PR, Häggström J, Fuentes VL, Oyama MA, Rush JE, Stepien R, Uechi M. ACVIM consensus guidelines for the diagnosis and treatment of myxomatous mitral valve disease in dogs. J Vet Intern Med. 2019; 33: 1127–1140

[13] Klide AM. Cardiopulmonary effects of enflurane and isoflurane in the dog. Am J Vet Res 1976; 37: 127–131

[14] Klide AM, Calderwood HW, Soma LR. Cardiopulmonary effects of xylazine in dogs. Am J Vet Res 1975; 36: 931–935

[15] Kuusela E, Vainio O, Short CE, Leppäluoto J, Huttunen P, Ström S, Huju V, Valtonen A, Raekallio M. A comparison of propofol infusion and propofol/isofluran anesthesia in dexmedetomidine premedicated dogs. J Vet Pharmacol Therapeut 2003; 26: 199–204

[16] Martinez EA, Hartsfield SM, Melendez LP, Matthews NS, Slater MR. Cardiovascular effects of buprenorphine in anesthetized dogs. Am J Vet Res 1997; 58: 1280–1284

[17] Muir W, Lerche P, Wiese A, Nelson L, Pasloske K, Whittem T. The cardiorespiratory and anesthetic effects of clinical and supraclinical doses of alfaxalone in cats. Vet Anaesth Analg 2009; 36: 42–54

[18] Muzi M, Berens RA, Kampine JP, Ebert TJ. Venodilation contributes to propofol-mediated hypotension in humans. Anesth Analg 1992; 74: 877–883

[19] Pascoe PJ. Anaesthesia for patients with cardiovascular disease. Proc AVA Spring meeting, Rimini, Italien 2005; 32–41

[20] Poliac LC, Barron ME, Maron BJ. Hypertrophic cardiomyopathy. Anesthesiol 2006; 104: 183–192

[21] Pypendop B, Verstegen J. Hemodynamic effects of medetomidine in the dog: a dose titration study. Vet Surg 1998; 27: 612–622

[22] Rivenes SM, Lewin MB, Stayer SA, Bent ST, Schoenig HM, McKenzie ED, Fraser CD, Andropoulos DB. Cardiovascular effects of sevoflurane, isoflurane, halothane, and fentanyl-midazolam in children with congenital heart disease: An echocardiographic study of myocardial contractility and hemodynamics. Anesthesiol 2001; 94: 223–229

[23] Robertson S. Advantages of etomidate use as an anesthetic agent. Vet Clin North Am Small Anim Pract 1992; 22: 277–280

[24] Savola JM. Cardiovascular actions of medetomidine and their reversal by atipamezole. Acta Vet Scand Suppl 1989; 85: 39–47

[25] Skarda RT, Bednarski RM, Muir WW, Hubbel JAE, Mason DE. Sedation und Narkose bei Hund und Katze mit Herzkreislaufkrankheit 1. Teil: Narkoseplanung nach Risikobeurteilung, hämodynamische Wirkung der Pharmaka, Monitoring. Schweiz Arch Tierheilk 1995; 137: 312–321

[26] Skarda RT, Muir WW, Bednarski RM, Hubbel JAE, Mason DE. Sedation und Narkose bei Hund und Katze mit Herzkreislaufkrankheit 2. Teil: Narkoseplanung an Hand der Pathophysiologie, Herzarrhythmien. Schweiz Arch Tierheilk 1995; 137: 543–551

[27] Skarda RT, Hubbel JAE, Muir WW, Bednarski RM, Mason DE. Sedation und Narkose bei Hund und Katze mit Herzkreislaufkrankheit 3. Teil: Ventilation, Überwachung der Atmung, postoperative Schmerzbehandlung. Schweiz Arch Tierheilk 1996; 138: 312–318

[28] Steinbacher R und Dörfelt R. Übersichtsarbeit: Anästhesie bei Hunden und Katzen mit Herzerkrankung – ein unmögliches Unterfangen oder eine Herausforderung mit überschaubarem Risiko? Wien Tierärztl Mschr 2012; 99: 27–43

[29] Tidholm A. Retrospective study of congenital heart defects in 151 dogs. J Small Anim Pract 1997; 38: 94–98

7.3 Interventions in and around the eyes

Eye/head surgery is a particular challenge for the anaesthetist. **Non-apparatus monitoring** is **limited** because the head is occupied by the surgeon. The **oculo-cardiac reflex** can trigger cardiac arrest. Adrenergic drugs injected into the ocular chamber can elevate blood pressure and heart rate. Good management and continuous monitoring of vital signs can be life-saving! This also applies to other operations on the head, such as dental cleanings or extractions, where the head often has to be held relatively firmly and therefore pressure is also exerted on the eye.

The aim is to sedate (large animals) or anaesthetise the patient in such a way that the following criteria are met:

• A quiet, fixed eye without blinking
• No unexpected movements by the patient
• Reduction of intraocular pressure (IOP) or prevention of pressure fluctuations due to e.g. gagging, coughing, vomiting
• Minimised risk of triggering the oculo-cardiac reflex
• Calm anaesthesia induction and recovery phase
• Postoperative analgesia and protection of the operated eye

Careful!

Oculo-cardiac reflex

The oculo-cardiac reflex is triggered by traction or pressure on the eye. Transmission via the trigeminal (afferent) and vagus (efferent) nerves results in bradycardia, hypotension, deep breathing and nausea. Bradycardia is extremely pronounced and seems to be observed more often in young animals (due to the higher vagal tone). In small and large animals (horses), cardiac arrest has been described as a consequence. This complication during eye surgery should therefore be taken very seriously!

If the reflex is triggered:

1. Immediately **stop** any **manipulation** of the eye!
2. Administer **atropine** (dog/cat: 0.02–0.04 mg/kg) IV OR
3. Administer **glycopyrrolate** (dog/cat: 0.01–0.02 mg/kg) IV

Caution with horses: Risk of colic (p. 336) with administration of parasympatholytic agents!

7.3.1 Preoperative management

To facilitate unrestricted access, the intravenous catheter can be placed in the hindlimb. For safety, the dosages of emergency drugs (atropine, adrenalin) should be individually calculated for the patient and the drugs should be ready. For enucleations, a retrobulbar or peribulbar block (p. 424) should be considered as a local anaesthesia technique.

7.3.2 Anaesthesia

If an increase in IOP would worsen the pathology, drugs that might increase IOP (e.g. ketamine) should be avoided. Rather, sedatives (midazolam, diazepam) and anaesthetics (propofol, etomidate, thiopental) that **lower IOP** should be used. Bradycardia (opioids, alpha2 agonists) should be avoided or treated before the start of the procedure. This does not mean that these drugs must not be used! The anaesthetist should only be aware that there is a risk of the oculo-cardiac reflex and that this could have a more fatal effect if the heart rate is already low at the beginning of the procedure.

Maintenance and perioperative analgesia

Maintenance of anaesthesia is usually performed with inhalation anaesthetics.

For analgesia, local anaesthesia is an option in addition to systemic administration of opioids and NSAIDs (if not contraindicated). Possible options are, for example, local anaesthetics (0.4% eye drops, active substance **oxybuprocaine**, duration of action 10–15 min) or, in case of surgery on the eyelid, tissue infiltration, e.g. with **lidocaine** 2%, around the surgical site but still at a distance.

II

Practice tip

Use of peripheral muscle relaxants

Peripheral muscle relaxants can be used to position the eye in a central position for procedures on the eye. It should be noted that all striated muscles are relaxed in a dose-dependent manner, including the respiratory muscles. Manual or mechanical ventilation of the patient is therefore essential. The depth of anaesthesia is no longer easy to assess.

When using e.g. **rocuronium** (dose dog/cat/horse 0.3–0.6 mg/kg slow IV) you get approx. 30 min muscle relaxation and a central globe position. Follow up with half the dose IV. Ventilation, blood pressure and heart rate must be monitored. In the recovery phase, oxygen should still be administered by mask to prevent possible hypoxaemia due to a residual block (= remaining muscle relaxation).

With the help of a nerve stimulator (TOF-guard), the neuromuscular blockade can be reliably and objectively monitored.

7.3.3 Postoperative management

Every "eye patient" should wear some kind of scratch protection (e.g. E-collar) early in the recovery phase to prevent scratching or rubbing the operated eye. Postoperative analgesia must be ensured, e.g. with NSAIDs (if not contraindicated) or opioids, depending on the type and degree of pain of the procedure.

7.3.4 Literature

[1] Loan PB, Paxton LD, Mirakhur RK, Connolly FM, McCoy EP. The TOF-Guard neuromuscular transmission monitor – A comparison with the Myograph 2000. Anaesthesia 1995; 50: 699–702

[2] Vann MA, Ogunnaike BO, Joshi GP. Sedation and anesthesia care for ophthalmologic surgery during local/regional anesthesia. Anesthesiol 2007; 107: 502–508

7.4 Dental and maxillofacial surgery procedures

Dental problems are among the most common reasons for presentation to the veterinarian in small animals. This fact is probably one of the contributing factors responsible for dental surgery being the third most common cause of mortality during anaesthesia (after exploratory laparotomy and laparotomy for pyometra). The reasons cited for the comparatively high mortality rate are

- Patients are mostly geriatric which can compensate less well
- There is a correlation between dental disease (periodontal disease burden) and systemic diseases, such as mitral valve insufficiency or pathologies of the liver or kidney
- Due to different stimuli, the depth of anaesthesia varies greatly (if local anaesthesia is not used)
- There is a risk of airway injury from the cuffed endotracheal tube due to manipulation of the head
- There is a higher risk of aspiration (and pneumonia)
- While dental procedures in large animals can often be performed under sedation, dogs and cats must be anaesthetised and intubated to ensure a full examination, further diagnosis and treatment within the oral cavity. This must be clearly communicated to the pet owner
- Risk of triggering the oculo-cardiac reflex

7.4.1 Preoperative management

In these patients, too, the **intravenous catheter** should be placed in the **hindlimb** to facilitate access on the one hand and to prevent contamination due to proximity to the oral cavity on the other. As mentioned, these are often geriatric patients (p. 267) who need to be cared for appropriately. In any case (and especially in the case of long procedures), the following aspects should be taken into account

- Comfortable, tension- and pressure-free positioning, soft bedding
- Active temperature management, maintaining normothermia
- Infusion management, maintain normovolaemia
- Protection of the cornea, apply eye ointment generously and repeatedly
- Mouth gags (especially those with strong springs or screw threads) should not be used continuously. Cerebral ischaemia and blindness may occur in the cat. If the use is unavoidable, e.g. in small mammals, then use as short as possible and with little force

During dental surgery, hyperaemia in the surgical area causes **bacteraemia** that lasts for several hours. For this reason, no other "sterile" surgery such as castration should be performed in the same anaesthesia period. Nevertheless, antibiotics are generally not indicated unless the patient suffers from e.g. a severe infection of the oral cavity or a systemic or recurrent disease. What helps in any case is **rinsing the oral cavity** with antiseptic-acting **chlorhexidine** 0.12% before and after dental cleaning.

Non-apparatus monitoring on the head is also **limited** in these patients. The sensor for the pulse oximeter should, if possible, not be attached to the tongue but at alternative places (needs to be re-attached constantly, causes frustration on both sides). Temperature should be taken rectally. The monitoring of vital signs should be complete and continuous, as the oculo-cardiac reflex (p. 297) can also be triggered in these patients.

Airway protection and protection against aspiration must be taken particularly seriously in these patients. The following measures can help:

- Position the head so that the tip of the nose is low and the larynx is at the highest point
- Intubation with a suitable endotracheal tube (p. 153)
- Proper inflation of the cuff

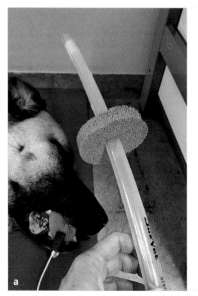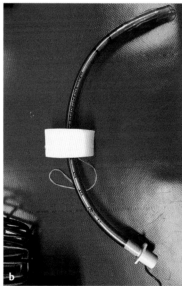

Fig. 7.4 Additional aspiration protection during oral surgery.
a Sponge as mechanical aspiration protection.
b Aspir-Guard as mechanical aspiration protection.

- Use of additional mechanical protection against aspiration such as wet swabs, sponge or Aspir-Guard (▶ Fig. 7.4). **It is very important to remove this mechanical barrier shortly before or with extubation**!!
- For hygienic reasons, a Heidelberg extension or perfusion line can be used instead of a gauze bandage or a cotton cord to keep the endotracheal tube in place

In small mammals, securing the airway can become an (almost) impossible challenge. Non-intubated rabbits and guinea pigs should be given oxygen via a nasal tube or mask.

7.4.2 Anaesthesia

In principle, there are no relevant specifics regarding the management of anaesthesia. Individual characteristics of the patient (including species, breed, age, temperament) and systemic diseases must be taken into account in the management. The invasiveness of the procedure must also be considered: Is it a simple tartar removal, an extensive dental surgery or the removal of half a jaw? Depending on this, the extent of analgesia and postoperative care will be lower or higher. In case of tumorous disease in the region of the oral cavity, it must be evaluated whether local anaesthesia is possible without displacing tumour cells.

Maintenance and perioperative analgesia

Maintenance of anaesthesia is usually performed with inhalation anaesthetics. The frequent changes of position of the intubated patient can be associated with complications such as injuries to the trachea. For this reason, it is particularly important to disconnect the ETT from the Y-piece before each change of position. Ideally, the order of events is as follows:
- Switch off oxygen at the flowmeter and inhalation anaesthetic at the vaporiser
- Disconnect ETT from the Y-piece
- Change position
- Reconnect the ETT to the Y-piece
- Switch on oxygen at the flowmeter and inhalation anaesthetic at the vaporiser again

This approach is particularly important in cats (and small dogs) as they have very delicate airways and tracheal trauma and rupture can be possible complications.

Analgesia should be administered according to the expected degree of pain and with appropriate duration. In small animals (p. 417) and horses (p. 442) it is possible to maintain excellent perioperative analgesia with local anaesthesia techniques, thereby keeping patients relatively light under anaesthesia (and therefore safer and with fewer complications). The effect of local anaesthesia usually lasts well into the recovery phase (depending on the drug used). In addition, NSAIDs are often used and, in very painful procedures, ketamine and opioids as well.

7.4.3 Postoperative management

In every dental patient, the **oral cavity should be examined** and **cleaned** from debris, blood coagula, etc. after the end of the procedure (there is usually a 3-way air-water-spray handpiece on the dental machine that can be used). The mechanical aspiration protection must also be removed at this point at the latest. Extubation should only take place when the patient can swallow reliably. The cuff may only be partially deflated in order to remove any particles that may have reached the upper airway. Immediate postoperative analgesia is usually assured if local anaesthesia techniques have been used. Depending on the severity of the procedure and the expected degree of pain, NSAIDS (if not contraindicated) and/or opioids or other analgesic drugs should be administered in time.

7.4.4 Literature

[1] Bellows J, Berg ML, Dennis S, Harvey R, Lobprise HB, Snyder CJ, Stone AES, Van de Wetering AG. 2019 AAHA- Dental care guidelines for dogs and cats. J Am Anim Hosp Assoc 2019; 55: 1–21

[2] Brodbelt DC, Blissitt KJ, Hammond RA, Neath PJ, Young LE, Pfeiffer DU, Wood JL. The risk of death: the confidential enquiry into perioperative small animal fatalities. Vet Anaesth Analg 2008; 35: 365–73

[3] Hardie EM, Spodnick GJ, Gilson SD, Benson JA, Hawkins EC. Tracheal rupture in cats: 16 cases (1983–1998). J Am Vet Med 1999; 15: 508–12

[4] Lockhart PB, Brennan MT, Sasser HC, Fox PC, Paster BJ, Bahrani-Mougeot FK. Bacteremia associated with tooth brushing and dental extraction. Circulation 2008; 117: 3118–25

[5] Pavlica Z, Petelin M, Juntes P, Erzen D, Crossley DA, Skaleric U. Periodontal disease burden and pathological changes in organs of dogs. J Vet Dent 2008; 25: 97–105

[6] Stiles J, Weil AB, Packer RA, Lantz GC. Post-operative cortical blindness in cats: twenty cases. Vet J 2012; 193: 367–73
Comment: This publication describes how the mouth gag can cause blindness in cats.

7.5 Dog/cat with epileptic seizures

Ideally, any patient with a history of epileptiform activity should be evaluated neurologically and any underlying disease identified and treated. If indicated, the patient can be kept seizure-free with orally administered barbiturates with or without additional gabapentin. The morning dose before anaesthesia should be administered.

Usually, induction and maintenance of anaesthesia only rarely causes a seizure in predisposed animals.

The general rules apply: Avoid stress, give oxygen, have dosages of emergency medication ready for the individual patient.

7.5.1 Preoperative management

The use of acepromazine has long been discussed as contraindicated in such patients as dogs (p. 304). The use of ketamine, which can potentially trigger convulsions, is also questionable – but it is primarily a question of dose!

Good to know

Acepromazine: seizure-inducing or seizure-terminating?
In human studies, chlorpromazine (from the same group of substances as acepromazine) has been shown to lower the seizure threshold and to produce a discharge pattern in the EEG similar to that of an epileptic seizure. In dogs with a history of seizures, acepromazine (p. 64) was used for sedation; none of the dogs had seizures in the following 16 h. In actively seizing dogs, it was also used and in 8 out of 11, the seizure could be stopped temporarily or permanently.

If the animal is acutely seizing, e.g. due to anti-slug pellet poisoning, monitoring should be started in parallel with attempts to stop the seizure. Here, particular attention should be paid to oxygen saturation (convulsions consume a lot of oxygen) and temperature (a lot of heat is produced by muscle work). In most cases, cooling must be started immediately because of the rapid increase in body temperature.

7.5.2 Anaesthesia

Good drugs for premedication are **midazolam** or **diazepam**, both of which are considered first-line anticonvulsant agents. For induction of anaesthesia, **thiopental**, which is second-line, or **propofol**, which is a third-line anticonvulsant agent, are suitable. Analgesics should not be forgotten if the procedure is painful.

Sedation

For calm, older or sick animals:

Dosage

- Combination of **Midazolam** IM, IV OR **Diazepam** 0.2–0.4 mg/kg IV AND
- **Butorphanol** 0.2 mg/kg IM, IV

For very agitated animals, a low dose of **medetomidine** or **dexmedetomidine** can be added to improve the quality of sedation and reduce agitation.

Dosage

- **Medetomidine** 0.01 mg/kg IM, 0.003–0.005 mg/kg IV OR **Dexmedetomidine** 0.005 mg/kg IM, 0.002–0.003 mg/kg IV

In fact, only a few micrograms are needed. That is a very small volume!

Induction

Induction of anaesthesia is done with **thiopental** or **propofol** after good sedation and preoxygenation. It is debated whether propofol itself also induces twitching and seizures, so it makes sense to reduce the induction dose as much as possible with good prior sedation, relaxation and a quiet environment.

Dosage

- **Thiopental** 10–15 mg/kg titrate strictly IV OR **Propofol** up to 4 mg/kg titrate IV

Maintenance

Maintenance of anaesthesia should be done with **isoflurane** or **sevoflurane** in O_2 with additional analgesia if a painful procedure is performed.

If an animal begins to have convulsions during anaesthesia…

1. Administration of **Midazolam** OR **Diazepam** 0.2–0.5, up to max. 1 mg/kg IV
2. Depending on what is available more quickly:
   - **Propofol** 2–8 mg/kg IV titrate until desired effect is achieved (**CAREFUL:** respiratory depression, probably needs ventilation) OR
   - **Phenobarbital** 2–4 mg/kg IV every 20–30 min up to a maximum dose of 20 mg/kg OR
   - **Pentobarbital** 6–15 mg/kg slowly IV as bolus, then CRI 0.5–2 mg/kg/h to effect

In any case, the clinical parameters must be well monitored and further measures may need to be taken.

7.5.3 Postoperative management

In the postoperative phase, seizure monitoring is performed over the next few hours (or days) that the patient is hospitalised.

In acutely convulsing animals (poisoning), medication is used to try to stop the convulsions. Drugs that are used for this purpose are again

- **Midazolam** or **diazepam** 0.05–0.2 mg/kg/h as CRI
- If this does not control seizures, a **barbiturate** can be added as a CRI as described for maintenance
- CRI with low-dose alpha2 agonists (**medetomidine** or **dexmedetomidine**) may also be useful in this situation: 2–5 µg/kg/h or less IV

Animals are then lightly to deeply sedated and must be subjected to intensive monitoring and complex intensive medical management. Especially if the animals still show (occasional) seizures, additional oxygen administration is beneficial.

Animals with a history of seizures should wake up calmly and with little stress after anaesthesia and be monitored closely for the next few hours. **Benzodiazepines** (midazolam/diazepam) should **not be antagonised** (for faster recovery) with flumazenil (p. 95).

7.5.4 Literature

[1] Platt SR, Adams V, Garosi LS, Abramson CJ, Penderis J, De Stefani A, Matiasek L. Treatment with gabapentin of 11 dogs with refractory idiopathic epilepsy. Vet Rec 2006; 159: 881–884

[2] Thomas WB. Idiopathic epilepsy in dogs. Vet Clin North Am Small Anim Pract 2000; 30: 183–206

[3] Tobias KM, Marioni-Henry K, Wagner R. A retrospective study on the use of acepromazine maleate in dogs with seizures. J Am Anim Hosp Assoc 2006; 42: 283–289
Comment: This study shows that, contrary to the opinion that dominated for many years, acepromazine is not contraindicated in seizing patients.

7.6 Traumatic brain injury/increased intracranial pressure in small animals

Traumatic brain injury is a common complication in small animals after a car accident, blow, fall or bite. Depending on the severity, supportive measures must be initiated immediately. As a rule, the immediate primary damage cannot be treated. The aim of therapy is therefore to reduce the extent of the secondary damage that develops in the following minutes and hours. The prognosis depends largely on the extent to which it is possible to keep the intracranial pressure within the normal range.

Clinical relevance

Structure of the intracranial space
Three different structures fill the intracranial space: The **brain** (approx. 80–90%), the **cerebrospinal fluid** (approx. 10%) and the **blood volume** (approx. 2–3%). Any enlargement of one or more of these structures leads to increased intracranial pressure, as the bony skull cannot give way. The only way for the brain to expand is through the *foramen magnum*, which (in the worst case) leads to entrapment of the *medulla oblongata* and thus to death by respiratory arrest.

▶ **Anamnesis.** Observed trauma, behavioural change, diagnosed space-occupying process in the brain

▶ **Clinical symptoms.** Occurrence immediately or up to days after trauma or progressive deterioration in tumour disease: Altered behaviour (depression, wandering, head pressing against the wall), impaired consciousness (stupor, coma). Progressive deterioration. Cushing's reflex.

Definition

Cushing's reflex or Cushing's triad

If **intracranial pressure** (ICP) increases, e.g. due to a cerebral trauma, the **mean arterial blood pressure** (MAP) must increase in order to keep the **cerebral perfusion pressure** (CPP) constant. This relationship is expressed by the formula:

CPP = MAP–ICP

The blood pressure can reach extremely high values (up to systolic 300 mmHg). This in turn increases the intracranial pressure, creating a vicious circle. The heart rate (HR) decreases until severe bradycardia is observed. The only appropriate therapy is to lower ICP, not to control the blood pressure or heart rate with medication.

Cushing's triad: ICP ↑, MAP ↑, HR ↓

7.6.1 Preanaesthetic or general management

The aim is to minimise secondary damage and restore or normalise perfusion of the brain. The following "sub-goals" or management measures contribute to achieving this goal:

- **Normotension** (circulatory support drugs e.g. dobutamine)
  - In case of hypotension with a mean arterial blood pressure < 60 mmHg, autoregulation no longer functions (▶ Fig. 7.5)

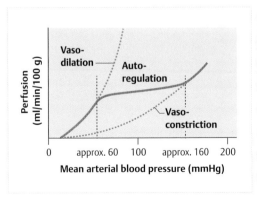

Fig. 7.5 Blood pressure to perfusion ratio in autoregulated organs (brain, heart, kidney).

- **Normovolaemia** (infusion of isotonic solutions)
  - Animals with cerebral damage are often dehydrated
  - Infusion therapy with the aim of correcting hypovolaemia and maintaining a physiological volume status
- **Normothermia**
  - Possibly allow mild hypothermia up to approx. 34 °C, does not reduce mortality, but can improve neurological outcome
  - Avoid hyperthermia or fever at all costs
- **Normoglycaemia**
  - Reduce hyperglycaemia by giving insulin, proven to improve outcome
- **Sedation**
  - Helps with agitation, helps to lower ICP
- **Improvement of venous return**
  - Elevation of the head at an angle of 30–45°, if necessary, place the patient on an inclined plane (reverse Trendelenburg position (p. 271), head up, butt down)
  - Avoid compression of jugular veins
- **Normoxaemia**
  - Oxygen therapy, maintenance of p_aO_2 above 80 mmHg, SpO_2 above 95%
- Maintenance of **normocapnia**
  - Positive pressure ventilation, if necessary, maintenance of p_aCO_2 below 35 mmHg
  - The concept of preventive continuous hyperventilation is outdated, but in transient ICP crises, ICP can be reduced in the short term by mild hyperventilation
- **Drainage of cerebral oedema**
  - Administration of hyperosmotic solutions (mannitol 0.5–2 g/kg over 20 min IV, use filter; repeat every 3–6 h, max. 3 × in 24 h, keep an eye on electrolytes), contraindicated in cerebral haemorrhage
  - Administration of furosemide (1–2 mg/kg IV) simultaneously
- **Anticonvulsive agents** against epileptiform activity
- **Avoid coughing and vomiting** (use antiemetics, sedation, do not use morphine or alpha2 agonists)
- **Analgesia**
  - Opioids, watch for potential respiratory depression
- Administration of **corticosteroids** is **not indicated**
  - No improved neurological outcome detectable with dexamethasone or methylprednisolone
  - Exception: Perifocal cerebral oedema in tumour disease
- **Surgical treatment** (possibly after CT diagnosis)

7.6.2 Anaesthesia

Hypoxia and hypercapnia are considered essential factors for the development and expansion of secondary brain damage. For this reason, patients should be ventilated if indicated and oxygen should be administered without interruption. Drugs that could additionally increase ICP or O_2 consumption should be avoided (e.g. ketamine). If possible, the head should always be elevated.

Clinical relevance

Intracranial pressure measurement

In human medicine, intraventricular ICP measurement is the gold standard for severe traumatic brain injury, as it enables an individual therapy based on the patient's status. In veterinary medicine, this procedure is only carried out in a few (university) intensive care units. For this reason, ICP diagnosis is oriented towards clinical symptoms: among others, nausea, vomiting, restlessness, fatigue, abnormal breathing types, congested pupil (= ophthalmoscopically detectable oedema at the junction of the optic nerve with the retina), later on, impaired consciousness.

Sedation

In some cases, sedation is not necessary because the animals already show slight sedation or impairment of consciousness. Attention should be paid to neuroprotective management at all times.

For calm or already impaired animals:

Dosage

- **Midazolam** OR **Diazepam** 0.2 mg/kg IV

Add **analgesics** as needed.

For painful procedures, e.g. craniotomy:

Dosage

- **Methadone** 0.1–0.5 mg/kg IV OR **Fentanyl** bolus 2–5 (up to 10) µg/kg IV with subsequent CRI 0.3–0.5 µg/kg/min as part of anaesthesia maintenance

For non-painful procedures, e.g. radiographs, MRI:

Dosage

- **Butorphanol** 0.2–0.4 mg/kg IV

At latest when the animal is sedated, oxygen should be administered, an intravenous access established and monitoring equipment applied.

Induction

Before intubation, deep anaesthesia should be ensured with the help of sedation and induction drugs. Lidocaine should be applied to the larynx to prevent coughing or gagging against the tube at all costs (causes increase in ICP).

After sedation:

Dosage

- **Propofol** 1–4 mg/kg IV OR **Thiopental** 10–15 mg/kg titrate strictly IV AND
- **Midazolam** OR **Diazepam** 0.2 mg/kg IV (if not already administered as part of premedication)

Titrate slowly and always administer oxygen.

If the animal is already obtunded and the procedure is painful, this is also possible:

Dosage

- **Fentanyl** 2–5 (up to 10) µg/kg AND
- **Midazolam** OR **Diazepam** 0.2 mg/kg IV
- Then immediately start continuous rate infusion of **Fentanyl** at 0.3–0.5 µg/kg/min AND (after intubation) **inhalation anaesthetics** in 100% oxygen

Expect **hypoventilation**! Normocapnia should be maintained by positive pressure ventilation.

Sevoflurane appears to be neuroprotective in patients with elevated ICP.

311

In the course of induction, 1 mg/kg **lidocaine** (without added vasoconstrictor) can be administered slowly IV before intubation. It reduces the response to intubation, lowers ICP and acts as a systemic analgesic. The duration of action is limited, but it can be further administered as a CRI if needed.

Maintenance

It is best to use a balanced anaesthesia technique with inhalation anaesthetics and opioids following good sedation.

Dosage

- **Isoflurane** OR **Sevoflurane** low dose in O_2 AND
- **Fentanyl** 0.3–0.5 µg/kg/min CRI

If possible, work with **local anaesthesia**.

However, total intravenous anaesthesia (TIVA) is also possible and is even preferred by some anaesthetists in dogs:

Dosage

- **Propofol** 0.1–0.4 mg/kg/min CRI in combination with
- **Fentanyl** 0.3–0.5 µg/kg/min CRI
- A CRI with **Lidocaine** 0.03–0.08 mg/kg/min can be added

Ketamine is contraindicated in high doses because it could increase ICP. However, as a low-dose CRI (5–10 µg/kg/min) it can have beneficial effects and contribute to multimodal analgesia.

Monitoring, complications and therapy

Full monitoring should be performed continuously. Particular attention should be paid to signs of increased ICP, i. e. Cushing's triad (p. 308).

The placement of a **central venous catheter** in the jugular vein is considered critical because it requires the vessel to be occluded, which briefly increases ICP. However, it is advantageous for measuring **central venous pressure** (CVP), taking regular blood samples to check laboratory parameters and administering infusion solutions or parenteral nutrition as needed. In case of doubt, it can also be placed peripherally and advanced. The neck bandage must not obstruct venous return under any circumstances. An **arterial catheter** enables continuous blood pressure measurement and arterial blood gas measurements.

Complications that may be **associated with an elevated ICP** are:

- **Hypertension**as part of the Cushing's triad; should not be controlled with antihypertensive treatment, as the increased blood pressure ensures perfusion of the brain, but measures should be taken to reduce ICP
- **Hypotension** must be controlled consistently
- **Hypoxaemia** due to compromised circulation and possible congestive lung disease
  - Administer oxygen
  - Maintain normoventilation
  - Administer diuretics, e.g. furosemide if indicated
- **Hypercapnia** due to central suppression or anaesthesia; ventilation should be monitored with capnography, the goal is normocapnia or mild hypocapnia
- Sudden **death**

7.6.3 Postoperative management

Depending on pathology and course of the surgical intervention, the recovery phase can be short and unspectacular (e.g. after craniotomy for removal of a small meningioma) or last for days. The goals discussed in the general management must also be considered in the postoperative phase. The goal is also to "normalise everything" and keep it there.

Further therapy can take weeks to months and the final outcome depends largely on the initial damage (trauma? tumour?), the extent of secondary damage and the peri- and postoperative care. Risk, cost and prognosis should be discussed in detail with the owner in order to provide a realistic assessment of the situation.

Depending on the severity of the disease, postoperative monitoring must be more or less intensive. Ideally, continuous full clinical and apparatus monitoring should be ensured. Ventilation should be continued (oxygen-air mixture) until the patient is able to maintain ventilation parameters within the physiological range. Ensure adequate analgesia for at least 3 days. It is known from human medicine that a craniotomy causes severe headaches. Parenteral or enteral nutrition should be started if the postoperative treatment lasts longer than a few days.

7.6.4 Literature

[1] Alderson P, Roberts I. Corticosteroids in acute traumatic brain injury: systematic review of randomized controlled trials. Br Med J 1997; 314: 1855–1859

[2] Battison C, Andrews PJD, Graham C, Petty T. Randomized, controlled trial on the effect of a 20% mannitol solution and a 7.5% saline/6% dextran solution on increased intracranial pressure after brain injury. Crit Care Med 2005; 33: 196–202

[3] Brain trauma foundation. Guidelines for the management of severe traumatic brain injury. J Neurotrauma 2007; 24: S1–S106

[4] Clifton GL. Is keeping cool still hot? An update on hypothermia in brain injury. N Engl J Med 2004; 10: 116–119

[5] Davis DP, Dunford JV, Poste JC, Ochs M, Holbrook T, Fortlage D, Size MJ, Kennedy F, Hoyt DB. The impact of hypoxia and hyperventilation on outcome after paramedic rapid sequence intubation of severely head-injured patients. J Trauma 2004: 57: 1–10

[6] Engelhard K, Werner C. Überwachung und Therapie des erhöhten intrakraniellen Drucks. Anästh Intensivmed 2008; 49: 258–268
Comment: Excellent German summary from human medicine

[7] Petersen KD, Landsfeldt U, Cold GE, Petersen CB, Mau S, Hauerberg J, Holst P, Skovgaard Olsen K. Intracranial pressure and cerebral hemodynamics in patients with cerebral tumors. Anesthesiol 2003; 98: 329–336

7.7 Patient with renal problems

A distinction is made between acute and chronic renal disease. Renal diseases often affect not only the kidneys themselves, but also other organ systems such as the cardiovascular system, the respiratory tract and the haematopoietic system. Over a long period of time, the failure of nephrons can be compensated for and no clinically recognisable symptoms occur. If the compensatory mechanisms are "challenged" by anaesthesia, this can lead to additional damage to the kidneys and even to renal failure. For this reason, an attempt should be made to identify patients with renal disease in advance by taking a thorough anamnesis, clinical examination and analysis of the relevant blood parameters (at least haematocrit, total protein, creatinine and electrolytes).

Among the **dog** breeds, Bernese Mountain dog, Shar Pei, Cocker Spaniel, Samoyed, Doberman and Basenji are affected. Among the **cat** breeds, Persians, Maine Coons, Abyssinians, Russian Blues, Burmese, Exotic Shorthairs, British Shorthairs, Cartesians and Norwegian Forest cats are predisposed.

▶ **Anamnesis.** Polyuria, polydipsia, anorexia, weight loss

▶ **Clinical signs.** Bad breath (*foetor ex ore*), dull coat, pale mucous membranes, hypothermia, occasional vomiting/diarrhoea, inflammation of the oral mucosa

▶ **Diagnosis.** Blood test (anaemia, hypoproteinaemia, hypoalbuminemia, increased SDMA and/or creatinine, deviation of electrolyte concentrations, possibly increased urea) and urine test (e.g. deviations in specific gravity, proteinuria)

7.7.1 Preoperative management

Good preoperative assessment and – if possible – therapy improve the chances of an anaesthesia period with few complications and a postoperative phase without additional damage to the kidneys. Patients with acute disease or obstruction are often faster and easier to treat because the damage is potentially reversible.

Plan and goals for anaesthesia in patients with renal disease:
- **Correct** acid-base abnormalities (p. 392) preoperatively
- **Normalise** electrolyte imbalances (p. 386), especially hyperkalaemia (p. 387)
  - A potassium value > 6 mmol/l should be corrected preoperatively; infusion with K-containing solutions, e.g. Ringer's lactate solution, **not NaCl 0.9%**, as this paradoxically worsens the hyperkalaemia by its acidifying effect
- Pre-operative examination of **blood pressure** (hypertension?) and **ECG** (signs of hyperkalaemia?)
- **Normotension**
  - Avoid hypotension at all costs so as not to decrease renal perfusion
  - Patients who were hypertensive preoperatively should be kept in their "normal range", i. e. slightly hypertensive if necessary
- **Restore/maintain normovolaemia** and physiological **hydration status**
  - Patients with renal disease may be hyperhydrated (oedema) if urine production is reduced; but they may also be dehydrated if they are polyuric
- Adjust dose of medication: **Reduce dose**
  - Hypoalbuminemia and -proteinemia result in an increased free (and therefore effective) fraction of many anaesthetics
  - In case of metabolic acidosis
  - Blood-brain barrier may be damaged by uraemia and is more easily permeable: this leads to a stronger effect at the same dose
- **Avoid hypoxia**
  - Many patients are anaemic, so a blood transfusion should be given if pre-operative haematocrit is less than 20%
  - Preoxygenation
  - Continuous oxygen administration and ventilation if necessary
- **Avoid hypercapnia**
  - Many patients suffer from metabolic acidosis, which they compensate for by an increase in ventilation (i. e. breathing off more CO_2); during anaesthesia, this compensation should be maintained by positive pressure ventilation

315

- **Decrease sympathetic tone**
  - With each stimulation, renal vessels become vasoconstricted, resulting in decreased perfusion
  - Provide a stress-free environment, sedation
  - Good analgesia (opioids)
- **Normothermia**
  - Active temperature management, especially important in small patients

---

Careful!

Avoid potentially nephrotoxic drugs:
- Aminoglycosides
- Non-steroidal anti-inflammatory drugs (NSAIDs)
- Radiocontrast media

7.7.2 Anaesthesia

The anaesthetic protocol should primarily support the management goals discussed above. This is less dependent on the choice of drugs, which – with a few exceptions (NSAIDs, alpha2 agonists) – can all be used without problems. However, as most anaesthetics decrease renal blood flow, glomerular filtration rate and urine output, a balanced protocol should be used. This allows a dose reduction of the individual drugs and thus lowers the amount of side effects.

Sedation

The aims of preanaesthetic sedation include stress-free handling and dose reduction of the induction and maintenance drugs. A combination of **opioids** and **benzodiazepines** is particularly well suited, but will hardly induce sedation, especially in (aggressive) cats.

In animals severely impaired by the disease:

Dosage

- Pure μ opioid agonists like **Morphine** OR **Methadone** 0.1–0.4 mg/kg OR **Butorphanol** 0.2 mg/kg or higher dose AND
- **Midazolam** OR **Diazepam** 0.2 mg/kg mixed in one syringe IM or IV

Ketamine 0.5–2 mg/kg or **alfaxalone** 1–5 mg/kg IM may be added for animals, especially cats, that would benefit from more sedation, e.g. very nervous/excited or aggressive/non-treatable animals.

Immediately when the animal is sedated, oxygen should be administered, intravenous access established and clinical and apparatus monitoring started.

II

Careful!

Avoid potentially harmful anaesthetics for the kidneys
- **NSAIDs** (e.g. carprofen, meloxicam) can reduce renal blood flow
- **Alpha2 agonists** (xylazine, dex-/medetomidine) cause severe vasoconstriction and thus greatly reduce renal blood flow. In VERY low doses sometimes useful, especially in aggressive cats
- **Mask induction with inhalational anaesthetics** causes major stress, thereby increasing sympathetic tone and subsequently also causing vasoconstriction of the renal vessels

Induction

Appropriate are these induction drugs, which should be titrated slowly IV and given after good sedation:

Dosage

- **Propofol** 1–4 mg/kg IV OR
- **Etomidate** 1–3 mg/kg IV OR
- **Alfaxalone** 1–5 mg/kg IV

Ketamine 1–2 mg /kg IV may be used in addition to the three induction drugs mentioned, or 2–5 mg/kg IV alone after sedation/muscle relaxation and for longer procedures.

In addition to the chosen induction drug(s), **midazolam** or **diazepam** 0.2 mg/kg IV can be administered if not already included in premedication. This reduces the induction dose, does not cause cardiovascular or respiratory side effects, prevents muscle tension or spasms and has other beneficial effects.

Maintenance

It is best to use a balanced anaesthesia technique based on inhalation anaesthesia in combination with analgesics.

Dosage

- **Isoflurane** OR **Sevoflurane** low dose in O_2 AND
- **Fentanyl** CRI 0.3–0.5 µg/kg/min IV
- For very painful procedures, additionally **Ketamine** CRI 10–30 µg/kg/min IV can be used

Work with **local anaesthesia** if possible.

Another suitable and quite efficient analgesic seems to be **metamizole** 25–50 mg/kg SC or slowly and diluted IV, which can be given when the patient is normotensive and has a physiological volume status.

Monitoring, complications and therapy

Monitoring should be continuous, with particular attention to cardiovascular parameters: ECG, pulse oximetry and blood pressure measurement, as well as assessment of volume status. It is helpful to measure central venous pressure (CVP) continuously in critically ill patients.

Expected problems and plan in **patients with impaired renal function**:

- **Hypotension**
  - Correct hypovolaemia
  - Perioperatively, a **dobutamine** continuous rate infusion with 1–5 µg/kg/min or a low-dose **dopamine** continuous rate infusion with 1–3 µg/kg/min can be used after all other measures such as reduction of the anaesthetic dose and infusion have been unsuccessful (▶ Table 8.1)
  - Let the patient breathe spontaneously, if possible, as long as the patient is normocapnic
- **Hypoventilation**
  - Positive pressure ventilation, with lung-protective ventilator settings: rather high frequency and low volume
- **ECG changes** or **arrhythmias** due to hyperkalaemia
  - Should already have been normalised preoperatively
- **Hypoxaemia** due to pulmonary oedema or uraemia-induced pneumonia
  - Oxygen administration
  - Positive pressure ventilation in case of hypoventilation

- **Oliguria/anuria**, check urine production
  - A urinary catheter should be placed
  - Urine output should be at least 0.5–1 ml/kg/h on average
  - If necessary, slowly increase diuresis with furosemide 1–2 mg/kg IV up to max. 8 mg/kg/24 h (especially in case of hyperhydration and hyperkalaemia)
- **Hypothermia**
  - Active temperature management

7.7.3 Postoperative management

Monitoring and treatment with analgesics and infusion should be continued in a similar way as pre- and perioperatively. Renal damage caused during surgery/anaesthesia may not be clinically apparent until days to weeks later. **Post-obstructive diuresis** with significantly increased urine output may occur in patients who have had an obstruction of the urinary tract surgically repaired and requires adequate infusion management. In patients at risk, renal function should therefore be monitored for at least 3 days postoperatively (clinically and by laboratory diagnostics). Additional gastric protection with medication is recommended for patients admitted to hospital.

7.7.4 Literature

[1] Bergmann HM, Nolte IJ, Kramer S. Effects of preoperative administration of carprofen on renal function and hemostasis in dogs undergoing surgery for fracture repair. Am J Vet Res 2005; 66: 1356–1363

[2] Bidwai AV, Stanley TH, Bloomer HA, Blatnick RA. Effects of anesthetic doses of morphine on renal function in the dog. Anesth Analg 1975; 54: 357–360

[3] Black HE. Renal toxicity of non-steroidal anti-inflammatory drugs. Toxicol Pathol 1986; 14: 83–90

[4] Boström IM, Nyman G, Hoppe A, Lord P. Effects of meloxicam on renal function in dogs with hypotension during anaesthesia. Vet Anaesth Analg 2006; 33: 62–69

[5] Burchardi H, Kaczmarczyk G. The effect of anaesthesia on renal function. Eur J Anaesth 1994; 11: 163–168

[6] Craig RG, Hunter JM. Recent developments in the perioperative management of adult patients with chronic kidney disease. Br J Anaesth 2008; 101: 296–310

[7] Di Bartola SP. Renal disease: clinical approach and laboratory evaluation. In: Textbook of veterinary internal medicine. 6th ed. Ettinger SJ, Feldmann EC. St. Louis: Elsevier 2005; 1716–1730

[8] Dörfelt R. Anästhesie und perianästhetisches Management von Kleintierpatienten mit Nierenerkrankungen. Wien Tierärztl Mschr 2001; 98: 226–231

[9] Dyson D. Anesthesia for patients with stable end-stage renal disease. Vet Clin North Am Small Anim Pract 1992; 22: 469–471

[10] Grauer GF. Prevention of acute renal failure. Vet Clin North Am Small Anim Pract 1996; 26: 1447–1459

319

[11] O'Malley CM, Frumento RJ, Hardy MA, Benvenisty AI, Brenzjens TE, Mercer JS, Bennett-Guerrero E. A randomized, double-blind comparison of lactated Ringer's solution and 0.9% NaCl during renal transplantation. Anesth Analg 2005; 100: 1518–24
Comment: This is one of the studies that prove that potassium-containing solutions are indeed more useful than saline in patients with hyperkalaemia.
[12] Petersen JS, Shalmi M, Christensen S, Haugan K, Lomholt N. Comparison of the renal effects of six sedating agents in rats. Physiol Behav 1996; 1996: 759–765
[13] Saleh N, Aoki M, Shimada T, Akiyoshi H, Hassanin A, Ohashi F. Renal effects of medetomidine in isoflurane-anesthetized dogs with special reference to its diuretic action. J Vet Med Sci 2005; 67: 461–465

7.8 Patient with liver problems: insufficiency and shunt

Due to the manifold functions of the liver, a variety of different symptoms as well as pathologically altered parameters can be seen in case of dysfunction. This needs to be taken into account before and during anaesthesia in order not to worsen the patient's condition.

Some of the most important **liver functions** are:
- Regulation of **glucose**, **protein** and **fat metabolism**
  - Bile production
- "Detoxification" and **metabolisation** (especially by the cytochrome P450 enzyme system), degradation of
  - Haemoglobin
  - Ammonia to urea
  - (Steroid) hormones
  - Drugs (anaesthetics!)
- **Protein synthesis**
  - Coagulation factors, antithrombin, plasminogen
  - Albumin
  - Transferrin
- **Production of erythrocytes**
- **Storage function**
  - Blood/erythrocytes
  - Glucose (glucagon)
  - Fat (lipoproteins)
  - Vitamins, minerals
- **Defence function**
  - Pathogens from the gastrointestinal tract

Liver insufficiency is a functional disorder associated with partial or total failure of its metabolic functions. The spectrum can range from minor deterioration of the functional parameters to life-threatening failure. In the most severe form, fulminant liver failure, there is a triad of symptoms: jaundice, clotting disorders and mental dullness (hepatic encephalopathy). The prognosis for these patients is poor. A distinction is also made between prehepatic (e.g. haemolysis), hepatic (e.g. intrinsic liver injury, tumour) and posthepatic (e.g. bile duct obstruction) causes.

The **portosystemic shunt** (**PSS**) is a vascular malformation in which the portal blood (coming from the stomach, intestine, pancreas and spleen) bypasses the liver and enters the systemic circulation via the shunt vessel. In this way, the liver is circumvented and cannot perform its function properly.

- In most cases, the PSS is a **congenital extrahepatic vascular** formation. Small dog breeds are predisposed (Yorkshire Terrier, Dachshund, Maltese, Shi Tsu, Miniature Schnauzer)
- **Intrahepatic shunts** are more common in large dog breeds (Labrador, Golden Retriever, Irish Wolfhound)
- One fifth of PSS in dogs are acquired, multiple, **extrahepatic shunts**

▶ **Anamnesis.** Fatigue, depression, anorexia, weight loss, vomiting, diarrhoea, dull coat (PSS often affects puppies)

▶ **Clinical symptoms.** All symptoms are consequences of liver dysfunction! Hepato-encephalic syndrome (seizures especially after eating, depression, unusual behaviour, aggression, weakness, ataxia, blindness, coma), gastrointestinal bleeding, diarrhoea, vomiting, ascites, polyuria/polydipsia, urinary tract problems (stone formation), salivation (cat)

▶ **Diagnostics.** Blood test (including anaemia, hypoproteinaemia, hypoalbuminemia, hypoglycaemia, in PSS often normal coagulation parameters), radiography (size, shape and extent of the liver), abdominal ultrasound (insufficiency: tissue density, cysts, tumour, bile stasis, stones), possibly biopsy, exploratory laparotomy, functional tests. In case of suspected PSS perform angiography

7.8.1 Preoperative management

Basically, the goal is to compensate for the hepatic dysfunction and to stabilise the patient as much as possible. Here, too, good preoperative assessment and (if possible) therapy improve the chances of an anaesthesia period with few complications and without a prolonged recovery phase.

Plan and goals for anaesthesia in **patients with liver dysfunction and porto-systemic shunt**, which can be worked on days before (scheduled) anaesthesia:

- **Correct acid-base, electrolyte** and **volume status abnormalities** preoperatively
  - Targeted infusion therapy with crystalloid and colloid solutions (possibly blood products such as fresh frozen plasma)
  - Restore/maintain normovolaemia and physiological hydration status
- **Prevent bleeding**
  - Determine blood group, organise donor animal
  - Treat coagulopathy by administration of blood products (fresh frozen plasma, fresh whole blood)
- **Normal glucose levels**
  - In case of hypoglycaemia substitute 2.5–5% glucose in balanced electrolyte solution, check perioperatively every 45–60 min
- **Reduce hepato-encephalic syndrome**
  - Reduce ammonia production and absorption with a low-protein diet prior to anaesthesia
  - Administration of lactulose
  - Reduce convulsions with anticonvulsant therapy; if possible, for up to 2 weeks: e.g. potassium bromide in dogs, phenobarbital in cats
- **Normotension**
  - Avoid hypotension at all costs so as not to deteriorate liver perfusion
  - Administer colloids (ideally: plasma) if low oncotic pressure due to hypoalbuminemia (< 2.2 g/dl)
- **Adjust drug dose**, possibly reduce dose
  - Hypoalbuminemia and -proteinemia result in an increased free (and thus effective) fraction of many anaesthetics
- **Avoid hypoxaemia**
  - Preoxygenation
  - Continuous oxygen administration and ventilation if necessary
- **Avoid hypoxia due to anaemia**
  - Determine blood group in time and look for donor animal
  - With a haematocrit of less than 20–25% administer a blood transfusion
- **Avoid hypercapnia**
  - Many patients suffer from metabolic acidosis, which they compensate for by an increase in respiration (i. e. breathe out more CO_2); during anaesthesia, this compensation should be maintained by ventilation
- **Normothermia**
  - Active warming, especially for small patients
- **Antibiosis**
  - To treat bacterial translocation from the gastrointestinal tract and bacteraemia

Immediately prior to surgery

- Check current **blood work** again (Hct, TP, albumin, glucose, lactate, electrolytes)
- Check **coagulation**: Prothrombin time (PT), partial thromboplastin time (PTT), activated clotting time (ACT)
  - If necessary and possible transfusion of whole blood or fresh frozen plasma
- If severe **ascites**
  - Drain ascites to reduce hypoventilation (pressure on diaphragm) and hypotension (pressure on *v. cava*)
  - Refill volume through infusion therapy
- Placement of a **central venous catheter** in the jugular vein (possible administration of blood products, parenteral nutrition and measurement of the central venous pressure)

7.8.2 Anaesthesia

The aim is to use, as far as possible, anaesthetics that are not or only very little metabolised by the liver, that have a very short effect or that can be antagonised. Drugs that are predominantly metabolised by the liver or have other adverse effects should be avoided.

  Less suitable are:

- **Acepromazine** is predominantly metabolised by the liver and is long acting
- **Barbiturates** are metabolised almost exclusively by the liver
- **Ketamine** can increase the risk of convulsions and even the first metabolite of ketamine also still has 30% effect
- **Midazolam/diazepam:** There are different opinions: It is possible that benzodiazepines worsen symptoms of hepatic encephalopathy; metabolites of diazepam are active, those of midazolam not – but benzodiazepines may also prevent seizures
- **Dex-/medetomidine/xylazine** are not recommended, because they are partially metabolised by the liver, cause vasoconstriction, but can be antagonised (dex-/medetomidine with atipamezole)
- **Morphine** can cause histamine release, which decreases liver perfusion
- **Lidocaine** can accumulate

In general, drugs will have a stronger and longer lasting effect in the patient with liver dysfunction, will accumulate more quickly and therefore need to be adjusted in dose and application intervals.

  Two IV catheters should be placed, one of them centrally.

Sedation

As animals with liver failure often already have a depressed level of consciousness, heavy sedation is often not necessary or should be avoided, if possible, because of the side effects. Opioids are a good option: either a pure µ opioid agonist such as **methadone** or alternatively **butorphanol**.

Dosage

- **Methadone** 0.1–0.4 mg/kg OR **Butorphanol** 0.2 mg/kg or higher doses IM, better IV

Careful!

Avoid potentially hepatotoxic drugs
- **Paracetamol**, an NSAID, has a liver toxic metabolite and is contraindicated in the cat (methaemoglobin formation)
- **Carprofen**, also an NSAID, can possibly cause hepatitis in the Labrador Retriever. This breed seems to be particularly sensitive
- **Halothane** and **Enflurane** are no longer on the market. Halothane is metabolised by up to 40% in the liver. This can cause acute halothane hepatitis or immunologically mediated delayed liver injury. Halothane is still occasionally used in laboratory animal science

Induction

Possible options are:

Dosage

- **Propofol** 1–4(–8) mg/kg titrated to effect IV + / –
- **Remifentanil** 1–5 µg/kg IV OR **Fentanyl** 1–5 µg/kg IV bolus and immediately start a CRI as part of balanced analgesia

Propofol (p. 131) is predominantly metabolised extrahepatically. Remifentanil (p. 133) is metabolised via plasma esterases and not at all by the liver.

After very good sedation, mask induction with **sevoflurane** or **isoflurane** is stressful but possible; only a very small proportion of these are metabolised by the liver (approx. 3% and 0.3% respectively).

Maintenance

It is best to use a balanced anaesthesia technique based on inhalation anaesthesia in combination with opioids as analgesics. Especially in PSS patients, anaesthesia time should be kept as short as possible.

- **Sevoflurane** or **isoflurane** in O_2 as needed, PSS patients seem to need less, they have lower MAC values
- **Remifentanil** or **fentanyl** CRI or **methadone** bolus as needed (but are likely to have longer duration of action!)
- Epidural anaesthesia with **morphine** or **methadone** (if no contraindications such as coagulation problems)

Monitoring, complications and therapy

As with any critical patient, monitoring should begin before induction! Pulse oximetry and ECG should be monitored and blood pressure taken. Capnography helps to assess the ventilatory status especially in case of ascites. Temperature should always be measured. Intraoperatively, Hct, TP and glucose should be assessed regularly.

The **main problems** to be expected are:
- **Hypotension**
  - Hypovolaemia, -proteinemia or -albuminemia
  - Perioperatively, a **dopamine** continuous rate infusion ($2–5\,\mu g/kg/min$ or more) can be used after all other measures such as reduction of the anaesthetic dose and infusion have been unsuccessful (▶ Table 8.1)
- **Hypoventilation** (due to ascites)
  - Positive pressure ventilation (p. 371), protective of the lungs: rather high frequency, low volume
- **Hypoxaemia**, also due to ascites
  - Oxygen administration
  - Positive pressure ventilation in case of hypoventilation
- **Hypothermia**
  - Active warming
- **Blood parameter deviations** (Hct, TP, glucose)
  - Correct deviations

7.8.3 Postoperative management

The most common and serious complication after occlusion of the PSS is the resulting portal hypertension, coagulopathy and neurological problems. A prolonged recovery phase should be expected and appropriate preparation for continuous care is recommended.

- **Analgesia** (based on opioid administration)
- Intravenous balanced electrolyte solution **infusion**, with 2.5–5% glucose supplementation if necessary
- Continue to **monitor**: Blood pressure (invasive if possible), laboratory values (Hct, TP, albumin, lactate, electrolytes), ECG
- Abdominal ultrasound or measurement of the **abdominal circumference** can give an early indication of the development of ascites
- **Seizure control** and preventive administration of antiepileptic drugs
- Patients at risk should be monitored several days postoperatively (clinically and by laboratory diagnostics)

7.8.4 Literature

[1] Hänel F, Werner C. Remifentanil. Anaesthesist 1997; 46: 897–908

[2] Raffe MR. Anesthesia for severe liver dysfunction. Vet Clin North Am Small Anim Pract 1992; 22: 478–480

[3] Shawcross D, Jalan R. Dispelling myths in the treatment of hepatic encephalopathy. Lancet 2005; 365: 431–433

[4] Yuan Z, Liu J, Liang X, Lin D. Serum biochmical indicators of hepatobiliary function in dogs following prolonged anaesthesia with sevoflurane or isoflurane. Vet Anaesth Anal 2012; 39: 296–300

7.9 Gastric dilatation-volvulus in dogs

Canine gastric dilatation-volvulus is an absolute **emergency** in which (surgical) therapy must be induced as soon as possible after a quick stabilisation of the patient.

▶ Anamnesis. Restlessness, attempts to vomit (mucus, food, unproductive), bloated abdomen

▶ Clinical symptoms. Dilated abdomen, tympanic sound on percussion, gagging, hypersalivation, low-grade to severe shock, severe (abdominal) pain

▶ **Diagnostics.** Clinical examination with emphasis on general condition, vital signs and percussion/palpation of the abdomen; electrocardiogram to detect premature ventricular extrasystoles (▶ Fig. 8.10). Radiographic images of abdomen (*sinistra-dextra*, possibly *ventro-dorsal*). Laboratory values should include haematocrit, total protein, glucose, lactate, blood gases and electrolytes (potassium, sodium, chloride) and creatinine

7.9.1 Preoperative management

The order must be adapted to the individual situation. Sometimes, as first emergency treatment, it may be necessary, for example, to decompress the stomach.

- **Oxygen administration** via mask
- Place at least one, preferably two, **large-lumen intravenous catheters** (18 G) in the cephalic vein
- Initial "shock" **infusion** (amount depending on the patient's condition and need)
  - 20–30 ml/kg balanced crystalloid solution, e.g. Ringer's solution or Sterofundin ISO over 15 min (repeat if necessary)
  - 4–6 ml/kg colloid solution, e.g. HES (Voluven) if crystalloid solution is not sufficient to improve perfusion parameters and blood pressure (repeat if necessary, but max. 30 ml/kg/24 h)
  - Once stabilised, continue with perioperative fluid infusion rates
- **Gastric decompression** (if necessary and possible) either via trocar technique, nasogastric tube or (only in intubated animals because of the risk of aspiration!) oral gastric tube; if necessary, administer the lidocaine bolus described below beforehand; the nasogastric tube should remain in place at least until the stomach is "untwisted"
- **Analgesia**
  - **Methadone** 0.2–0.5 mg/kg very slowly IV (very good analgesia, works for approx. 3–4 h, repeat if necessary) or
  - **Butorphanol** 0.2 mg/kg IV (either if no pure μ agonist is available or as preoperative sedation with quite good visceral analgesia, acts briefly, only approx. 30–40 min, can then be followed intraoperatively by e.g. fentanyl bolus and CRI)
- Other drugs
  - **Lidocaine** acts 1. as (preventive) therapy against premature ventricular extrasystoles, 2. as systemic analgesic, 3. +/– radical scavenger and 4. as prokinetic. Bolus 1–2 mg/kg IV over 10 min (equivalent to 0.05–0.1 ml/kg for 2% lidocaine), then CRI 0.03–0.08 mg/kg/min further perioperatively
  - **Omeprazole** 1 mg/kg before surgery orally, then every 12 h IV – proton pump inhibitor, inhibits gastric acid production, increases gastric pH

- ○ +/− **Maropitant** 1–2 mg/kg at least 2 h before surgery SC or PO, better over several days, against nausea and vomiting
- ○ +/− **Metoclopramide** 0.1–0.3 mg/kg every 8 h as prokinetic support
- ○ Antibiotic treatment: e.g. **cefazolin** 20 mg/kg slow IV every 8 h

7.9.2 Anaesthesia

As this is an absolute emergency and time plays a major role for the outcome, sedation or anaesthesia should be started quickly (after necessary stabilisation).

Sedation

Sedation is not usually necessary; rather, immediate analgesic treatment is indicated for this highly painful disease. Ideally, pure μ agonists are used.

Dosage

- **Methadone** 0.2–0.5 mg/kg very slowly IV OR **Fentanyl** 2–5 μg/kg or more very slowly IV +/−
- **Midazolam** OR **Diazepam** 0.2 mg/kg IV (then omit at induction)

Induction

After preoxygenation, induction of anaesthesia and intubation should be performed rapidly to avoid regurgitation and aspiration into the unprotected airways.

Dosage

- **Propofol** draw up 4–6 mg/kg in syringe, titrate slowly for induction. Often only half the dose is needed
- Can be combined with **Ketamine** 0.5–2 mg/kg depending on the patient's condition. Well suited as a bolus if it is given as a CRI afterwards. Has an analgesic effect in higher doses, reduces the dose of propofol, is generally protective of the cardiovascular system +/−
- **Midazolam** OR **Diazepam** 0.2 mg/kg. Hardly any cardiovascular or respiratory side effects, has many positive effects (relaxing, dose-reducing, amnesia, anxiolysis)

In practice, one would give about 1 mg/kg of propofol (i.e. a quarter of the dose), then ketamine (and midazolam), wait a little and then titrate further with propofol until an anaesthetic depth is reached at which intubation can be performed. Immediately connect to the breathing system of the anaesthesia machine, give 100% oxygen and inflate the cuff of the endotracheal tube. Ensure adequate ventilation; often the distended abdomen impairs physiological oxygenation and ventilation of CO_2. Positive pressure ventilation may be necessary.

Maintenance

Anaesthesia maintenance is based on inhalation anaesthesia plus analgesia.

Dosage

- **Isoflurane** OR **Sevoflurane** in O_2 titrated to effect AND
- **Fentanyl** initial bolus 2–5 μg/kg then CRI 0.2–0.5 μg/kg/min OR **Methadone** bolus 0.2–0.4 mg/kg IV every 3–4 h AND
- **Lidocaine** initial bolus 1–2 mg/kg very slow IV then CRI 0.03–0.08 mg/kg/min +/–
- **Ketamine** CRI 0.01–0.03 mg/kg/min

After "untwisting" the stomach, stabilise circulation with rapid bolus infusion (if necessary) and then start a perioperative maintenance dose: 10 ml/kg/h balanced electrolyte solution and, if necessary, continued administration of a colloid solution, i.e. HES. A continuous rate infusion with **methadone, lidocaine and ketamine** (**MLK**) is suitable for postoperative analgesic care. The mixture and dosages can be found in the box below. If the MLK drip is to be continued postoperatively, a different concentration in the analgesic mixture should be used, as the volume administered should be lower.

MLK: Methadone-Lidocaine-Ketamine as perioperative continuous rate infusion
NaCl 0.9% 500 ml PLUS
- **Methadone** 1 ml (= 10 mg, 1 ml with 10 mg/ml)
- **Lidocaine** 9 ml (= 180 mg, with 2% lidocaine containing 20 mg/ml)
- **Ketamine** 0.6 ml (= 60 mg, with 10% ketamine containing 100 mg/ml)
Mix well and label.

This mixture can be given **during surgery** at up to 10 ml/kg/h (titrate amount as needed) and ensures multimodal analgesia. One bag lasts approx. 1 h in the classic large gastric dilatation-volvulus patient. Therefore, several bags should be mixed at once if necessary. Shock infusion must be administered separately with balanced electrolyte solution (without additional drugs).

A **perioperative administration** of the MLK mixture of 10 ml/kg/h corresponds approximately to a dosage of methadone 0.2 mg/kg/h, lidocaine 0.06 mg/kg/min and ketamine 0.02 mg/kg/min. Titrate the dose down as needed over time. Of course, this type of analgesia can also be used for other painful procedures in small animals.

Monitoring, complications and therapy

In addition to the usual non-apparatus monitoring, vital signs should be monitored with the following apparatus monitoring: Pulse oximetry, ECG, (ideally invasive) blood pressure, capnography and core body temperature.

Problems to be expected in **patients with gastric dilatation-volvulus**:
- **Hypotension**
  - General risk, severe hypotension possible after "untwisting" the stomach
  - Keep **dopamine** continuous rate infusion (2–10 μg/kg/min or more) ready, should be used after all other measures such as reduction of anaesthetic dose and infusion have been unsuccessful (▶ Table 8.1)
- **Hypoventilation** due to pressure of the dilated stomach on the diaphragm
  - Positive pressure ventilation: Careful! Use a higher frequency and smaller volume!
  - Support circulation (reduced circulation due to shock or endotoxin release also reduces ventilation)

- **Hypoxaemia** due to pressure of the dilated stomach on the diaphragm
  - Continuous oxygen administration
  - Positive pressure ventilation in case of hypoventilation
- **ECG changes** or **arrhythmias** (premature ventricular extrasystoles)
  - Prevention or therapy should already be started preoperatively
  - Lidocaine bolus and CRI
- **Hypothermia**
  - Active temperature management
  - Lavage of the abdomen with **warm** (!) flushing solution
- Aspiration (p. 396) risk due to distended stomach and exploration/flushing of the stomach
  - Ensure that the cuff of the endotracheal tube is adequately inflated
  - If necessary, wash out the oral cavity and oesophagus after surgery (warm water with or without added bicarbonate)
  - If extubation is necessary, potentially leave cuff slightly inflated in order to pull out regurgitated stomach contents or reflux material

7.9.3 Postoperative management

Depending on the condition of the patient preoperatively and the surgical findings, the postoperative care is adapted. In addition to continuous monitoring (comparable to perioperative monitoring), the following should be considered:
- Administer **oxygen** continuously
- **Volume status** is checked and adjusted (infusion)
- **Vital signs** such as heart rate and blood pressure as well as oxygenation are checked
- Continuous **ECG monitoring** is ensured (▶ Fig. 7.6), in case of increasing numbers of premature ventricular extrasystoles, an additional bolus of lidocaine (1 mg/kg slow IV) may help
- Ensure a **calm and stress-free environment**
- Administer sufficient **analgesics** or **antiarrhythmics** (**opioids**, **ketamine** and **lidocaine** CRI)
- Check and balance out **acid-base balance** and **electrolyte concentrations**
- **Continue** as before
  - **Omeprazole** 1 mg/kg every 12 h IV
  - **Maropitant** 1–2 mg/kg SC or PO once a day OR
    Ondansetron 0.1–0.2 mg/kg IV every 8 h
  - **Metoclopramide** 0.1–0.3 mg/kg every 8 h IV or 1 mg/kg over 24 h as CRI
  - Antibiotic treatment: e.g. **cefazolin** 20 mg/kg slow IV every 8 h

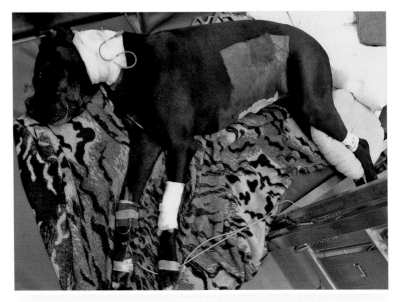

Fig. 7.6 Great Dane postoperatively after gastric dilatation-volvulus surgery: Two large lumen venous accesses in the cephalic vein with continuous infusion, oesophageal feeding tube, continuous monitoring (electrocardiogram and non-invasive blood pressure measurement).

Practice tip

Calculation of the lidocaine CRI dose

A syringe pump is required for the controlled and continuous administration of drugs.

- Lidocaine 2% equals 20 mg/ml
- Postoperative dose approx. **0.03**–0.06 mg/kg/min, maximum 8 mg/kg/24 h

Example calculation:
Dog weighs 35 kg

$$0.03 \,(mg) \times 35 \,(kg) \times 60 \,(min) = 63 \,(mg/h)$$
$$63 \,(mg/h) : 20 \,(mg/ml = Lidocaine\ concentration) = 3.15\ ml/h$$

So, 3.15 ml/h must be administered to this patient. If arrhythmias occur, the dose can be doubled (0.06 mg/kg/min) = 6.3 ml/h

7.9.4 Literature

[1] Bruchim Y, Itay S, Shira BH, Kelmer E, Sigal Y, Itamar A, Gilad S. Evaluation of lidocaine treatment on frequency of cardiac arrhythmias, acute kidney injury, and hospitalization time in dogs with gastric dilatation volvulus. J Vet Emerg Crit Care 2012; 22: 419–427

[2] Figueiredo, JP, Green, TA. Gastrointestinal disease In: Snyder & Johnson (Eds.), Canine and feline anaesthesia and co-existing disease, 1. edition, Wiley Blackwell, 105–110, 2015

[3] Glickman LT, Glickman W, Pérez CM, Schellenberg DB, Lantz GC. Analysis of risk factors for gastric dilatation and dilatation-volvulus in dogs. J Am Vet Med Assoc 1994; 204: 1465–1471

[4] Green TI, Tonozzi CC, Kirby R, Rudloff E. Evaluation of initial plasma lactate values as a predictor of gastric necrosis and initial and subsequent plasma lactate values as a predictor of survival in dogs with gastric dilatation-volvulus: 84 dogs (2003–2007). J Vet Emerg Crit Care. 2011; 21: 36–44

[5] Mackenzie G, Banhart M, Kennedy S, DeHoff W, Schertel E. A retrospective study of factors influencing survival following surgery for gastric dilatation-volvulus syndrome in 306 dogs. J Am Vet Med Assoc 2010; 46: 97–102

7.10 Patient with diabetes mellitus

Diabetes mellitus (DM) is most common in dogs and cats. A similar disease, equine metabolic syndrome (similar to DM type 2), is also frequently diagnosed in horses. Sporadically, DM occurs in large and small ruminants, ferrets, rabbits, guinea pigs, chinchillas and pigs. The management of a patient with DM for anaesthesia highly depends on preanaesthetic preparation of the patient. Glucose levels should be largely within normal limits and ketones should be low so that there is no risk of sliding into diabetic ketoacidosis.

Feline DM often affects older, male, neutered cats that are kept indoors and are overweight. This DM is similar to DM type 2 in humans, in which there is a relative, later absolute insulin deficiency.

Canine DM is similar to DM type 1 in humans. Older, female, neutered, obese animals are most often affected.

▶ **Anamnesis.** Polyuria, polydipsia, polyphagia, weight/muscle loss

▶ **Clinical symptoms**
• **Cat:** Shaggy, dull coat, polyneuropathy
• **Dog:** Cataract, cushingoid appearance

▶ **Diagnostics.** Blood test (hyperglycaemia, hyperfructosaminaemia, ketonaemia) and urine test (glucosuria, ketonuria)

7.10.1 Preoperative management

Ideally, it is already known that the patient suffers from DM and glucose values are controlled within the normal range with the help of regular insulin administration by the owner. On the morning of surgery, **half the usual insulin dose** is administered to the fasting animal.

If DM is an incidental finding during the preoperative blood test, it must be considered whether surgery must be performed immediately (emergency) or whether the patient can (ideally) be adjusted beforehand.

Stress and pain should be avoided as much as possible to avoid causing additional stress hyperglycaemia (especially in cats). The following should be prepared for perioperative management:

- Flushing and infusion solutions: **NaCl 0.9%** and Ringer's lactate or other **balanced electrolyte solution**
- **Potassium maleate** as an additive to the infusion solution
- **50% glucose** solution as an additive to the infusion solution
- (Norm-)Insulin
- Glucometer

The DM patient's surgery should be scheduled as **first thing in the morning** to avoid fasting the patient for too long, to give them time to recover and feed, and to ensure postoperative monitoring.

7.10.2 Anaesthesia

In general, all sedatives and anaesthetics can be used. Only the use of alpha2 agonists such as xylazine (p. 145), dexmedetomidine (p. 86) and medetomidine (p. 111) is controversial because they interfere with glucose levels (cause hyperglycaemia).

Careful!

Use of alpha2 agonists in patients with diabetes mellitus is controversial
Alpha2 agonists inhibit insulin secretion and therefore contribute to hyperglycaemia.

Sedation

Particularly low-stress handling of the patient should be emphasised in order not to increase glucose levels unnecessarily. It is even recommended to sedate the patient before placing the IV catheter or to place the catheter the day before (this ideally allows infusion therapy and glucose monitoring overnight).

Monitoring, complications and therapy

In addition to the usual non-apparatus monitoring, blood glucose should be measured at regular intervals (approx. every 30–60 min). All that is needed to obtain blood is a needle prick on the footpad or ear, and a glucometer can then be used to measure glucose. If the glucose level is below normal, glucose should be added to the infusion solution (e.g. Ringer's lactate solution) to get a 2.5% solution (5 ml 50% glucose in 95 ml Ringer's lactate solution). If the glucose level continues to fall, the concentration can be increased to 5% (10 ml of 50% glucose to 90 ml of Ringer's lactate solution). Infusion rates depend on the individual patient and range from 2 to 10 ml/kg/h. If glucose concentration increases, there should be no added glucose in the infusion solution. If it continues to increase, about a quarter of the otherwise used daily dose of normal insulin SC can be administered.

Good to know

Normal values glucose
- **Dog:** 60–110 mg/dl
- **Cat:** 70–150 mg/dl

Conversion: mmol/l × 18 = mg/dl resp. mg/dl × 0.0555 = mmol/l

Electrolytes – especially sodium (p. 390) and potassium (p. 386) – and acid-base status (p. 392) should be measured before and at least once during anaesthesia and corrected if necessary. Hydration status (p. 163) should be assessed based on clinical findings (▶ Table 5.2).

Possible complications (and ways to avoid them) are:
- Risk of aspiration (p. 396) due to possible polyneuropathy (in any case intubate and inflate the cuff of the endotracheal tube properly)
- **Haemodynamic instability:** Prepare infusion therapy, possibly cardiovascular support drugs such as dopamine (▶ Table 8.1)
- **Problems with positioning** of cachectic animals: Position gently to avoid pressure lesions or nerve damage

- **Risk of infection/wound healing disorder**: Work cleanly, possibly antibiotics if indicated; the placement of a urinary catheter should be avoided if possible

7.10.3 Postoperative management

Attention should be paid to adequate pain management at all times to minimise additional stress and the associated influence on glucose levels.

Glucose, electrolytes, acid-base and hydration status should be checked and corrected at least once postoperatively. Once the animal has fully recovered from anaesthesia and is eating again, insulin therapy can be continued as preoperatively.

7.10.4 Literature

[1] Cook AK. Monitoring methods for dogs and cats with diabetes mellitus. J Diabetes Sci Technol 2012; 6: 491–495

[2] Reusch CE, Tschuor F, Kley S, Boretti F, Sieber-Ruckstuhl N. Diabetes mellitus bei der Katze: Ein Überblick. Schweiz Arch Tierheilkd 2006; 148: 130–138

7.11 Colic in horses

Anaesthesia of horses with colic is demanding and costly, especially if the animals are already endotoxaemic or have severely dilated intestinal loops. The colic patient is extremely painful and multimorbid with abnormalities in volume status, haemodynamic parameters, blood-gas analysis and electrolyte and acid-base balance. Extensive stabilisation of the patient before induction of anaesthesia is usually not possible due to the urgency of the surgery. Work should therefore be concentrated, rapid and ideally well-prepared in order to get the patient "on the table" in a reasonable time.

7.11.1 Preoperative management

Preparation: To save time, it would be ideal if the rooms for induction of anaesthesia and surgery, including the anaesthesia machine and ventilator, were prepared before the arrival of the colic patient; all equipment should be checked and fully functional

History and clinical examination: The duration of colic symptoms, previous treatment (drugs: dose, time of last administration and reaction of the animal), any medical conditions (orthopaedic, laryngeal paralysis, etc.) and known problems/reactions with previous anaesthesia should be enquired about; a full clinical examination should be performed

Further diagnostics: A blood test including haematocrit, total protein, acid-base parameters as well as lactate, creatinine, electrolytes (sodium, potassium, chloride, ionised calcium) and glucose should be performed

Stabilisation of the patient: After placing at least one 10–14 G IV catheter in the jugular vein (rather two in severely ill animals!), infusion therapy should be started immediately to normalise volume status and balance acid-base status and electrolytes; provide adequate analgesia, possibly start lidocaine CRI at this stage to counteract endotoxaemia

Practice tip

Basic information on fluid therapy for colic patients

1. Calculate the fluid deficit and replace as much as possible before induction of anaesthesia; example: a 500 kg horse that is 10% dehydrated means a deficit of 50 litres. Hypertonic NaCl solution, isotonic NaCl or balanced electrolyte solutions and additional colloidal solutions can be used for infusion
2. Calculate the maintenance rate per hour; example: 2 ml/kg/h for this 500 kg horse, means 1 l/h – add that rate on
3. Add additional losses; example: haemorrhage, reflux, etc. – estimate the lost volume and add that on

During anaesthesia, 2 and 3 are often combined as the "anaesthesia maintenance rate" at 5–10 ml/kg/h. This rate is intended to replace the actual maintenance requirements as well as a small deficit and additional losses.

Clinical relevance

Which infusion solution should you chose for (fast) rehydration?

It is not entirely clear which infusion solution is best to use for initial rehydration. There is some evidence in favour of **hypertonic saline (NaCl 7.5%)**. The effect lasts about 20–30 min in the horse and the effect is achieved faster than with **isotonic solutions**. It is recommended to combine NaCl 7.5% with **colloidal solutions (HES)** to reduce redistribution into the tissue and therefore the formation of oedema.

One recommendation is:

Initial 2–4 ml/kg NaCl 7.5% IV as soon as possible, combined with or subsequently isotonic (balanced) electrolyte solution and if total protein and/or blood pressure are low additionally colloidal solutions (HES), max. 20 ml/kg/24 h.

If the animal allows it, the surgical field can be clipped and washed before induction. Do not forget to rinse out the mouth!

Plan and objectives for anaesthesia of a **horse with colic** are:

- **Correct acid-base deviations** and **electrolyte changes, keep glucose** within a **normal** range
- **Normotension**
  - Avoid hypotension (MAP < 70 mmHg)
  - Restore normovolaemia and physiological hydration status, restore colloid osmotic pressure
  - Cardiovascular support with positive inotropic or vasoconstrictive drugs (▶ Table 8.1)
- **Address arrhythmias**
- **Avoid hypoxaemia/hypoxia**
  - Continuous administration of 100% oxygen
  - Ventilation: Ultimate goal is always tissue oxygenation, mode of ventilation (frequency, volume, alveolar recruitment) and cardiovascular parameters (blood pressure, perfusion) must be weighed against each other
- **Avoid hypercapnia**
  - Ventilation with consideration of cardiovascular parameters: Do not ventilate at all costs, e.g. if blood pressure is poor; keyword: permissive hypercapnia, i.e. possibly allow slightly higher CO_2 values
- **Normothermia**
  - Active warming; many colic horses are already hypothermic before induction of anaesthesia
- **Analgesia**

7.11.2 Anaesthesia

The choice of anaesthetics is much more limited for horses than for small animals and unfortunately there is no one, correct protocol! The protocol for the colic horse differs little from that for a healthy horse with a planned surgery. The main difference is in the preparation phase and the complex perioperative management. If this is done well, the likelihood that the patient will get through this severe illness and surgery increases.

Sedation

Premedication consists of a combination of an alpha2 agonists and an opioid.

Dosage

- **Xylazine** 0.5–0.7 mg/kg IV, potentially less. Wait a few minutes for the effect, THEN
- **Butorphanol** 0.01–0.03 mg/kg OR a pure μ opioid agonist (**Morphine** or **Methadone**) 0.1 mg/kg slowly IV

If the animal is already heavily sedated after the administration of xylazine or wants to go down, the opioid can also be given later under controlled conditions during anaesthesia. Acepromazine should be avoided especially in the hypovolaemic patient.

Induction

Ketamine in combination with a benzodiazepine or other muscle relaxant IV is suitable as an induction drug:

Dosage

- **Ketamine** up to 2 mg/kg IV AND
- **Midazolam** OR **Diazepam** 0.05–0.1 mg/kg IV

Whether ketamine or the benzodiazepine is administered first probably makes no difference. In **very sick animals**, the **ketamine dose should be significantly reduced** (down to ⅓ of the normal dose).

Intubation and cuff inflation should be done as soon as possible after induction of anaesthesia. Before transport to the operating table, check that the depth of anaesthesia is adequate and eye ointment can be applied at this stage. Then connect to the breathing system of the anaesthesia machine as soon as possible to be able to provide oxygen, attach monitoring equipment and place an arterial catheter.

Maintenance

It is best to use a balanced anaesthesia technique based on inhalation anaesthesia in combination with analgesics. Dosages of continuous rate infusions need to be continuously titrated down over time!

Dosage

- **Isofluran** (p. 102) in 100% O_2 as low a dose as possible (1 MAC for horses 1.3%) AND
- **Ketamine** (p. 105) CRI 0.01–0.05 mg/kg/min IV AND
- **Lidocaine** (p. 108) bolus 1–2 mg/kg over 15 min followed by CRI 0.05 mg/kg/min. CRI should be switched off 20 min before the end of general anaesthesia, otherwise there will be increased ataxia in the recovery phase.

Practice tip

Viennese double-drip for colics

1. Prepare a 500 ml NaCl 0.9% bag with 10 ml Ketamine (100 mg/ml) and 3 ml Midazolam (5 mg/ml), mix well and label!
2. Administer 0.6 ml/kg/h from the start of anaesthesia using an infusion pump; MAC isoflurane is significantly reduced, maintenance phase is rather stable
3. Reduce the dose over time
4. Switch off double-drip 10–15 min prior to the end of the administration of the inhalation anaesthetic
5. Antagonise midazolam with flumazenil at the earliest after 15 min in recovery when the horse already shows signs of waking up

Monitoring, complications and therapy

As with any anaesthesia, vital signs should be continuously monitored and documented. It is important in large animals to constantly monitor the depth of anaesthesia! Invasive blood pressure measurement, arterial blood gases as well as control of the ventilator setting or ventilation are among the most important parameters.

Good to know

Anaesthesia time = complication time
Every possible effort should be made to keep the anaesthesia time as short as possible!

The **most important complications** to be expected and their therapy are:
- **Hypotension**
  - Compensate for hypovolaemia or low colloid osmotic pressure (infusion of crystalloid and colloid solutions)
  - Perioperatively, a **dobutamine** CRI 0.5–5 µg/kg/min can be used after all other measures such as reduction of the anaesthetic dose and infusion have failed to achieve the desired result (▶ Table 8.1)
  - In horses that are not yet tachycardic, **ephedrine** can also be given as a bolus 0.05–0.2 mg/kg slowly IV to increase blood pressure
  - Bolus **norepinephrine** or CRI 0.01–1 µg/kg/min will produce severe vasoconstriction, resulting in higher blood pressure but also drastically reduced perfusion; use cautiously
  - If possible, allow spontaneous ventilation as long as there is normocapnia and normoxaemia; consider on the basis of the clinical situation whether ventilation is necessary immediately or whether it can/must be waited for
- **Hypoventilation**
  - Positive pressure ventilation; hypercapnia can often be tolerated if hypotension does not permit more aggressive ventilation and as long as oxygenation is within a tolerable range
- **ECG changes** or **arrhythmias**
  - Often premature ventricular extrasystoles, then give lidocaine as CRI
- **Hypoxaemia** due to low V/Q ratio and cranial displacement of the diaphragm
  - Reduce pressure on diaphragm as soon as possible; surgeon should gain access and deflate intestines quickly
  - Regular monitoring by pulse oximetry and arterial blood gas analysis
  - Give 100% oxygen
  - Positive pressure ventilation; try to achieve the best possible oxygenation through different ventilator settings: Tidal volume, respiratory rate, inspiration to expiration ratio, maximum inspiratory pressure, recruitment manoeuvre, positive end-expiratory pressure (PEEP)
  - Possibly use bronchodilator (salbutamol as aerosol)
  - Possibly use reverse Trendelenburg position (p. 272): Tilt the table so that the head is high and the back is low
- **Deviations in acid-base** and **electrolyte balance**
  - Targeted balancing
- **Full urinary bladder**
  - This causes stress and pain for the animal, especially in the recovery phase, and may cause the horse to try to get up too early, so it is best to place a urinary catheter at the beginning of anaesthesia

- **Hypothermia**
  - Ideally active warming (warm air blower)
  - Passive warming (rescue blanket)
- **Pain**
  - Administer analgesics in time

7.11.3 Recovery and postoperative management

The recovery box should be dry, clean, warm and quiet. The patient should continue to be monitored during the recovery phase as there is a continuing risk of the animals getting worse both haemodynamically and in terms of blood gases, acid-base balance and electrolytes.

- **Monitoring**
  - Pulse oximeter
  - Temperature
  - In very sick animals possibly blood pressure
- Horses, especially those that were hypoxaemic during anaesthesia, should continue to be ventilated with **100% O_2**
  - Ventilate with a **demand valve** until they breathe spontaneously
  - From then on with insufflation of O_2 via the tube or after extubation via the nose
- Continue **infusion**
- Give phenylephrine 0.15% in each nostril in time to **decongest nasal mucosa** (horses are obligate nasal breathers)
- **Reduce hypothermia**, even while the animal is still lying down
  - Dry with towels or similar
  - Warm air blower and possibly a sweat blanket
  - Prevent air draft
- **Pull out urinary catheter**
- If possible, (smaller) horses should be placed in **sternal recumbency**
  - Improves oxygenation
  - Helps reduce swelling of the nasal mucosa
- **Analgesia,** more options see chapter "Postoperative pain management concepts: Horse" (p. 411)
  - **Flunixin meglumine** 1.1 mg/kg slow IV every 12 h already start preoperatively
  - Continue CRI **lidocaine** after getting up
  - Possibly CRI **butorphanol** 0.013 mg/kg/h (relatively expensive, but very effective!) or **methadone** or **morphine** 0.1–0.2 mg/kg slow IV every 4 h +/–
  - **Ketamine** CRI

Animals are often weak and attempts to stand up are uncoordinated. Support with head and tail ropes can be helpful. If the patient is not standing after several hours, it should be encouraged to get up. If this does not help, it may be useful to cover the floor of the recovery box with straw and continue postoperative care on site.

7.11.4 Literature

[1] Blaze CA, Robinson NE. Apneic oxygenation in anesthetized ponies and horses. Vet Res Commun 1987; 11: 281–291

[2] Boesch JM. Anesthesia for the horse with colic. Vet Clin North Am Equine Pract 2013; 29: 193–214

[3] Clutton RE. Opioid analgesia in horses. Vet Clin North Am Equine Pract 2010; 26: 493–514

[4] Corley KT. Inotropes and vasopressors in adults and foals. Vet Clin North Am Equine Pract 2004; 20: 77–106

[5] Doherty TJ, Seddighi MR. Local anesthetics as pain therapy in horses. Vet Clin North Am Equine Pract 2010; 26: 533–549

[6] Gleed RD, Dobson A. Improvement in arterial oxygen tension with change in posture in anaesthetized horses. Res Vet Sci 1988; 44: 255–259

[7] Kelmer G. Update on treatments for endotoxemia. Vet Clin North Am Equine Pract 2009; 25: 259–270

[8] Koenig J, McDonell W, Valverde A. Accuracy of pulse oximetry and capnography in healthy and compromised horses during spontaneous and controlled ventilation. Can J Vet Res 2003; 67: 169–174

[9] Lee YH, Clark KW, Alibhai HI, Song D. Effects of dopamine, dobutamine, dopexamine, phenylephrine, and saline solution on intramuscular blood flow and other cardiopulmonary variables in halothane-anesthetized ponies. Am J Vet Res 1998; 59: 1463–1472

[10] Rezende ML, Wagner AE, Mama KR, Ferreura TH, Steffey EP. Effect of intravenous administration of lidocaine on the minimum alveolar concentration of sevoflurane in horses. Am J Vet Res 2011; 72: 446–451

[11] Sellon DC, Roberts MC, Blikslager AT, Ulibarri C, Papich MG. Effects of continuous rate intravenous infusion of butorphanol on physiologic and outcome variables in horses after celiotomy. J Vet Intern Med 2004; 18: 555–563

[12] Villalba M, Santiago I, Gomez de Segura IA. Effects of constant rate infusion of lidocaine and ketamine, with or without morphine, on isoflurane MAC in horses. Equine Vet J 2011; 43: 721–726

[13] Wendt-Hornickle EL, Snyder LB, Tang R, Johnson RA. The effects of lactated Ringer's solution (LRS) or LRS and 6% Hetastarch on the colloid osmotic pressure, total protein and osmolarity in healthy horses under general anesthesia. Vet Anaesth Analg 2011; 38: 336–343

7.12 Foals

Anaesthesia of foals up to 4 weeks of age can be challenging even for the experienced practitioner. Mortality is more than $7\times$ higher than in adult horses. The physiological and pharmacological characteristics of the neonatal patient (p.262) must be considered. In particular, the increased oxygen requirement must be taken into account by administering oxygen continuously.

7.12.1 Preoperative management

History and clinical examination: The induction of anaesthesia should be preceded by a thorough clinical examination with special attention to the cardiovascular system. A machine murmur on auscultation of the heart in the 1st week of life indicates an as yet unoccluded ductus arteriosus (p. 287), which may be of haemodynamic significance.

The basic blood values haematocrit, total protein and glucose should be measured.

The foal should be allowed to suckle until shortly before anaesthesia. The mare and foal should always be handled calmly and together; only shortly before induction of anaesthesia should the mare be led away. In the case of suckling foals, the mouth does not need to be rinsed out before induction of anaesthesia.

Sedate the mare!
Many mares react extremely distraught when the foal is taken away from them. It helps to leave the mother with the foal as long as possible, if possible until sedation or anaesthesia induction of the foal. A tried and tested combination to sedate a mare (approx. 500 kg) is:
- **Acepromazine** (10 mg/ml) 1 ml AND
- **Detomidine** (10 mg/ml) 1 ml

mixed in one syringe and then give half the amount of IV, half the amount of IM.

If the mare does not calm down, half the dose can be re-administered.

Plan and objectives for anaesthesia of a foal:
- **Normotension**
  - Cardiac output is predominantly dependent on heart rate, therefore, it should be kept within the physiological range (foals: 70–100 beats/min) and bradycardia avoided (do not use alpha2 agonists such as xylazine in very young or hypovolaemic animals); if invasive blood pressure measurement is not possible, oscillometric blood pressure measurement (cuff proximal to the fetlock joint) can also be used
- **Avoid hypoxaemia and hypercapnia**
  - Continuous administration of 100% oxygen; this is particularly important because consumption is approx. 2–3 times higher than in adult animals

- Ventilation: For longer procedures, manual or mechanical ventilation should be used, as the respiratory muscles tire over time; ventilation should be adapted to the physiological respiration of the foal: Higher respiratory rate (20–50 breaths/min, the younger the faster) and lower tidal volume
- **Normothermia**
  - Active warming, foals cool down quickly due to their large surface area compared to their small mass; shivering in the recovery phase increases the oxygen requirement considerably
- **Analgesia**
  - Buprenorphine 0.01 mg/kg IV every 6 h and/or phenylbutazone 2.2–4.4 mg/kg PO/IV every 12–24 h in foals > 1 month of age

7.12.2 Anaesthesia

Good preparation helps to minimise the risk of complications. Depending on the size and weight of the animal or the size of the endotracheal tube, a small animal (up to approx. 150 kg body weight) or large animal anaesthesia machine (from approx. 150 kg) is used. Before the foal is anaesthetised, different tube sizes, suitable adapters and the appropriate anaesthesia machine and breathing system should have been set up and tested. If no anaesthesia machine is used, oxygen should be supplied with a mask via the nostrils or a tube in the ventral nasal passage (flow rate approx. 5–10 l/min).

One should always place an **IV catheter** for the administration of drugs and infusion solutions. The jugular vein is the most suitable. If this is not possible while awake, IM sedation helps. A small depot of local anaesthetic in the puncture area also helps to minimise defensive reactions.

As foals have a higher body water content than adults, they are particularly susceptible to fluid loss. **Perioperative infusion** should be given, e.g. Ringer's lactate solution 5–10 ml/kg/h. If anaesthesia is prolonged, the bladder should be emptied before the recovery phase at the latest, but it is better to place a urinary catheter at the beginning of the procedure.

After induction of anaesthesia, **orotracheal intubation** is performed blindly with the head fully extended, as in the adult horse. Another possibility is **nasotracheal intubation**, which can also be performed in the cooperative awake or already sedated foal. For this, the tube is coated with lubricant containing lidocaine and inserted into the ventral nasal passage. The head must be extended considerably in order to be able to advance the tube through the larynx into the trachea. The correct fit must be checked (fogging of the inner wall of the tube with expiration, capnography). For animals weighing approx. 50–80 kg, tube sizes of 8–12 mm ID are used.

345

Especially in cold weather or under field conditions, the foal should be protected from heat loss or better **actively warmed** from the beginning. Legs can be bandaged for protection.

Sedation

The choice of premedication depends primarily on age and condition of the foal.

For foals up to the 1st week of life:

Dosage

- **Midazolam** IM or IV OR **Diazepam** IV (do not mix) 0.05–0.2 mg/kg can be combined very well to deepen sedation and as an analgesic component AND
- **Butorphanol** 0.1–0.2 mg/kg IM or IV

In normovolaemic foals from the 2nd to the 4th week of life:

Dosage

- **Xylazine** IM or IV 0.3–1 mg/kg can be combined very well WITH
- **Butorphanol** 0.1 mg/kg IM or IV

In normovolaemic foals between the 4th week and the 3rd month of life:

Dosage

- **Acepromazine** 0.01–0.04 IM or IV causes mild sedation lasting several hours (caution: vasodilation → hypotension and cooling), wait approx. 30 min, THEN
- **Xylazine** IM or IV 0.5 mg/kg can be combined very well WITH
- **Butorphanol** 0.1 mg/kg IM or IV

If the animal is already very sedated after the administration of xylazine and has settled down, the opioid can also be given later under controlled conditions during anaesthesia.

Induction

Appropriate induction drugs are include ketamine in combination with a benzodiazepine.

Dosage

- **Isoflurane** OR **Sevoflurane** in 100% O_2 via the endotracheal tube if the foal, awake or sedated, could already be intubated nasotracheally OR
- **Propofol** 2–4 mg/kg IV OR **Ketamine** 2 mg/kg IV AND
- **Midazolam** OR **Diazepam** 0.05–0.1 mg/kg IV, if it has not already been administered as part of premedication

Maintenance

It is best to use a balanced anaesthesia technique based on inhalation anaesthesia in combination with analgesics.

Dosage

- **Isoflurane** in 100% O_2 dosed as low as possible (about 1–1.5%) AND
- **Ketamine** CRI 0.05 mg/kg/min IV AND/OR
- **Butorphanol** bolus 0.05 mg/kg IV every 60 min as needed

Analgesia: One should always check whether local anaesthesia is possible for surgical interventions. **Lidocaine** can be used up to a dose of 4 mg/kg per 24 h. In foals > 1 month, the NSAIDs **phenylbutazone** 2.2–4.4 mg/kg every 12–24 h PO or IV or **carprofen** 0.7 mg/kg IM can be given.

Monitoring, complications and therapy

As with any anaesthesia, vital signs should be continuously monitored and documented. In addition, haematocrit, total protein and glucose should be checked at regular intervals. In foals with a ruptured bladder, additionally check electrolytes. Deviations from physiological values should be treated immediately.

The **most common complications** to be expected and their treatment are:
- **Hypotension**
  - Compensate for hypovolaemia or low colloid osmotic pressure

- Ringer's lactate solution 10–30 ml/kg/h and (if necessary)
- Colloid solution, e.g. HES 5–10 ml/kg/h and (if necessary)
- Dobutamine CRI 0.5–2 µg/kg/min or more
- If possible, let the patient breathe spontaneously as long as there is normocapnia and normoxaemia so as not to impair venous return to the heart

- **Hypoventilation/hypercapnia**
  - Positive pressure ventilation; try to simulate physiological breathing: Tidal volume rather small (10 ml/kg or less), respiratory rate rather high (approx. 20 breaths/min), maximum inspiratory pressure (10–20 cmH$_2$O)

- **Hypoxaemia**
  - Regular monitoring by pulse oximetry and arterial blood gas analysis
  - Administration of 100% oxygen

- **Acid-base and electrolyte balance abnormalities**
  - Targeted balancing

- **Full urinary bladder** (particularly after administration of xylazine)
  - Causes stress and pain for the animal, especially in the recovery phase; it is best to place a urinary catheter at the beginning of anaesthesia

- **Hypothermia**
  - Active warming (warm air blower, heating mat, warm infusion solution)
  - Passive warming (blanket, keep clipped area small, keep body surface dry, use bandages on legs)

- **Pain**
  - Administer analgesics in time

7.12.3 Recovery and postoperative management

The recovery environment should be dry, clean, warm and calm. The foal should continue to be monitored during the recovery phase, checking temperature, pulse quality and rate, respiratory rate and oxygenation using a pulse oximeter would be ideal. If deviations from normal values are measured, appropriate therapy should be initiated (including active warming, infusion therapy, oxygen administration) to return parameters to the physiological range.

Phenylephrine 0.15% should be given in each nostril in time to decongest the nasal mucosa (foals are also obligate nasal breathers).

Analgesia must not be neglected after surgical procedures (especially) in foals: The keyword is pain memory. Opioids (e.g. **buprenorphine** 0.01 mg/kg IV) are primarily used after painful procedures, and NSAIDs are also used in older foals. Ideally, animals should be supported by one person at a time when standing up by the halter and tail. The mother mare should be allowed near as soon as the foal is standing. The foal should start to suckle again as soon as it is able to swallow.

7.12.4 Literature

[1] Carter SW, Robertson SA, Steel CJ, Jourdenais DA. Cardiopulmonary effects of xylazine sedation in the foal. Equine Vet J 1990; 22: 384–388

[2] Johnston GM, Eastment JK, Wood JLN, Taylor PM. The confidential enquiry into perioperative equine fatalities (CEPEF): mortality results of phases 1 and 2. Vet Anaesth Analg 2002; 29: 159–170

[3] Tranquilli WJ, Thurmon JC. Management of anesthesia in the foal. Vet Clin North Am Equine Pract 1990; 6: 651–663

[4] Robertson SA. Sedation and general anaesthesia of the foal. Equine Vet Educ 2005; 7: 94–101

II

8 Anaesthetic incidents and complications

Before performing any anaesthesia, one should think about anticipated complications. It is best to **sort thoughts** so that preparation is as good as it can be and then keeps the risk manageable and predictable:

1. **Complications that may occur with this individual animal**, species and breed (p.150)
2. **Complications that may occur with this procedure** (p.271)
3. **Complications that may occur with the anaesthesia** or the chosen anaesthetics (p.63)

During anaesthesia there is (almost) always a depression of cardiovascular function and respiration as well as a decrease in core body temperature. Less frequently, there are shifts in acid-base or electrolyte balance or regurgitation/aspiration of foreign material into the trachea or lung. The better one can 1. recognise possible complications, 2. assess their consequences, 3. avoid them and 4. treat them, the more relaxed anaesthesia will be for both, anaesthetist and patient.

8.1 Cardiovascular system

Veterinarians usually have to deal with **hypotension** (in contrast to human medicine, where hypertension is the bigger problem) with their anaesthetised patients. It is important to understand what physiological conditions influence blood pressure so that the cause of hypotension can be identified and treated as specifically as possible (▶ Fig. 8.1). Rarely **hypertension** does occur, the approach is similar. The most common perioperative **arrhythmia** is sinus bradycardia, which is often easy to treat once the cause is identified.

An assessment of the circulatory situation is made with the help of clinical (non-apparatus) monitoring of perfusion parameters (p.41) and blood pressure measurement (p.47).

8.1.1 Hypotension/cardiovascular failure

Perioperative hypotension is defined as a mean arterial blood pressure (MAP) below 65–70 mmHg (small animal) or 70–75 mmHg (horse). When the MAP falls below this value, the autoregulation of the vital organs (brain, kidneys, heart) and therefore their adequate supply with oxygen can no longer be guaranteed.

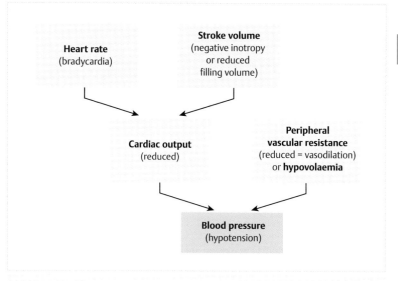

Fig. 8.1 Parameters responsible for the development of blood pressure. The classic causes of hypotension during anaesthesia are in brackets.

Possible causes

- Level of anaesthesia too deep
- Bradycardia (e.g. due to hypothermia)
- Hypovolaemia
- Vasodilation (e.g. due to inhalation anaesthetics, propofol)
- Negative inotropy (= reduced stroke volume)
- Positive pressure ventilation (reduces venous return to the heart)
- Deviations in electrolyte concentrations or acid-base balance

Complications/consequences

- Reduced perfusion/oxygenation of the periphery or, in the worst case, of vital organs
  - ◦ Temporary or permanent blindness
  - ◦ Temporary or permanent deafness
- Acute renal failure
- Myopathy (especially in large animals)
- Cardiac arrest, death

Prophylaxis/therapy

- Know the causes of hypotension in advance and avoid/treat them
- Adjust depth of anaesthesia
- Infusion/bolus with crystalloid, then colloidal solutions
- Circulatory support drugs (▶ Table 8.1); efficacy only fully given if patient is normothermic
- Administration of atropine or glycopyrrolate to treat vagally mediated bradycardia
- (Partial) antagonisation of alpha2 agonists
- Positive inotropic drugs: Dobutamine, dose-dependent dopamine
- Drugs that cause vasoconstriction: Dopamine, noradrenalin, phenylephrine
- Correction of electrolyte imbalances and metabolic abnormalities
- Adjustment of ventilation parameters (possibly less pressure, higher frequency)
- Start resuscitation

A list of drugs that support circulation, including dosages, can be found in ▶ Table 8.1. Emergency drugs and their dosages according to weight can be found in ▶ Table 10.1.

8.1.2 Hypertension

That a patient becomes hypertensive during anaesthesia is rather the exception, provided that a balanced anaesthetic regime is used. The term severe hypertension is used to describe a blood pressure at which the autoregulated organs can no longer maintain constant perfusion, i. e. at a mean arterial blood pressure of > 160 mmHg.

Possible causes

- Too light anaesthesia
- Insufficient analgesia
- Sympathetic stimulation (release of catecholamines due to e.g. pain stimulus or pheochromocytoma)
- Administration of drugs: Adrenalin, noradrenalin, ephedrine, phenylephrine, the initial phase after alpha2 agonist administration
- Indirectly via tachycardia e.g. iatrogenically caused by atropine/glycopyrrolate (especially when administered to treat bradycardia caused by alpha2 agonists)
- Primary disease (e.g. hyperthyroidism)

Table 8.1 Overview of receptor binding, mechanism of action, dose and exemplary indication of the circulatory supportive drugs

Drug	Receptor	Mechanism of action	Dose IV	Example for indication
Atropine (Parasympatholytic)	Muscarinic receptor antagonist	Positive chronotropic effect	0.02–0.04 mg/kg	Vagally mediated bradycardia (opioids, oculo-cardiac reflex or as part of resuscitation)
Glycopyrrolate (Parasympatholytic)	Muscarinic receptor antagonist	Positive chronotropic effect	0.01–0.02 mg/kg	Vagally mediated bradycardia (opioids, oculo-cardiac reflex or as part of resuscitation)
Adrenalin (Sympathomimetic)	Alpha 1 (and 2) Beta 1 (and 2)	Positive inotropic and chronotropic effect, vasoconstriction	Low dose: 0.01 mg/kg High dose: 0.1 mg/kg	Resuscitation or when nothing else helps (poor prognosis)
Noradrenalin (Sympathomimetic)	Alpha 1 (and 2) Beta 1	Vasoconstriction	Low dose: 0.01–0.05 μg/kg/min High dose: 0.1 mg/kg/min	Hypotension in septic patient
Ephedrine	Indirect Alpha 1 and Beta 1	Releases noradrenalin, weaker and longer lasting	Bolus: 0.03–0.1 mg/kg	Hypotension that is otherwise unresponsive (no syringe pump needed)
Phenylephrine	Alpha 1	Severe vasoconstriction	1–3 μg/kg/min	Hypotension (due to severe vasodilation) that is otherwise unresponsive
Dopamine	Dopa effect: 0.5–2 μg/kg Beta 1 effect: 2–10 μg/kg Alpha effect: >10 μg/kg	Dose-dependent: first positive inotropic effect, then vasoconstriction	1–20 μg/kg/min	Hypotension (due to vasodilation) in small animals
Dobutamine	Beta 1	Positive inotropic and chronotropic effect	1–20 μg/kg/min	Hypotension in horses; dilated cardiomyopathy or mitral valve insufficiency in small animals

II

Complications/consequences

- Cell damage, if prolonged

Prophylaxis/therapy

- Balanced anaesthesia with appropriate analgesic component
- Cautious and smart use of sympathomimetic drugs

8.1.3 Arrhythmias

The most important arrhythmias in anaesthesia, intensive care and emergency medicine are presented below. The characteristics and possible causes are explained and treatment options are suggested. For a more comprehensive study of this topic, relevant textbooks are recommended.

Normal ECG in small animals, respiratory sinus arrhythmia

Respiratory sinus arrhythmia (▶ Fig. 8.2) occurs physiologically in many animal species. It disappears with increasing heart rate.

Characteristics of arrhythmia

- Recurrent periods of faster and slower heart rates, usually associated with breathing
- Increased heart rate with inspiration
- Lower heart rate with expiration and during respiratory pause
- Normal P-QRS-T complexes
- More pronounced with increased vagal tone

Therapy is not indicated as it is a physiological arrhythmia.

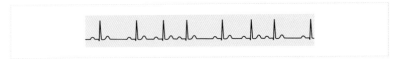

Fig. 8.2 Respiratory sinus arrhythmia in the dog. Morphology of the complexes is identical, heart rate varies synchronously with respiration.

Normal ECG horse

The physiological ECG lead of the horse (▶ Fig. 8.3) shows some special characteristics:

- Morphology of the P wave is very variable, it can be "dented" or biphasic
- Successive P waves often look different; this is caused by a "wandering pacemaker" i. e. the excitation is generated in the sinus node or elsewhere in the atrium
- T waves can also look very diverse

When horses show bradyarrhythmia, they are usually physiological and caused by high vagal tone. If they show tachyarrhythmia, it is usually pathological.

Sinus bradycardia

Sinus bradycardia is physiologically common in trained animals with high vagal tone (well exercised dog, horse) and does not require any therapy (▶ Fig. 8.4). However, it also occurs in the course of anaesthesia and can have many causes. It is necessary to decide on a case-by-case basis whether therapy is indicated. It should be treated if hypotension is present at the same time.

Characteristics of arrhythmia

Regular rhythm, too slow for the given situation (e.g. heart rate of < 60 /min in an awake dog that is just being examined by the vet).

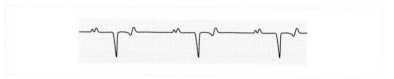

Fig. 8.3 Normal ECG in the horse.

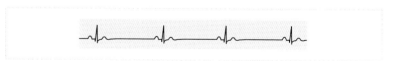

Fig. 8.4 Sinus bradycardia. Slow frequency, normal morphology.

Possible causes

- Too deep anaesthesia, coma
- After administration of certain drugs
  - Opioids (via vagal stimulation, small animals)
  - Alpha2 agonists (reflex bradycardia due to vasoconstriction and consecutive hypertension)
  - B receptor blocker
  - Digoxin
- Increased vagal tone
  - Good training condition
  - Young animal
  - Brachycephalic dog
  - Manipulation on the ventral neck or eyes, e.g. oculo-cardiac reflex
  - Severe gastrointestinal or respiratory disease
- Increased intracranial pressure
- Hypothermia
- Hypertension
- Hyperkalaemia
- Severe hypothyroidism

Therapy

- Stop the stimulus
- Find the cause and treat it!
- Always try to reduce the depth of anaesthesia
- If opioid administration is the cause, give atropine/glycopyrrolate
- If alpha2 agonists are the cause, (partially) antagonise

Sinus tachycardia

Sinus tachycardia (► Fig. 8.5) leads to increased myocardial work and an increase in O_2 consumption. The myocardium itself can no longer be sufficiently perfused and supplied with O_2.

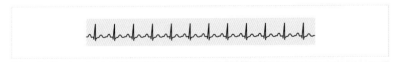

Fig. 8.5 Sinus tachycardia. Fast rate, normal morphology.

Characteristics of arrhythmia

Regular rhythm over 30% above normal (e.g. heart rate of > 160 /min in dogs, > 180 /min in cats, > 50 /min in horses, > 100 /min in cattle)

Possible causes

- Insufficient depth of anaesthesia or inadequate analgesia
- Hypotension, shock
- Hypoventilation or hypoxaemia
- Administration of certain drugs
  - Atropine or glycopyrrolate
- Hyperthermia
- Hypokalaemia
- Full urinary bladder

Therapy

- Find and treat the cause!
  - Adjust depth of anaesthesia, optimise analgesia
  - Infusion, volume substitution
  - Improve ventilation and oxygenation
  - Cooling
  - Compensate for changes in electrolyte balance
- Short-term episodes of tachycardia (< 15 min) do not require treatment if no cause can be found and treated

1st, 2nd and 3rd degree AV blocks

In general, it can be argued that AV blocks become more pathological and dangerous from degree to degree, so a 1st degree AV block is usually much more "harmless" than a 3rd degree AV block.

1st degree AV block

With this block, the conduction time between the atria and the ventricles is delayed (> 0.13 s in dogs and > 0.09 s in cats, ► Fig. 8.6). It is not really an arrhythmia. The prognosis depends on the cause.

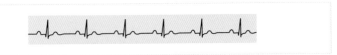

Fig. 8.6 1st degree AV block. Normal morphology, the distance between P wave and QRS complex is prolonged.

Characteristics of arrhythmia

The interval between P wave and QRS complex is prolonged. This arrhythmia cannot really be diagnosed with a 3-lead anaesthetic ECG.

Possible causes

- Administration of drugs
  - Opioids
  - Alpha2 agonists
  - Digitalis
  - B receptor blocker
  - Calcium channel blocker
- Electrolyte abnormalities (hyperkalaemia)
- Increased vagal tone (young animal, trained animal)

Therapy is not indicated.

2nd degree AV block

This block occurs when some electrical conductions are passed from the atria to the ventricles via the AV node and some are not. In dogs, especially puppies and horses, 2nd degree AV block is physiological in most cases and disappears with exercise.

A distinction is made between 2nd degree AV block type 1 (or Wenckebach periodicity) and type 2.

Characteristics of arrhythmia

- In 2nd degree AV block type 1, the interval from P wave to QRS complex becomes progressively longer before the QRS complex drops out (▶ Fig. 8.7)
- In 2nd degree AV block type 2, the interval from P wave to QRS complex is always of the same duration (▶ Fig. 8.8)

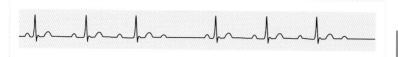

Fig. 8.7 2nd degree AV block type 1.

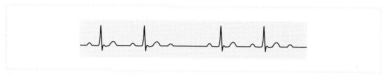

Fig. 8.8 2nd degree AV block type 2.

Possible causes

- Physiological, high vagal tone (more likely type 1)
- Administration of drugs (more likely type 1)
  - Opioids
  - Alpha2 agonists
  - Digitalis
  - Atropine (initial effect)
- Disease in the AV node (more likely type 2)

Therapy

- Usually, no therapy is indicated unless the arrhythmia causes hypotension or the block progresses to the severe form where multiple beats are missed in succession
- If a 2nd degree AV block becomes severe or affects blood pressure, the cause determines therapy
  - High vagal tone, administration of opioids: Stop stimulus and administer atropine/glycopyrrolate
  - Alpha2 agonists: Partially antagonise with atipamezole IM
- In type 2, therapy may not be effective and the arrhythmia may progress to a 3rd degree AV block; the patient should be referred to a cardiologist

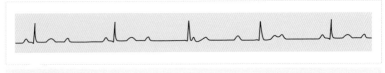

Fig. 8.9 3rd degree AV block.

3rd degree AV block

This block is also called complete heart block and occurs when there is no conduction whatsoever between atria and ventricles (▶ Fig. 8.9).

Characteristics of arrhythmia

- Sinus node excitation occurs in its rhythm and produces P waves in the ECG through atrial conduction
- AV node or ventricular pacemaker initiates excitation in its comparatively slower rhythm and generates the QRS complex, ventricular rhythm
- If the QRS complex is generated in the **AV node or above, it is narrow**
- If the QRS complex is generated in a **ventricular** pacemaker, it is **wide and bizarre**
- P waves and QRS complexes are completely **independent** of each other seen in the ECG
- Distance of the P waves from each other is often regular
- Distance of the QRS complexes from each other is often regular

This complete heart block can occur during anaesthesia and is then potentially caused by **a very high vagal tone**, which temporarily or permanently prevents conduction. An attempt at therapy with atropine is possible and often successful.

If a "real" complete block is present, the cause is unknown in most cases. Degenerative processes are discussed. An attempt at therapy with atropine can be made. If a permanent therapy is desired or indicated, the only option is the implantation of a pacemaker.

Premature ventricular extrasystoles

This is one of the most common arrhythmias in veterinary medicine. In general, it is not life-threatening and is easily treated. The situation becomes more serious when there is a pulse deficit, when isolated premature extrasystoles are multifocal and/or progress to ventricular tachycardia.

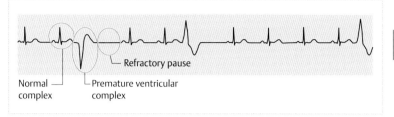

Fig. 8.10 Premature ventricular extrasystoles.

Characteristics of arrhythmia

- The normal rhythm is prematurely interrupted by a QRS complex, which is often wide, bizarre and of large amplitude (▶ Fig. 8.10)
- These QRS complexes are not preceded by a P wave
- T wave runs in the opposite direction to the QRS complex
- Often refractory pause after the extrasystole
- One speaks of unifocal when the QRS complexes look morphologically identical and of multifocal when they have a different morphology

Possible causes

- Congestive heart failure
- Myocarditis
- Ischaemia (e.g. gastric dilatation-volvulus)
- Pancreatitis
- Uraemia
- Administration of atropine
- Pain, stress

Therapy

- Find and treat the cause
- Basic measures are:
  - Ensure oxygenation and ventilation
  - Adjust the depth of anaesthesia
  - Correct electrolyte shifts or deviations in acid-base balance
- Optimise analgesia
- Lidocaine (p. 108) bolus and continuous rate infusion, adhere to maximum dosages and watch for signs of overdose

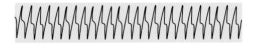

Fig. 8.11 Ventricular tachycardia.

Ventricular tachycardia

Isolated premature ventricular extrasystoles may progress to ventricular tachy-cardia (▶ Fig. 8.11). The effects on the cardiovascular system become more seri-ous and therapy more difficult.

Characteristics of arrhythmia

- QRS complexes are often wide, bizarre, and have a large amplitude
- QRS complexes have no connection to the P wave

Possible causes

- Cardiac disease e.g. dilated cardiomyopathy (dog), hypertrophic cardiomyop-athy (cat)
- Myocardial ischaemia (temporary or permanent) e.g. due to
  ○ Gastric dilatation-volvulus
  ○ Trauma
  ○ Endotoxaemia, pyometra
- Electrolyte shifts or deviations in acid-base balance

Therapy

- Oxygen administration
- Lidocaine (p. 108) bolus and continuous rate infusion, adhere to maximum dosages and watch for signs of overdose

Bigeminy

This arrhythmia is often seen in the first minutes after induction of anaesthesia with thiopental (p. 140).

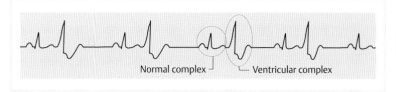

Normal complex — — Ventricular complex

Fig. 8.12 Bigeminy.

Characteristics of arrhythmia

- Any normal P-QRS-T complex is followed by a premature ventricular extra-systole (no P wave, QRS complex wide, bizarre and with large amplitude, ▶ Fig. 8.12)
- In some cases followed by supraventricular extrasystole (QRS complex narrow)
- Refractory pause after the extrasystole, ventricle has a long time to fill; strong systole following
- Premature extrasystole often generates only a weak pulse (ventricular filling volume is small because there is no time for filling)
- May present as pulse deficit (heart rate 180 /min, pulse rate 90 /min)

Possible causes

- Induction of anaesthesia with thiopental, more common with high thiopental concentration
- Digitalis overdose

Therapy

- Often not necessary, arrhythmia disappears after a few minutes
- Monitor oxygen saturation and ventilation
- Adjust depth of anaesthesia
- Lidocaine (p. 108) bolus and continuous rate infusion, if necessary, stay below maximum dosages and watch for signs of overdose

Sinus arrest/sinus node arrest

Sinus arrest is a failure of the primary pacemaker, the sinus node. If none of the secondary pacemakers (such as the AV node or His bundle) jump in, acute cardiac arrest occurs.

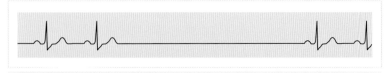

Fig. 8.13 Temporary sinus arrest/sinus node arrest.

Characteristics of arrhythmia

- Rhythm pauses lasting longer than two R-R intervals (▶ Fig. 8.13)
- Morphology of P-QRS-T is normal

Possible causes of the missing excitation in the sinus node

- Congenital heart defect
- Cardiac disease such as the sick sinus syndrome
- Bacterial endocarditis
- Increased vagal tone

Therapy

- Often not necessary, especially if it occurs only sporadically
- Anticholinergics (atropine, glycopyrrolate) can be given as a therapy attempt, but often have no/very little effect
- If therapy is necessary, implantation of a pacemaker is recommended

Escape rhythm

If the sinus arrest is prolonged, a secondary pacemaker may intervene to "save" the patient. This escape rhythm maintains circulation and is life-saving.

Characteristics of arrhythmia

- After a longer sinus pause, a ventricular QRS complex appears (delayed), which is wide, bizarre and with a large amplitude (▶ Fig. 8.14)
- Since each pacemaker has its own frequency, it may be possible to determine where the excitation is generated

Logically, this escape rhythm should not be "treated", as it at least partially secures circulation.

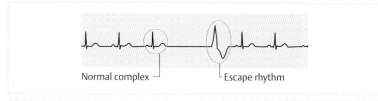

Normal complex — ⌐Escape rhythm

Fig. 8.14 Ventricular escape rhythm.

Cause and therapy: As described under "Sinus arrest/sinus node arrest" (p. 363)

Careful!

Premature ventricular extrasystoles (VES) vs. escape rhythm
Although these two arrhythmias look very similar on ECG, they have virtually nothing in common. Premature VES are relatively benign and can be treated with lidocaine if necessary. Administering lidocaine to a patient with an escape rhythm would be a fatal mistake! For this reason, the arrhythmia must be diagnosed before any therapy:

In **premature VES**, ventricular excitation occurs BEFORE normal rhythm would generate excitation.

In an **escape rhythm**, the ventricular excitation occurs AFTER a sinus pause longer than the normal R-R interval.

Atrial fibrillation/atrial flutter

In atrial fibrillation/flutter, there is an increased number of electrical conductions across the atria, which are transmitted absolutely irregularly to the ventricles (▶ Fig. 8.15).

Characteristics of arrhythmia

- Irregular ventricular rhythm
- P waves are replaced by so-called F waves (F for fibrillation), which may be relatively large or small
- QRS complexes may be normal or wide and bizarre
- Auscultatory absolute arrhythmia can be detected ("like shoes in the dryer")

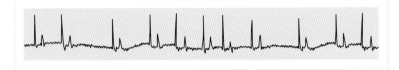

Fig. 8.15 Atrial fibrillation in a horse. Irregular rhythm, jagged baseline.

Possible causes

- Multiple ectopic foci in the atrium (from which discharges originate)
- Atrial enlargement
- Chronic atrio-ventricular valve regurgitation (mitral valve regurgitation)
- Dilated cardiomyopathy (dog), congestive (decompensated) heart failure (horse)
- Congenital heart defects (persistent ductus arteriosus Botalli, congestive heart failure)

Therapy

- Often no therapy is needed during anaesthesia but anaesthesia time should be kept as short as possible
- Establish treatment plan to slow down atrio-ventricular conduction, e.g. digoxin in dogs, quinidine in horses or attempt cardio-conversion (= restoration of normal sinus rhythm) by drugs or electrical impulse. Often only successful if the arrhythmia has only existed for a short period of time

Ventricular fibrillation

This arrhythmia is life-threatening and must be treated immediately, otherwise cardiac arrest is imminent. In general, the prognosis is poor.

Characteristics of arrhythmia

- Irregular bizarre waves that can be of different heights (▶ Fig. 8.16)
- Usual P-QRS-T complexes are not recognisable

Possible causes

- Trauma
- Cardiac disease

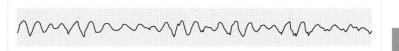

Fig. 8.16 Ventricular fibrillation.

- Severe shifts in electrolyte concentrations (especially potassium and calcium)
- Severe abnormalities in acid-base balance
- Anaesthetic overdose
- Direct manipulation of the heart during surgery
- Administration of catecholamines (overdose to support circulation in massively impaired animals)

Therapy

- Defibrillation (external 2–4 joules/kg), increasing the dose each time
- Start resuscitation (p. 471) according to the ABC scheme
- Find cause and treat (electrolytes, acid-base balance)

ECG changes with hyperkalaemia

With hyperkalaemia, more or less classical ECG changes are found with increasing K^+ concentration in the blood (▶ Fig. 8.17). However, it has only recently been shown that these abnormalities do not necessarily occur even at high K^+ concentrations.
- Decrease in P wave amplitude until the P wave disappears completely
- High, tented T waves
- Prolongation of the QRS complex
- Bradycardia (not characteristic in cats)

Without therapy, the QRS complex continues to widen until it appears sinusoidal and eventually progresses to asystole.

Possible causes

- Obstruction of the urethra (especially common in male cats and goats)
- Urinary bladder rupture, failed bladder puncture
- Renal insufficiency

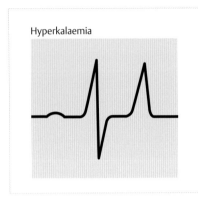

Hyperkalaemia

Fig. 8.17 Classic ECG changes with hyperkalaemia.

- Diabetic ketoacidosis
- Addisonian crisis
- Excessive K^+-infusion

Therapy

- Start to normalise serum potassium concentration immediately
- If surgery is planned, be sure to stabilise before induction of anaesthesia (anaesthesia increases K^+ levels due to fluid shifts)
- Infusion therapy (after the obstruction has been removed)
- Detailed procedure is described under "Hyperkalaemia" (p. 387)

8.1.4 Literature

[1] Chen HC, Sinclair MD, Dyson DH. Use of ephedrine and dopamine in dogs for the management of hypotension in routine clinical cases under isoflurane anesthesia. Vet Anaesth Analg. 2007; 34: 301–311

[2] Gordon AM, Wagner AE. Anesthesia-related hypotension in a small-animal practice. Veterinary Medicine 2006: 22–6

[3] Mazzaferro E, Wagner AE. Hypotension during anesthesia in dogs and cats: recognition, causes, and treatment. Compend Contin Educ Pract Vet 2001; 23: 728–37

[4] Redondo JI, Rubio M, Soler G, Serra I, Soler C, Gómez-Villamandos RJ. Normal values and incidence of cardiorespiratory complications in dogs during general anaesthesia. A review of 1281 cases. J Vet Med A Physiol Pathol Clin Med. 2007; 54: 470–477

[5] Silverstein DC, Kleiner J, Drobatz KJ. Effectiveness of intravenous fluid resuscitation in the emergency room for treatment of hypotension in dogs: 35 cases (2000–2010). J Vet Emerg Crit Care. 2012; 22: 666–673

8.2 Respiration

The biggest fear that young anaesthetists have, is that the patient will stop breathing during anaesthesia or in an emergency situation. Therefore, in addition to clinical monitoring, various monitoring devices are very important to diagnose and detect problems (early). Capnography and pulse oximetry are essential for monitoring ventilation and oxygenation. Spirometry can be helpful, but will not be discussed here. Further information can be found in the relevant literature.

8.2.1 Hypoventilation/apnoea

Hypoventilation is when the arterial partial pressure of CO_2 (p_aCO_2) rises **above** the physiological normal value. This varies from species to species and is in the **awake animal between 30–45 mmHg** (▶ Table 2.3). It can be assumed that almost every patient hypoventilates during general anaesthesia. For this reason, some increase in p_aCO_2 may be tolerated in the anaesthetised animal. Depending on the situation, an **increase of up to 60 mmHg may be tolerated**.

Diagnosis

The diagnosis of hypoventilation can only be made by measuring p_aCO_2 or etCO$_2$ (▶ Fig. 8.18). If this is not possible or is too time-consuming, an assessment can be made based on clinical findings. There are some indications which suggest that the patient is hypoventilating:

- Low respiratory rate
- Low tidal volume (weak thoracic movement)
- Hypoxaemia (to be measured with the pulse oximeter) may be present

Possible causes

Apart from the fact that there are central and other causes of hypoventilation, in anaesthetised patients the (**side**) **effects of the anaesthetics** are usually responsible:

- Muscle relaxation
- Decreased respiratory drive due to increased tolerance to increasing arterial CO_2
- Increased respiratory resistance (e.g. endotracheal tube too small)
- Reduced distensibility of the lungs (e.g. pregnancy)
- Unphysiological body position (e.g. dorsal recumbency)

369

Consequences/complications

Hypoventilation inevitably leads to **hypercapnia** (which is how hypoventilation is defined!). This leads directly to:
- Respiratory acidosis
- Vasodilation (throughout the body, except in the lungs, where vasoconstriction occurs)
- Increase in blood pressure, tachycardia
- Pulmonary hypertension
- Hypoxaemia
- Complete respiratory arrest, death

Clinical relevance

The hydration of carbon dioxide
Carbon dioxide (CO_2) acts like an acid in the body. The reason lies in the equation below. If CO_2 increases, the equation is shifted to the right and more hydrogen ions (H^+) are released.

$$CO_2 + H_2O \leftrightharpoons H_2CO_3 \leftrightharpoons H^+ + CO_3^-$$

Therapy

In general, a balanced anaesthesia technique can be used from the beginning to try to keep respiratory depression as low as possible. Specifically, this means using anaesthetics that are particularly respiratory depressants (such as propofol or iso-/sevoflurane) in the **lowest possible dose**.

If hypoventilation occurs despite precautionary measures, the most effective and simplest therapy is to take over ventilation in the intubated animal with **intermittent positive pressure ventilation** (**IPPV**).

Doxapram in case of respiratory depression/apnoea?

Doxapram is a CNS stimulant, which leads to a temporary increase especially in respiratory volume and less in respiratory rate. Since O_2 consumption and CO_2 production are increased at the same time, there is hardly any increase in arterial O_2 saturation when the animal is breathing room air. Arrhythmias, hypertension and seizures may occur after repeated administration of high doses. It may be used as a short-term aid to bridge severe hypoventilation or an apnoea phase in an emergency situation, but **positive pressure ventilation is much more sensible, effective and has fewer side effects**.

Manual positive pressure ventilation

If the patient is intubated and no anaesthesia machine is available, small animals can be ventilated using an **AMBU bag**. If not already done, the cuff on the endotracheal tube (p. 153) must be inflated properly beforehand.

When pressure is applied to the bag (inspiration), thoracic excursion should look physiological; expiration occurs passively by releasing the bag. The ratio of inspiration to expiration time should be 1:2 to 1:3. The ventilation rate should be appropriately physiological depending on the species (small animal approx. 8–12 × /min, large animal slower approx. 4–8 × /min).

There is a small adapter on each AMBU bag for connecting an oxygen supply. This can be used with an oxygen cylinder with pressure reducer or an oxygen concentrator (p. 31). In order to ventilate with the highest possible oxygen concentration, an additional reservoir bag attached to the AMBU bag should be used.

Do not leave an AMBU bag on a spontaneously breathing animal!

Rebreathing of CO_2 or hypoxaemia can easily occur even though the animal is breathing spontaneously! As soon as the animal is breathing on its own again, the AMBU bag should therefore be removed. This also decreases the resistance to breathing.

If the animal is connected to an **anaesthesia machine** but no ventilator is available, manual ventilation can be used. Proceed as follows:
- If not already done, turn on the oxygen on the flowmeter
- Close the APL valve
- Manually press the breathing bag on the device until a peak airway pressure of approx. 10 cmH_2O (small animal) or 20–30 cmH_2O (large animal) is reached or the thorax excursion looks physiological
- Ventilation frequency should be physiological for the respective animal species, the frequency should be counted deliberately, as ventilation is often inadvertently too fast, especially in an emergency (▶ Table 2.1)
- Time ratio inspiration to expiration is 1:2 or 1:3 – this means that at a respiratory rate of 10 breaths /min, one breath takes about 6 sec. Of this, 2 sec for inhalation and 4 sec for exhalation
- Release the bag completely in between breaths (no pressure in the system)
- **Important:** After completion of positive pressure ventilation, the **APL valve must be fully opened again**!

Mechanical positive pressure ventilation

The anaesthesia machine must be checked for leaks before starting. If the patient is connected to the anaesthesia machine and a ventilator is available, set the ventilation parameters before starting. Depending on the setting options of the ventilator, pressure- or volume-controlled ventilation can be used.

The advantage of **pressure-controlled ventilation** (PCV) is that the peak airway pressure is limited to a predefined value. The volume of breaths can vary depending on the stiffness or compliance of the chest. The advantage of **volume-controlled ventilation** (VCV) is the administration of a predefined volume of breaths. However, depending on the condition of the chest or other influences, the pressure administered may vary. It is best to set a value (e.g. pressure) and check the dependent variable (e.g. volume) to see if it is also within the physiological range or appropriate for the individual patient. Modern ventilators have many other ventilation modes that can, for example, support the patient in breathing on its own. It is worth getting to know your ventilator better in order to be able to use it optimally.

▶ Basic settings on the ventilator
- Peak inspiratory pressure approx. 8–12 cm H_2O for small animals, 20–30 cmH_2O for large animals
- Tidal volume 8–15 ml/kg (applies to all animal species)

- Respiratory rate (adapted to animal species and case, usually between 4–8 breaths/min for large animals and 8–20 breaths/min for small animals)
- In animals without respiratory pathologies, a minute ventilation of approx. 100–150 ml/kg/min should be aimed for

II

Practice tip

Lung protective ventilation
Strategies to minimise ventilation-induced lung injury
1. Keep ventilation time as short as possible
2. Reduce the oxygen concentration (if possible), but O_2 saturation should always remain in the physiological range
3. Keep the maximum ventilation pressure as low as possible (approx. 6 cmH$_2$O) and compensate by increasing the respiratory rate (in small animals up to approx. 20 breaths/min)
4. If necessary, apply a slight positive end-expiratory pressure (PEEP between 2 and 5 cmH$_2$O) to prevent the lungs from collapsing completely

In essence, (physiological) spontaneous breathing is always preferable to manual or mechanical ventilation. It protects the lung tissue and supports the circulation by promoting venous return to the heart through the negative pressure in the thorax during inspiration. It is important to always consider the overall concept of ventilation and oxygenation of the tissue and **not to treat individual numbers** on the monitor (i. e. "CO$_2$ is high, therefore I have to ventilate"). Positive pressure ventilation should only be considered when mean arterial blood pressure is > 65 mmHg (small animal) or > 75 mmHg (large animal). Otherwise, severe hypotension may occur, which may negate the benefit of improved ventilation.

In non-intubated small mammals with apnoea, a form of ventilation can be achieved by swaying the animal (p. 211).

8.2.2 Hyperventilation

Hyperventilation occurs when the arterial partial pressure of CO$_2$ (p_aCO_2) falls below the physiological value (▶ Table 2.3). When using a balanced anaesthesia technique, it is rather rare.

Diagnosis

Analogous to hypoventilation, the diagnosis of hyperventilation can only be made by measuring p_aCO_2 or $etCO_2$ (▶ Fig. 8.19). Again, one can get an idea from the clinical findings. There are some indications that suggest that the patient is hyperventilating:

• High respiratory rate
• High tidal volume

$\rightarrow$ overall high minute ventilation

Hyperventilation ≠ panting

Hyperventilation involves a decrease in the arterial partial pressure of CO_2. Panting, on the other hand, is predominantly dead space ventilation, the main aim of which is to get rid of heat. CO_2 partial pressure remains within the normal range.

Possible causes

There are other triggers for hyperventilation in addition to central causes. Apart from these, the following causes are probable in anaesthetised patients:
• Too light anaesthesia
• Inadequate analgesia
• Iatrogenic (too excessive manual or mechanical ventilation)
• Hypoxaemia
• Administration of drugs
  ○ CNS stimulants such as doxapram
  ○ Bicarbonate (rather in awake patients)

Consequences/complications

Hyperventilation inevitably leads to **hypocapnia** (definition of hyperventilation!). The consequences are:
• Respiratory alkalosis
• Vasoconstriction (body, brain), vasodilation (lungs)
• Muscle spasms
• Unconsciousness (in awake patients)

Therapy

Basically, the cause must be identified and treated:
- Adjust depth of anaesthesia
- Optimise analgesia regime
- Check and correct ventilation parameters
- O_2 administration

8.2.3 Abnormal waveforms in capnography

Capnography measures the partial pressure of CO_2 in the inhaled and exhaled air and can be used to assess the patient's **ventilation**. The shape of the capnography waveform provides additional information about possible complications. The most common abnormal waveforms in anaesthesia are shown and interpreted below as examples.

In **hypoventilation, CO_2 is increased** and/or rises continuously (▶ Fig. 8.18). Often the respiratory rate and/or tidal volume is decreased. The waveform shown could also be an indication of circulatory improvement with **increased perfusion**.

In **hyperventilation, CO_2 is deceased** or decreases continuously (▶ Fig. 8.19). Often the respiratory rate and/or tidal volume is increased. The waveform shown could also be an indication of circulatory depression with **reduced perfusion**.

Normally there is **no (or very little) CO_2 in the inspiratory air**. If there is CO_2 in the inspiratory air, i. e. if there is **CO_2 rebreathing** (▶ Fig. 8.20), this may indicate the following problems:

- Too little fresh gas flow especially when using a non-rebreathing system (p. 22)
- Too much (apparatus) dead space, e.g. endotracheal tube too long, too many/large volume adapters between ETT and Y-piece
- Exhausted or non-functional CO_2 absorber lime (p. 28) in the circle system
- Missing, open or leaking valve disc in the one-way valve (p. 26) of the expiratory or inspiratory limb

High inspiratory CO_2 partial pressures are tolerated very well for a short time. However, the cause should be found and corrected.

When the respiratory rate is slow, a **wavy descending line** can sometimes be seen in the capnography curve after the end of expiration. This pattern is called **cardiogenic oscillation** (▶ Fig. 8.21). This waveform occurs physiologically when, with "deflated" lungs and zero pressure in the airways, the heart rhythmically beats against the lungs with each contraction.

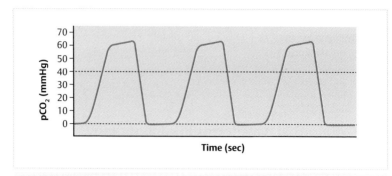

Fig. 8.18 Hypoventilation.

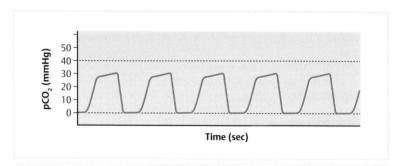

Fig. 8.19 Hyperventilation.

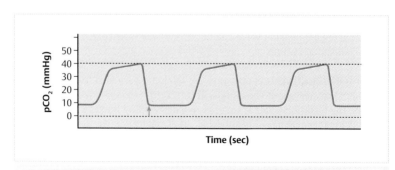

Fig. 8.20 Rebreathing: Inspiratory CO_2 (increase in baseline).

If the patient is ventilated with the help of a ventilator, but the waveform is not very regular, but there are occasionally "dents" in the curve (▶ Fig. 8.22), the patient breathes spontaneously in between (= **curare cleft**, as this waveform can appear when the effect of a peripheral muscle relaxant wears off and the patient begins to breathe again). One should not tolerate the condition, but look for the cause: Wrong ventilator setting? Patient too light in anaesthesia? Hypercapnia? Hypoxaemia? and correct it.

This is only a small selection of classical waveforms that can be identified on the capnograph. It is worthwhile to study the further literature.

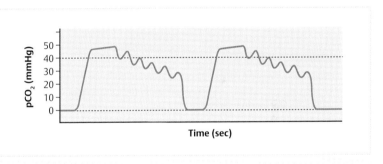

Fig. 8.21 Cardiogenic oscillation with slow respiratory rate.

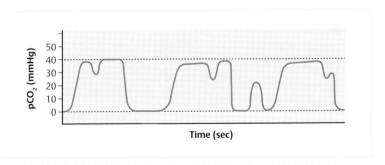

Fig. 8.22 Spontaneous breathing of the patient on the ventilator.

8.2.4 Hypoxaemia

A patient is hypoxaemic when the p_aO_2 is less than 80 mmHg, which corresponds to a haemoglobin oxygen saturation measured with the pulse oximeter of 95%. **Severe hypoxaemia** is defined as a p_aO_2 below 60 mmHg, which corresponds to a saturation of 90%.

Using a rule of thumb and the inspiratory O_2 concentration, the expected p_aO_2 can be calculated as follows:

Inspiratory O_2 concentration $\times 5$ = expected p_aO_2

Thus, for a patient who inhales 100% O_2, one expects a p_aO_2 of about 500 mmHg. If you perform a blood gas analysis (BGA) on this patient and the measured p_aO_2 is below but still above 80 mmHg, you are dealing with "**relative**" **hypoxaemia**. The partial pressure of O_2 is not as high as it should be, but is still above the value of absolute hypoxaemia. In this case, too, one should try to find the cause and take therapeutic steps if necessary. Hypoxaemia leads to **hypoxia**, an insufficient supply of oxygen to the tissues.

Diagnosis

The diagnosis of hypoxaemia is most accurately made by arterial BGA. The calculated O_2 saturation, which is estimated with the pulse oximeter, also provides important information. However, the significance is limited if the inspiratory fraction of oxygen (F_iO_2) is > 0.21 (i.e. room air containing 21% oxygen). Clinical parameters can also be used for diagnosis, but they should only complement the diagnosis by BGA and/or pulse oximetry.

- **Clinical indications for hypoxaemia can be:**
  - Cyanosis (only if patient is not anaemic), generally a very late sign
  - Hyperventilation (not possible when very deeply anaesthetised)
  - First hyper- then hypotension
  - First tachy- then bradycardia
  - Acute hypoxaemia must be distinguished from chronic (and usually compensated) hypoxaemia

Clinical relevance

Cyanosis with anaemia?
The blue colouring when hypoxaemic only becomes visible when more than
5 g/dl haemoglobin (Hb), which corresponds to a haematocrit of approx. 15%,
is desaturated. This means that cyanosis will never be visible in an animal that
has a Hb concentration below 5 g/dl or correspondingly a haematocrit below
approx. 15%, even if there is absolute oxygen deficiency. Conversely, an animal
with very high Hb values may show cyanosis and still not suffer from hypoxia.

Possible causes

There are **5 reasons** why a patient may become hypoxaemic:
1. **Low F_iO_2** (inspiratory O_2 concentration too low, e.g. breathing system is not
   connected to the anaesthesia machine) or **low pO_2** (partial pressure of O_2
   too low, e.g. at high altitude)
2. **Hypoventilation** (often caused by anaesthetics and position)
3. **Diffusion barrier** (history? pneumonia, pulmonary oedema, fibrosis, etc.)
4. **Pathological shunt** (young animal? persistent ductus arteriosus Botalli, ventricular septal defect, foramen ovale)
5. **Ventilation-perfusion (V/Q) mismatch** of the lungs (usually caused by atelectasis during anaesthesia = decreased ventilation). It is usually a low V/Q
   ratio causing hypoxaemia (a high V/Q ratio can even lead to improved oxygenation). The maximum manifestation of a low V/Q ratio is shunt, the maximum manifestation of a high V/Q ratio is dead space ventilation
   (▶ Fig. 8.23).

In **small animals**, the most common cause for hypoxaemia during anaesthesia
is **hypoventilation**.
   In **large animals**, especially in dorsal recumbency, the most likely cause is
ventilation-perfusion (V/Q) mismatch (▶ Fig. 8.24).
   In hypoxaemic **young animals**, a **congenital shunt** should always be considered.

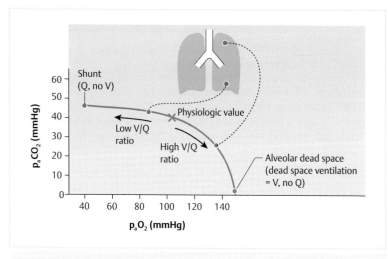

Fig. 8.23 Distribution of ventilation and perfusion in the lungs. V = Ventilation; Q = Perfusion.

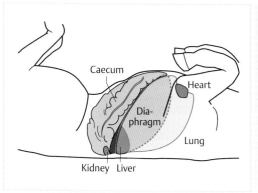

Fig. 8.24 Schematic of a horse in dorsal recumbency.

Consequences/complications

The risk of causing permanent cellular damage increases with the degree and duration of hypoxaemia. The brain in particular is extremely sensitive to O_2 deficiency, as there are practically no O_2 reserves in the tissues.

Therapy

As always, it makes sense to find the cause and take targeted therapeutic measures. Especially in case of hypoxaemia, a structured approach is important because the consequences could be fatal.

Basically:
- Keep anaesthesia time as short as possible
- Use a balanced anaesthesia regime
- Get patient back to sternal recumbency as soon as possible

Careful!

Oxygen intoxication
If a patient is ventilated with a high O_2 concentration (> 50%) for a longer period of time (> 14 h) due to severe respiratory insufficiency with simultaneous reduced O_2 uptake, oxidative damage to the alveolar membrane may already occur. At > 24 h with 100% O_2, a deterioration in lung function tests can be observed. The reason is that alveolar cells type 2 are destroyed by free radicals. These cells produce surfactant, which reduces surface tension. If surfactant is missing, atelectasis (collapse of the alveoli) occurs. For the average anaesthesia patient, oxygen intoxication does not really play a role, as anaesthesia times are usually much shorter.

8.2.5 Literature

[1] Alef M, Oechtering G. Nichtinvasive Patientenüberwachung in der Tiermedizin: Pulsoxymetrie und Kapnographie. Teil II: Kapnographie [Non-invasive patient monitoring in veterinary medicine: pulse oximetry and capnography. II. Capnography]. Tierarztl Prax. 1995;23: 1–16

[2] Bonikos DS, Bensch KG, Northway WH Jr. Oxygen toxicity in the newborn. The effect of chronic continuous 100 percent oxygen exposure on the lungs of newborn mice. Am J Pathol 1976; 85: 623–650

[3] Calice I, Moens Y. Modern spirometry supports anesthetic management in small animal clinical practice: A case series. J Am Anim Hosp Assoc 2016; 52: 305–11

[4] Henao-Guerrero N, Riccó CH. Comparison of the cardiorespiratory effects of a combination of ket-amine and propofol, propofol alone, or a combination of ketamine and diazepam before and after induction of anesthesia in dogs sedated with acepromazine and oxymorphone. Am J Vet Res. 2014; 75: 231–239

[5] Hess D, Kacmarek RM. Essentials of mechanical ventilation. New York: Mc- Graw-Hill Medical 2014

[6] Hopper K, Powell LL. Basics of mechanical ventilation for dogs and cats. Vet Clin North Am Small Anim Pract. 2013; 43: 955–69

[7] Valente T. Capnography, King of the ABC's: A systematic approach for paramedics. New York: iUniverse 2010

[8] West JB. Respiratory Physiology: The essentials. 8th edition. Philadelphia: Wolters Kluwer/Lippincott Williams & Wilkins 2008

8.3 Temperature

Both hypo- and hyperthermia can have profound impact on the well-being and health of the patient. Despite this, temperature management (i.e. measuring core body temperature and maintaining it within the normal range) is often neglected in small and large animals. This is surprising because the measurement is simple, the measurement device inexpensive and the time invested is small. You just have to do it!

The description of how to carry out the measurement and the standard values of the different animal species can be found under "Temperature measurement" (p.58).

8.3.1 Hypothermia

Hypothermia is any temperature deviation below the normal value. A distinction can be made between mild, moderate or severe hypothermia. The absolute values assigned to this grading system vary greatly depending on the literature. Starting at a deviation of **–1°C from the physiological temperature**, one speaks of **perioperative hypothermia** and should perceive this as a complication.

Possible causes

Temperature is lost by radiation, conduction, convection and evaporation. Examples:
- In small animals, unfavourable ratio between body mass (small) and body surface area (large)
- Open body cavities
- Cold ambient temperature, cold contact surface (metal table)
- Cold, dry respiratory gases (especially with high flow rates)
- In neonates, thermoregulation mechanisms are still insufficiently developed

- Vasodilatation (e.g. through acepromazine administration, high isoflurane or sevoflurane concentration)
- Mechanisms for preserving heat (vasoconstriction) or generating heat (shivering) are not functional during anaesthesia

Complications/consequences

- Increases the effect of anaesthetics (for every 1 °C of hypothermia, MAC isoflurane (p. 102) is reduced by approx. 5%)
- Prolonged duration of action of all anaesthetics, prolonged recovery phase
- Therapy-resistant bradycardia and hypotension
- Metabolic acidosis (pH decreases by 0.017 per 1 °C hypothermia)
- Coagulation is impaired (greater blood loss)
- Increased risk of wound infection/wound healing disorder
- Impaired immune system, increased risk of infection (pneumonia)
- Shivering when the animal wakes up
- High level of discomfort
- Decreased O_2 consumption, however, increased O_2 consumption with shivering
- Decreased CO_2 production, however, increased CO_2 production with shivering

Prophylaxis/therapy

- Passive temperature management
  - Socks
  - Blanket or bubble wrap
  - Emergency blanket
  - Keep clipped area as small as possible/use alcohol sparingly as a disinfectant
- Active temperature management
  - Warm air blower (most effective)
  - Heating mat (not as effective, effectiveness depends on position and type of mat)
  - Heating lamp (e.g. during anaesthesia preparation)
  - Warming of infusion or irrigation solutions
  - Use of heated infusion line pumps
  - Disposable gloves filled with warm water or similar (for very small animals)
  - Increase room temperature

Perioperative hypothermia can of course also be used deliberately, e.g. to reduce O_2 consumption in the brain or to reduce the risk of ischaemic damage after clamping off supplying vessels. It is important to consider the disadvantages and possible complications.

If an animal is admitted as an emergency with severe hypothermia, rewarming should be performed very slowly (about 1 °C/h), controlled and intensively monitored (apparatus monitoring). This is in contrast to animals that have cooled down perioperatively, which should be warmed up as fast as possible.

8.3.2 Hyperthermia

Hyperthermia is defined as a core body temperature above the normal value. Hyperthermia is to be distinguished from the symptom fever!

Possible causes

- Iatrogenic, especially in small mammals, due to "too much" warming
- Increased muscle work and thus heat production
- Malignant hyperthermia
- Convulsions, epileptic seizures
- High ketamine dose without or not enough co-administered muscle relaxant agent
- Particularly good heat insulation due to dense fur, e.g. Newfoundland or St. Bernard dogs
- High ambient temperature, limited possibility of compensation (e.g. brachycephalic breeds)
- Excitement during recovery phase

Complications/consequences

- Panting in the awake animal, may cause oedematous swelling of the upper respiratory tract, especially in brachycephalic breeds
- Increased O_2 consumption
- Increased CO_2 production
- Cell damage, protein denaturation

Prophylaxis/therapy

- Switch off heating, if necessary, start active cooling (wrap ice in plastic bag and towel, use cool packs, ▶ Fig. 8.25)
- Air blower, fan

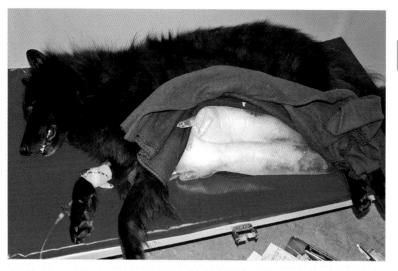

Fig. 8.25 Cooling with ice packs of a dog with thick, long fur.

- Cool paws
- Possibly clip the fur on the belly if nothing else helps and after agreement from the owner

Especially in convulsing animals (poisoning, epileptic seizures), animals with high muscle tone (e.g. after administration of ketamine or opioids during recovery in cats) or strong muscle work (e.g. brachycephalic patient with increased respiratory work), core body temperature can rise very quickly. Temperature should be measured routinely during the initial examination and regularly or better continuously during anaesthesia. A measurement in the recovery phase will guide further management.

8.3.3 Literature

[1] Kowalczyk L, Steinbacher R, Dörfelt R. Hypothermie während der Anästhesie – eine unterschätzte Komplikation. Tierärztl Umschau 2010; 65: 384–391

[2] Posner LP, Pavuk AA, Rokshar JL, Carter JE, Levine JF. Effects of opioids and anesthetic drugs on body temperature in cats. Vet Anaesth Analg 2010; 37: 35–43

[3] Steinbacher R, Mosing M, Eberspächer E, Moens Y. Der Einsatz von Infusionswärmepumpen vermindert perioperative Hypothermie bei Katzen. Tierärztl Prax (K) 2010; 38: 12–22

8.4 Electrolytes and acid-base balance

This chapter discusses the deviations of two electrolytes (potassium and sodium) and the acid-base balance and their therapy. Potassium was chosen because the anaesthetist is probably most concerned with its normalisation and balancing. Sodium seems to be the second most important electrolyte for the anaesthetist. However, balancing it is not easy and is often left to colleagues trained in intensive care medicine. Under no circumstances should one forget to determine the calcium concentration and treat deviations, especially in critically ill patients. It is worthwhile to study „Further reading" (p.491), as only a very compact overview can be presented here.

First of all, it is important to know the normal values in order to recognise deviations (▶ Table 8.2).

8.4.1 Potassium

Potassium (K) can be found 99% in the cell (concentration approx. 140 mEq/l) and only a small part is found in the plasma (this is the part we measure and "treat": approx. 4 mEq/l, see ▶ Table 8.2). A normal K concentration is crucial for normal neuromuscular function as it is responsible for the maintenance of the resting membrane potential. Both hyper- and hypokalaemia occur frequently in practice. Especially in cases of hyperkalaemia, rapid and correct therapeutic intervention can be life-saving!

Table 8.2 Normal values of sodium and potassium concentration in different animal species

Species	Sodium (mEq/l)	Potassium (mEq/l)
Dog	140–155	3.5–5.1
Cat	145–158	3.0–4.8
Rabbit	138–155	3.7–6.3
Ferret	139–166	3.8–5.5
Horse	125–150	2.8–4.5
Cattle	130–157	3.5–5.3
Sheep	139–152	3.9–5.4
Goat	142–155	3.5–6.7
Llama	147–158	4.0–5.5
Alpaca	148–155	4.0–5.3
Pig	134–153	3.5–7.5
mEq milliequivalent, l litre		

Hyperkalaemia

Hyperkalaemia requiring treatment is present when the plasma K concentration exceeds 5.5 to 6.0 mEq/l. It becomes life-threatening at concentrations above 7.5 mEq/l. Because of fluid shifts (and therefore possibly increasing K concentration) during anaesthesia, it is recommended that a patient which has a preoperative plasma K concentration of 6.0 mEq/l or higher be treated first and only then induce anaesthesia. Hyperkalaemia causes, among other things, muscle weakness and ECG changes due to prolonged de- and repolarisation phases, which may progress to arrhythmias (p. 350) such as ventricular fibrillation or ventricular flutter and asystole.

Good to know

ECG changes with hyperkalaemia

ECG changes do not correlate directly with the level of K concentration! There are also patients with severe hyperkalaemia worthy of treatment without ECG changes and the other way around (▶ Fig. 8.17)!

- Decrease in P wave amplitude until the P wave disappears completely
- Tall, tented T waves
- Lengthening of the QRS complex
- Bradycardia (not characteristic in cats)

Clinical relevance

Causes of hyperkalaemia

- Diabetes mellitus with ketoacidosis
- Urinary retention disorders, ruptured urinary bladder
- Iatrogenic (administration of an old blood transfusion)
- Addison's disease
- Tissue destruction
- Redistribution of potassium from intracellular to extracellular
- HYPP: Hyperkalaemic Periodic Paralysis, genetic defect in the Quarter Horse
- Pseudohyperkalaemia: Potassium is released more frequently in thrombocytosis or leukocytosis

Therapy

Ideally, therapy should be carried out under constant ECG control. In fact, in this situation, K-containing infusion solutions help better than e.g. NaCl 0.9% in order not to drive the potassium level up further. In case of life-threatening elevated plasma K concentration (with ECG changes), treatment should initially be started with calcium gluconate (stabilises membrane potential) followed by insulin and glucose (drives K into the cells). Otherwise, therapy with insulin and glucose alone, which can take up to 30 minutes to take effect, is sufficient (▶ Table 8.3).

Plasma electrolyte concentrations as well as glucose levels should be checked regularly (initially every hour, then at longer intervals when K starts to decrease) and the therapy adjusted.

Hypokalaemia

In general, there is less concern about hypokalaemia than about hyperkalaemia. But even with this electrolyte abnormality, there can be serious consequences due to generalised muscle weakness: Stiff gait, plantigrade stance and a drooping head as well as reduced motility of the gastrointestinal tract. This may be followed by CNS depression and, due to reduced cardiac contractility, hypotension and hypoperfusion.

Table 8.3 Therapy of life-threatening hyperkalaemia

Drugs	Dose	Mechanism of action	Onset of effect after
Calcium gluconate 10% as immediate emergency treatment	0.5–1.0 ml/kg over 10 min IV	Does not change K concentration in plasma, but stabilises membrane potential	3–5 min
Bicarbonate	1–2 mEq/l over 15 min IV	Controversial, increases extracellular pH, translocation of K into the cell	>15 min
5% glucose with insulin = "real" therapy because K migrates into the cell	Standard insulin 0.2–0.5 IU/kg IV plus 2 g glucose per IU insulin IV over 30–60 min	Translocation of K into the cell	15–30 min

IV intravenous, K potassium, IU international unit, mEq milliequivalent

Clinical relevance

Causes of hypokalaemia
- Abnormal losses (vomiting, diarrhoea, diuresis, anorexia)
- Decreased intake
- Diabetes mellitus
- Chronic kidney disease (especially cat)
- Dehydration (high urine K concentration)
- Redistribution of potassium from extracellular to intracellular
- Iatrogenic (administration of infusion solutions low in K)

Therapy

Therapy is actually quite simple and is achieved by K substitution (e.g. 1 molar KCl solution, 1 ml = 1 mEq) strictly according to ▶ Table 8.4.

Good to know

Increase K concentration SLOWLY!
The increase in K concentration should be at a **maximum rate of 0.5 mEq/kg/h**. Always close the IV line to the patient while mixing the solution with potassium and then mix and label well!

Table 8.4 Guideline of potassium substitution in hypokalaemia

Serum potassium concentration (mEq/l)	Add to 500 ml infusion solution (mEq)	Add to 1000 ml infusion solution (mEq)	Maximum infusion rate (ml/kg/h)
< 2	40	80	6
2.1–2.5	30	60	8
2.6–3.0	20	40	12
3.1–3.5	14	28	18
3.6–5.0	7	14	25

mEq milliequivalent

8.4.2 Sodium

The extracellular concentration of sodium (Na) is important for the transcellular fluid flow and is usually controlled by the kidney. In chronic diseases (> 24 h) with water losses, hypernatraemia can occur, and with e.g. very high water consumption, hyponatraemia can occur. Both hyper- and hyponatraemia can change neuronal cell volume and function and therefore damage them.

Hypernatraemia

Acute hypernatraemia is usually not caused by too much sodium, but by too little free water. It causes cellular dehydration in the brain, which is compensated for within approx. 24 h by the formation of intracellular "osmoles". The volume of neurons is restored. If hypernatremia is now compensated by rapid fluid intake, cellular oedema occurs, which can cause severe damage, especially in the brain. For this reason, compensation should always be done **slowly**!

Clinical relevance

Causes of hypernatraemia
- Loss of low-sodium fluids (diarrhoea, vomiting)
- Lack of access to water
- Iatrogenic (e.g. wrong infusion solution)
- Osmotic diuresis (treatment with mannitol)
- Diabetes insipidus – polyuria of low-sodium urine

Therapy

Patients with hypernatremia therefore have a free water deficit. Free water must be replaced carefully and under constant control (e.g. with the help of 5% glucose solution). This solution is administered in addition to the maintenance infusion solution.

Good to know

Reduce Na concentration SLOWLY!
The plasma sodium concentration should **not be reduced faster than 1 mEq/l/h**! 1 mmol/l corresponds to 1 mEq/l sodium.

The free water deficit is calculated as follows:

Free water deficit (in l) = (patient's plasma Na concentration [mEq/l]
÷ normal plasma Na concentration)
− 1 × (0.6 × body weight in kg)

The result is an amount in kg that indicates the volume of 5% glucose (= free water) in litres that must be substituted. This volume must now be infused over the calculated time period.

Example: If the patient's current Na level is 170 mmol/l and it should be 150 mmol/l, the 20 mmol/l must be compensated in 20 hours. In addition, of course, a maintenance solution with electrolyte concentrations as similar as possible to those of the patient should be administered.

The patient's Na level should be checked every 4 h and the infusion rate or the electrolyte composition of the infusion solution should be adjusted.

Hyponatraemia

This electrolyte imbalance is rather rare. Affected patients usually suffer from water retention and/or increased water intake. The electrolyte imbalance must again be corrected slowly because otherwise free water is "pulled out" of neurons too quickly and cells shrink, leading to myelinolysis. Clinical signs only become visible after days, so one cannot assume that the patient has tolerated rapid compensation well just because one does not observe any clinical deterioration on day 1 and 2 after start of treatment.

Clinical relevance

Causes of hyponatraemia
- Decreased effective circulating blood volume (e.g. congestive heart failure, gastrointestinal losses, polyuria, body cavity effusions such as ascites)
- Excessive water intake (e.g. psychogenic polydipsia)
- Hypoadrenocorticism
- Thiazides and loop diuretics
- Insufficient ADH secretion

Therapy

If (mild) hyponatraemia (> 130 mmol/l) is due to a low effective circulating volume, the value is usually corrected by therapy of the underlying pathology. Often, it is also sufficient to restrict the drinking quantity. However, if symptoms appear and a Na concentration of < 120 mmol/l is reached, therapeutic intervention is recommended carefully without worsening the clinical symptoms. However: "If you do not know what to do, do nothing" (Plato). The wrong therapy for hyponatraemia can be fatal.

Good to know

Increase Na concentration SLOWLY!
The increase in Na concentration must be even slower than the decrease, with a **maximum of 0.5 mEq/l/h**! Another recommendation is to correct even slower with a maximum 10 mEq/l in the first 24 h.

If the patient's condition permits, a dual approach can be chosen: On the one hand, the excretion of free water can be promoted (use of diuretics such as mannitol and furosemide; especially if oedema exists) and on the other hand, Na-containing infusion solutions can be administered. 0.9% NaCl solution (154 mEq/l, equivalent to 0.15 mEq/ml) or 3% hypertonic NaCl solution (514 mEq/l, equivalent to 0.5 mEq/ml) can be used as correction fluid.

The sodium deficit is calculated as follows:

Sodium deficit (in l) = (sodium plasma concentration [mEq/l]
approx. 10–15% higher than the current
patient sodium plasma concentration
– patient sodium plasma concentration)
× (0.6 × body weight in kg)

If the patient's plasma sodium concentration is 120 mEq/l, the first "target" should be a concentration of approx. 135 mEq/l.

8.4.3 Acid-base balance and blood gas analysis

The body regulates its acid-base balance through three mechanisms:
- The regulation of pCO_2 via ventilation (p. 369)
- The buffering of acids by bicarbonate and other buffering systems
- The excretion of acids or bases by the kidneys

Table 8.5 Normal values related to acid-base balance in the arterial blood

Parameter	Normal ranges (varies by species!)
pH	7.35–7.45
pCO_2	30–45 mmHg (▶ Table 2.3)
HCO_3^-	20–27 mEq/l (Carnivores slightly lower, herbivores slightly higher)
BE	−3 to + 3 (Herbivores up to + 5)

pCO_2 partial pressure of carbon dioxide, HCO_3^- bicarbonate concentration, BE base excess

Table 8.6 Simple acid-base disorders and how to recognise them using pH, pCO_2 and HCO_3^-

Acid-base disorder	pH	Primary disorder	Compensation
Respiratory acidosis	↓	↑ pCO_2	↑ HCO_3^-
Respiratory alkalosis	↑	↓ pCO_2	↓ HCO_3^-
Metabolic acidosis	↓	↓ HCO_3^-	↓ pCO_2
Metabolic alkalosis	↑	↑ HCO_3^-	↑ pCO_2

pCO_2 partial pressure of carbon dioxide, HCO_3^- bicarbonate concentration, ↑ increase, ↓ decrease

Basically, it can be simplified that pCO_2 represents the respiratory component and bicarbonate the metabolic component. Normal values are found in ▶ Table 8.5.

Definition

- pCO_2 = Partial pressure of carbon dioxide in mmHg
- HCO_3^- = Bicarbonate in mEq/l or mmol/l
- **BE** = Base excess = amount of acid or base to be added to the blood to maintain a pH of 7.4 (at 37 °C and pCO_2 of 40 mmHg)

The body will always try to maintain the pH value in its physiological optimum around 7.4 or to bring it back there. If, for example, pCO_2 (= acid) increases due to hypoventilation, then the bicarbonate (= base) balancing system will also increase in order to compensate for the resulting acidosis and bring the pH back towards the normal value (▶ Table 8.6).

Table 8.7 Expected degree of compensation to a simple disorder

Primary disorder	Expected degree of compensation
Respiratory acidosis (acute)	↑ [HCO_3^-] by 0.15 mEq/l per 1 mmHg ↑ pCO_2
Respiratory acidosis (chronic)	↑ [HCO_3^-] by 0.35 mEq/l per 1 mmHg ↑ pCO_2
Respiratory alkalosis (acute)	↓ [HCO_3^-] by 0.25 mEq/l per 1 mmHg ↓ pCO_2
Respiratory alkalosis (chronic)	↓ [HCO_3^-] by 0.55 mEq/l per 1 mmHg ↓ pCO_2
Metabolic acidosis	↓ pCO_2 by 0.7 mmHg per 1 mEq/l ↓ [HCO_3^-]
Metabolic alkalosis	↑ pCO_2 by 0.7 mmHg per 1 mEq/l ↑ [HCO_3^-]

pCO_2 partial pressure of carbon dioxide, HCO_3^- bicarbonate concentration, ↑ increase, ↓ decrease

To see if it is a simple acid-base disorder with normal compensation, one can look at the expected degree of compensation (▶ Table 8.7) and compare with the values of the patient.

If the compensation is more or less as expected, it can be assumed to be a simple disorder. If the compensation is different than expected, one must assume that it is a mixed disorder. This means that there are primary disorders in both the respiratory and metabolic systems.

Blood gas analysis

There are various ways to perform blood gas analysis, the only important thing is to do it in an orderly and complete manner. Of course, in the clinical setting, the **analysis of the partial pressure of oxygen (pO$_2$)** is also an **important** part of the process.

For example, the following scheme is recommended:

1. Evaluation of **pH**
   - Within normal limits
   - If low: Acidaemia
   - If increased: Alkalaemia
2. Evaluation of **pCO$_2$** as a **respiratory** component
   - Within normal limits
   - If low (hyperventilation): Alkalosis
   - If increased (hypoventilation): Acidosis
3. Evaluation of **HCO$_3^-$** or **BE** as a **metabolic** component
   - Within normal limits
   - If HCO$_3^-$ low or BE negative: Acidosis
   - If HCO$_3^-$ increased or BE positive: Alkalosis

4. **Define the primary disturbance**. In other words: Which disorder (respiratory or metabolic) causes the deviation of the pH value in the same direction?
5. Check if the compensation is as expected
6. Establish your diagnosis based on the overall picture of the patient's acid-base balance

The most common changes in acid-base balance encountered by the anaesthetist are:

1. **Hypoventilation** during anaesthesia (= **respiratory acidosis**)
2. **Hypoperfusion** and therefore retention of waste products such as lactate in the body (= **metabolic acidosis**, which is often accompanied by an additional respiratory acidosis, resulting in a mixed disorder that can lead to severe acidaemia).

Therapy of deviations in the acid-base balance

Basically, one should always look for the underlying cause and address it.

Respiratory acidosis and alkalosis

During anaesthesia there are many reasons for hypo- (p. 369) or hyperventilation (p. 373).

Metabolic acidosis

This abnormality occurs in more than 40% of all dogs and cats in which a blood gas analysis is performed at a veterinary university. In horses, it may result from losses of bicarbonate with hypochloraemia or retention of acids.

Apart from a variety of gastrointestinal problems that can cause this condition, the cause during anaesthesia is often hypoperfusion and hypoxia of the peripheral tissues with accumulation of lactate as acid. This leads to the therapeutic options: Administration of oxygen, ventilation, correction of volaemic status, normalisation of blood pressure and core body temperature to improve perfusion.

The additional administration of bicarbonate is controversial. If it is indicated in selected cases (e.g. uraemic acidosis), then dosing should be done quite carefully according to the following formula:

Na-bicarbonate (mEq) = $0.3 \times$ body weight (kg) $\times$ base deficit (mEq/l)

This amount is often calculated, but treatment then started with half of the calculated value. The amount should be infused slowly over at least 30 minutes. Exhalation of the resulting CO_2 should be ensured.

395

Metabolic alkalosis

This deviation is relatively rare, the reason is often a gastrointestinal problem (e.g. gastrointestinal obstruction) or iatrogenically caused (e.g. loop diuretics, suctioning of the gastric tube).

8.4.4 Literature

[1] Diercks DB, Shumaik GM, Harrigan RA, Brady WJ, Chan TC. Electrocardiographic manifestations: electrolyte abnormalities. J Emerg Med 2004; 27: 153–160

[2] Gennari JF. Hypokalemia. N Engl J Med 1998; 339: 451

[3] Hengrave Burri I, Tschudi P, Martig J, Liesegang A, Meylan M. Neuweltkameliden in der Schweiz. II. Referenzwerte für hämatologische und blutchemische Parameter. Schweiz Arch Tierheilk 2005; 147: 335–343

[4] Rhee KH, Toro LH, McDonald GG, Nunnally RL, Levin DL. Carbicarb, sodium bicarbonate, and sodium chloride in hypoxic lactic acidosis. Effect on arterial blood gases, lactate concentrations, hemodynamic variables, and myocardial intracellular pH. Chest 1993; 104: 913–918

8.5 Reflux/regurgitation/aspiration

The most common cause of perioperative aspiration pneumonia is inhalation of gastric contents. The decisive factor here seems to be the low pH: The more acidic the aspirate, the worse the consequences. But aspiration of (contaminated) blood, saliva, mucus or pus can also have problematic consequences. Some predisposing factors for perioperative regurgitation and/or aspiration are:

- Patients with a full stomach (not fasting or unable to empty stomach, e.g. in ruminants)
- Drugs/anaesthetics that relax the lower oesophageal sphincter (e.g. opioids)
- Delayed gastric emptying, e.g. due to anxiety, pain, shock or drugs
- Increased intraabdominal pressure, e.g. pregnancy, obesity, distended gastrointestinal tract/colic
- As pathology associated with brachycephalic syndrome
- Oral surgery, dental cleaning
- Anaesthesia, especially if it lasts longer than 2 h

8.5.1 Small animals

When the patient is under anaesthesia, passive or active **reflux** of stomach contents may occur due to unconsciousness and impaired function of the protective reflexes. If **regurgitation** occurs, the liquid greenish-brownish stomach contents can often be seen in and around the muzzle. However, reflux can happen completely unnoticed.

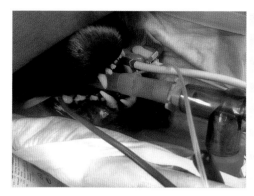

Fig. 8.26 Regurgitation in a dog after several hours of anaesthesia.

- **Preventive measures**
  - Fast animals for an appropriate period of time preoperatively
  - Especially in animals with predisposing factors, rapid induction and intubation with inflation of the cuff (previously tested for leaks)
  - Possibly pre-treatment with metoclopramide and/or ranitidine/famotidine and/or omeprazole
- **Therapy** for reflux/regurgitation during anaesthesia (▶ Fig. 8.26)
  - Ensure that the endotracheal tube is properly placed and properly cuffed
  - Position the head in a way so that reflux can drain out
  - Aspirate and clean out regurgitated material from the oral cavity, pharynx and oesophagus
  - Flush the oesophagus with 0.9% NaCl solution with added sodium bicarbonate and wash out the oral cavity
  - If reflux/regurgitation is expected, place a gastric tube
  - Before extubation, inspect the oral cavity and wash it out if necessary
  - Potentially keep cuff slightly inflated during extubation

The prognosis is quite good in small animals depending on pH and material aspirated, extension in the lungs and therapeutic intervention. However, the main focus should always be on prevention.

8.5.2 Large animals

In horses that have to be operated on because of colic, it is important to remove most of the stomach contents before anaesthesia with a nasogastric tube.

- **Preventive measures**
  - Fast animals for an appropriate period of time preoperatively
  - In patients with colic, place nasogastric tube and attempt to remove gastric contents before induction of anaesthesia
  - After induction (especially if predisposing factors are present) intubate as soon as possible, inflate cuff to seal trachea
  - Keep cuff slightly inflated during extubation

The prognosis of horses with aspiration pneumonia is not considered as favourable as that of small animals, even with attempted therapy (antibiosis).

8.5.3 Literature

[1] Kogan DA, Johnson LR, Sturges BK, Jandrey KE, Pollard RE. Etiology and clinical outcome in dogs with aspiration pneumonia: 88 cases (2004–2006). J Am Vet Med Assoc 2008; 233: 1748–1755

[2] Ovbey DH, Wilson DV, Bednarski RM, Hauptmann JG, Stanley BJ, Radlinsky MG, Larenza MP, Pypendop BH, Rezende ML. Prevalence and risk factors for canine post-anesthetic aspiration pneumonia (1999–2009): a multicenter study. Vet Anaesth Analg 2014; 41: 127–136

[3] Tart KM, Babski DM, Lee JA. Potential risks, prognostic indicators, and diagnostic and treatment modalities affecting survival in dogs with presumptive aspiration pneumonia: 125 cases. J Vet Emerg Crit Care 2010; 20: 319–329

9 Pain and pain therapy

Every vertebrate is capable of feeling pain. A distinction is made between acute and chronic pain, as well as between different types and qualities, e.g. rather sharp/stabbing or rather dull/throbbing.

Clinical pain can be divided into **nociceptive pain** and **neuropathic pain**, which differs from physiological pain by a pathological hypersensitivity. Nociceptor pain occurs predominantly in tissue and can be caused by trauma, inflammation or tumour. Neuropathic pain is localised in and around damaged nerve cells. The consequences of chronic or recurring pain are **allodynia**, as well as primary and secondary **hyperalgesia**.

Definition

Central sensitisation and chronic pain

A long-term pain stimulus can lead to adaptive changes at the cellular level in the CNS ("neuroplasticity"). This leads to the so-called "wind-up" phenomenon, which is expressed in increased pain sensation. **Chronic pain is difficult to diagnose and difficult to treat**. Therefore, if possible, pain should ideally be avoided rather than treated after it has occurred. Chronic neuropathic pain can manifest itself in different ways:

- **Allodynia:** Pain sensation triggered by stimuli that are **normally perceived as not painful**
- **Primary hyperalgesia: Excessive pain sensitivity** and reaction to a painful stimulus (especially heat stimulus), often due to local sensitisation
- **Secondary hyperalgesia: Sensitivity** to pain that occurs through neuronal connections even **in places that were not originally injured**

In veterinary medicine, the appropriate treatment of pain is often neglected for various reasons. These are among others:
- Difficulties in recognising the signs of pain
- Inaccurate "knowledge" (e.g. "4 days old puppies cannot feel pain because the nerves are not fully grown yet" or the use of opioids or lidocaine in cats is avoided by many veterinarians due to old and misinterpreted studies)
- Too few or no approved analgesics for certain species
- Fear of possible side effects

▶ **What are the consequences of pain?** Pain affects almost all areas of the body. In short, pain causes a pain and a stress reaction that manifests itself as follows:

- Hyper- or hypoventilation
- Tachycardia, increased cardiac output
- Impaired gastrointestinal motility
- Decreased urine production and excretion
- Increased metabolism
- Decreased immune response
- Tendency to higher blood clotting activity
- Tendency to gastric ulcers
- Transition to a chronic pain state

9.1 Signs of pain

The signs of pain vary considerably from species to species (▶ Table 9.1) and sometimes differ even within a species from breed to breed!

However, some **general signs** are seen across species:

- Often increased respiratory rate with/without breath sounds
- Weight loss due to inappetence, among other things
- Dehydration due to reduced water intake
- Hypothermia
- Dull, ruffled, shaggy, partly unkempt fur
- Half-closed or closed eyes, sometimes also eyes wide open
- Seclusion from other animals of the same species
- Seeking out shadows/darkness, avoiding light

Especially in animal species that are subject to threats from predators, no signs of pain are obvious for a long time, because otherwise (in the wild) the enemy could be attracted. Therefore, these animals tend to suffer silently and a close look must be taken to detect signs of pain or suffering (▶ Fig. 9.1).

It is helpful to study the physiological, **normal behaviour** of a species in order to recognise deviations more quickly. So-called **grimace scales** are available for several species, with which one can recognise pain on the basis of facial expression.

For practical use, **numerical rating scales** with a scale from 1 (not painful) to 10 (extremely painful) have proven to be useful for assessing the current condition and the course of the disease. However, **composite scales** seem to be the best option, as they include several components.

Table 9.1 Signs of pain in different animal species

Species	General	Behaviour	Abnormal activity	Posture	Vocalisation
Dog	Signs of appeasement (licking, yawning, smacking), reduced appetite	Unusually calm, aggressive when approached, later apathetic	Unwillingness to move, insecurity, protective posture, lameness, licking/biting at certain parts of the body	Change in lying and resting behaviour (e.g. lying on one side)	Barking, yelping or moaning
Cat	Often rather subtle, can be easily overlooked	Protective behaviour, unusually quiet or aggressive, withdrawal into the corner	Particularly quiet, lack of movement, sometimes increasingly looking for attention	Crouched, huddled, back arched up, head down, half-closed eyes	No meowing or strong meowing, even screaming
Rabbit	Deviations often very difficult to recognise, as painful conditions are often endured without noticeable reactions	Reduced environmental responses, disturbed exploratory behaviour	–	Crouching posture, unusual stretching of the body, tilted head	Normally hardly any, in acute pain piercing, shrill pain sounds
Guinea pig	Apathy, often motionless on examination, hair loss, often inappetence is the only sign	Typical avoidance behaviour, initially increased, later apathy	Gnawing at own fur	Tucked up abdomen, curved back with abdominal pain, lameness, cautious gait, reduced muscle tone	Normal, reduced when in pain

Table 9.1 continued

Species	General	Behaviour	Abnormal activity	Posture	Vocalisation
Ferret	Painful conditions are often endured stoically	Change in behaviour, aggressive (sudden biting) or withdrawal behaviour	–	Ruffled fur, curling up	Varies individually, none or whimpering
Rat	Signs difficult to recognise, apathy	Aggressive or withdrawal behaviour, automutilation	–	Ruffled coat, arched back	Squealing
Mouse	Apathy, often turned away from light source	Defensive reactions increased, biting or later withdrawal behaviour, seclusion from the group	Automutilation, cautious, unsteady gait	Ruffled fur, arched back	High-pitched squeals when grasping, decreases with increasing weakness
Hamster	Wet tail (diarrhoea), increasing sluggishness	Increased aggression, depression, i.e. reduced behaviour despite external stimuli, restricted exploration behaviour	Strongly altered sleeping times	Curled up position, inhibited locomotion	Possibly squeals
Horse (▲ Fig. 9.1)	Sweating, apathy, tired, absent or fixed gaze or widened eyes, looking at the painful part of the body	Seclusion from others, loss of rank, restlessness, increased anxiety, sudden aggression or conspicuous attention	Trembling, lips pressed together, tense jaw muscles, teeth grinding, foaming, head and tail flapping	Restricted mobility, lying down or stays standing	Moaning

Table 9.1 continued

Species	General	Behaviour	Abnormal activity	Posture	Vocalisation
Cattle	Are stoic for a very long time, very subtle signs, lack of movement, reduced food intake	–	Teeth grinding, foaming	Restricted movement, evasion, retraction of the painful body part	Moaning
Sheep/ goat	Very subtle signs of pain, restlessness, looking at the affected body part	Changed behaviour, seek the protection of the group	Striking with legs against affected region, lack of movement	Striking posture, arched back	Screaming only in acute cases
South American camelids	Very stoic, show hardly any signs, lack of movement	Initially restlessness, later depression and apathy	Smacking, foaming, teeth grinding	Arched back, stiff gait	Moaning
Pig	Restlessness, defensive reactions, kicking, inappetence	Aggression or withdrawal behaviour	Turning away, isolation from other animals	Increased lying down phases	In acute cases, piercing, loud screaming

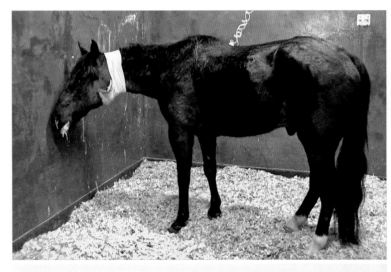

Fig. 9.1 Horse with severe pain.

9.2 Peri- and postoperative pain

Even in human medicine, perioperative and posttraumatic acute pain therapy is insufficient according to several studies. There is a "striking underuse and misuse of care" (S3 guideline, DIVS). One may hardly imagine what the situation is like in small and large animal practice, let alone in practice with food-producing animals.

Besides medical and additional non-medical therapy, a quiet, warm, dry environment should be provided, especially during recovery phase. If surgery permits, food and water should be offered again soon. Occasional "TLC" (tender loving care) or sedation helps especially restless and anxious animals. Regeneration occurs mainly during sleep: the patient should therefore be given the opportunity or the environment should be created so that sleep is possible (rest, lights off, no hourly vital signs check unless indicated).

The best time to start pain therapy is BEFORE the actual pain stimulus in order to avoid sensitisation of the central nervous system and therefore increased pain sensation or the development of chronic pain states. It is important to provide analgesia in the **correct dose** via an **appropriate mode of administration** at the **required application intervals** and over an **appropriate period of time**. Often, a combination of different analgesics is used (= **multi-**

modal analgesia) in order to increase the desired effect (analgesia) analogous to balanced anaesthesia while simultaneously reducing the risk of side effects.

Basically, therapy should be based on the pain ladder of the World Health Organization (WHO): Pain is classified according to its degree and treated accordingly. This is to prevent both overuse and underuse of pain medication. The following are some examples of degrees, although the degree must be adapted according to the individual case:

- **No/short-term pain:** Fixation of the animal, removal of sutures, applying bandages
- **Minor pain:** Skin suture, debridement, placement of a urinary catheter, abscess splitting
- **Moderate pain:** Removal of skin tumours, castration, cystotomy, tooth extraction
- **Severe pain:** Fracture treatment, amputation, thoracoscopy
- **Extreme pain:** Thoracotomy lateral/sternal, laminectomy, total ear canal ablation

Good to know

Pain in the emergency patient

Emergency patients often suffer from pain. This pain should not be overlooked in the heat of the moment! Pain therapy should already be integrated as a step during the stabilisation phase. Often, analgesia can be provided relatively easily with opioids.

In dogs and cats, methadone 0.2–0.4 mg/kg IV or IM is a good choice. At this dosage, good analgesia with manageable side effects can be expected.

9.3 Analgesics and postoperative pain management strategies

Analgesic care with drugs can be provided by systemic administration of analgesics, by local anaesthesia or, ideally, by a combination of the two.

The following is an overview of frequently used drugs with analgesic effects. Perioperative use is described under "Species-specific anaesthesia" (p. 150), and in other chapters of the book. In the corresponding chapter, the individual drugs (p. 63) mentioned are also discussed in detail. There you will find, among other things, desired effects and side effects as well as dosages for different animal species. A discussion of suitable non-pharmacological options (p. 466) is given at the end of the chapter.

9.3.1 Local anaesthetics

The effects, side effects and dosages of the drugs **bupivacaine** (p.76), **lidocaine** (p.108) and **ropivacaine** (p.137) have already been discussed. Local anaesthetic techniques should be used whenever possible. The quality of analgesia is unmatched, the transmission of the pain signal to the (spinal cord and) brain is practically "cut off".

9.3.2 Non-steroidal anti-inflammatory drugs (NSAIDs) and similar analgesics

This group includes an increasing number of COX2-selective drugs (keyword "coxibs") that are approved as analgesics in animals; as an example, **cimicoxib** (p.82) is discussed in this book. In the drug section, two classic representatives of NSAIDs are also discussed in more detail: **carprofen** (p.81) and **meloxicam** (p.114). Piprants intervene very far down the arachidonic acid cascade. **Grapiprant** (p.100) is a representative of these highly modern analgesics. **Metamizole** (p.117), an active substance from the group of non-acidic non-opioid analgesics, which is however often classified as an NSAID, must not be forgotten as a very good analgesic.

NSAIDs are considered analgesics in small animals suitable for treating low to moderate pain. They have anti-inflammatory, antipyretic and some other positive effects, but one must also consider the side effects. NSAIDs can be given for a longer period of time if needed. They are very good drugs to give postoperatively to the owner, who can then administer them to the patient orally over a few days.

In ruminants and horses, NSAIDs are also good analgesics for low to moderate pain. **Flunixin meglumine** or **phenylbutazone** can be used in horses, and **ketoprofen** in ruminants.

9.3.3 Opioids

Among the opioids described in this book, all except the κ agonist/μ antagonist **butorphanol** in some countries and **tramadol** are scheduled drugs and must be treated accordingly. However, this should not discourage one from having these very good analgesics available on clinics and from using them. Pure μ agonists are excellent emergency analgesics, e.g. **methadone** (p.119), **morphine** (p.123) or **pethidine** (p.129), and can also be used routinely for perioperative pain control. Some easy to titrate opioids such as **fentanyl** (p.92), **remifentanil** or **sufentanil** are particularly suitable for perioperative use. **Buprenorphine** (p.77) as a partial μ agonist is particularly suitable for use postoperatively and in small mammals due to its long duration of action.

9.3.4 Dissociative anaesthetics: Ketamine

Ketamine has anti-hyperalgesic (low dose) and analgesic (high dose) effects in addition to the dissociative/hypnotic effect, which appear to be particularly well suited to treat orthopaedic pain or pain associated with skin, muscles and bones. It is very useful to support cardiovascular stability during general anaesthesia. It is used as a bolus and CRI in dogs (p. 329), cats (p. 184) and horses (p. 336). The anti-hyperalgesic effect reduces hypersensitisation.

9.3.5 Alpha2 agonists

The drugs in this substance group, which are discussed in more detail in the drug section, are **dexmedetomidine** (p. 86) and **medetomidine** (p. 111), **xylazine** (p. 145), **detomidine** (p. 84) and **romifidine** (p. 135). Alpha2 agonists are primarily sedatives or hypnotics that also have an analgesic and muscle relaxing effect. They are not primarily used as analgesics. In terms of structure, they are similar to local anaesthetics and therefore have a local analgesic effect. They are used in combination with local anaesthetics or opioids for epidural or spinal analgesia. In very low doses, they can be given to calm agitated animals that have already received analgesic care, e.g. medetomidine 2–3 µg/kg IV.

9.3.6 Other drugs with analgesic effects

Our pets are getting older and are increasingly suffering from age-related orthopaedic chronic pain conditions. In dogs, but also in cats, two drugs are available, among others, that can help alleviate neuropathic pain: **Gabapentin** (p. 97) and **amantadine** (p. 68). Anti-neuronal growth factors (NGF) antibodies (**bedinvetmab**, LIBRELA for dogs and **frunevetmab**, SOLENSIA for cats), which are increasingly used for osteoarthritis, use a completely different but very effective mechanism of action.

9.3.7 Postoperative pain management concepts: Dog and cat

Ideally, analgesics are used perioperatively prior to the painful stimulus and according to the expected type and degree of pain. Depending on the severity of pain, the appropriate drug and route of administration should also be chosen postoperatively. Of course, **analgesic management should be tailored to the individual patient** and pain evaluations should be performed regularly.

After interventions that can cause **mild to moderate** (inflammatory) **pain**, it is usually sufficient to administer an **NSAID** for a few days with the option to add on other analgesics. NSAIDs can also be administered as a "first step" in case of moderate or severe pain, if the patient's condition/illness allows it.

After procedures involving **severe pain**, the animal should be hospitalised and given **opioids** either regularly or as continuous therapy. In dogs and cats, methadone 0.2–0.5 mg/kg every 3–4 h IV is suitable, but in cats buprenorphine, e.g. 0.02 mg/kg IV, IM or orally transmucosal every 6 h is also suitable.

In case of severe pain, long-term therapy with methadone in combination with ketamine and lidocaine can be started in dogs admitted to the hospital.

Practice tip

MLK: Methadone-Lidocaine-Ketamine as postoperative continuous rate infusion for dogs
NaCl 0.9% 100 ml PLUS
- **Methadone** 1 ml (= 10 mg, 1 ml with 10 mg/ml)
- **Lidocaine** 5 ml (= 100 mg, 2% lidocaine with 20 mg/ml)
- **Ketamine** 0.3 ml (= 30 mg, ketamine with 100 mg/ml)
Mix well and label.

This mixture can be started **postoperatively with 1–2 ml/kg/h** and ensures balanced and multimodal analgesia. The higher dose should be chosen at the beginning or in very painful conditions. It is **very important to evaluate the patient closely and regularly and to adjust the dose** to the need – this usually means **reducing the dose over time**! Depending on the size of the patient, the appropriate amount should be mixed (a large dog weighing 30 kg needs a total of 3 × 500 ml NaCl 0.9% mixed with MLK for 24 h at a rate of 2 ml/kg/h)!

A postoperative administration of **2 ml/kg/h** corresponds approximately to a dosage of methadone 0.2 mg/kg/h, lidocaine 0.03 mg/kg/min and ketamine 0.01 mg/kg/min. The **dosages are chosen fairly high**, the mixture can also be mixed in **half the concentration**, especially if regular monitoring of the patient is not guaranteed. The **rate must be adapted to the patient's condition continuously**. The condition should – as already mentioned – be checked at regular intervals (e.g. every 4 h). If animals are sedated with MLK, the dose should be reduced. Hypothermia can be prevented with active temperature management.

The postoperative MLK drip described in the box above can also be used in a slightly modified way for the **cat**: **Lidocaine is omitted** and the **dose of methadone and ketamine is halved**. Instead of 10 mg methadone, 5 mg is added, and instead of 30 mg ketamine, 15 mg is added. The infusion rate remains the same.

Practice tip

FK: Fentanyl-Ketamine as a postoperative continuous rate infusion for cats

NaCl 0.9% 100 ml PLUS
- **Fentanyl** 5 ml (= 0.25 mg, 10 ml with 0.05 mg/ml)
- **Ketamine** 0.15 ml (= 15 mg, ketamine with 100 mg/ml)

Mix well and label.

This mixture can be given **postoperatively at 1–2 ml/kg/h** and ensures balanced and multimodal analgesia.

A postoperative administration of **2 ml/kg/h** corresponds approximately to a dosage of fentanyl 0.005 mg/kg/h and ketamine 0.005 mg/kg/min. The patient's condition should be monitored at regular intervals. In very painful conditions, the dose of fentanyl can be doubled, i. e. the drip mixed with 10 ml instead of 5 ml.

If necessary, a **ketamine CRI can also be used with the addition of opioid boluses**, e.g. methadone 0.2–0.5 mg/kg IV every 4 h or buprenorphine 0.02 mg/kg IV every 6 h.

As an additional analgesic component, especially for chronic orthopaedic pain, gabapentin or amantadine can be used as long-term therapy. Either one can be administered with good success and few side effects in dogs, cats and rabbits.

If the animal is discharged home with severe pain, options are limited. Tramadol can be given, often in combination with an NSAID. This opioid-like drug is the only one that can be taken orally. The analgesic effect is largely dependent on metabolisation and highly variable.

9.3.8 Postoperative pain management concepts: Small mammals

Appropriate pain management in small mammals is a particular challenge. The reasons are:

- Dosages and administration intervals are often adopted from other (larger) pets, but have not been evaluated for the respective pet species; it is obvious that the published and generally accepted dosages for small mammals are too low and application intervals too long

Table 9.2 Overview of dosages and application intervals of various analgesics in rabbits, guinea pigs, mice, hamsters and rats

Species	Carprofen	Meloxicam	Metamizole	Buprenorphine	Lidocaine	Bupivacaine
Rabbit	4 mg/kg SC, IV	0.4–0.6 mg/kg SC, PO	20–50 mg/kg SC, IM, PO q4	0.01–0.05 mg/kg SC, IV BID–QID	Max. 4 mg/kg SC*	1–2 mg/kg SC*
Guinea pig	4 mg/kg SC	0.5–1 mg/kg SC, PO	80 mg/kg SC, IM, PO q4–QID	0.01–0.05 mg/kg SC BID–QID	Max. 4 mg/kg SC*	1–2 mg/kg SC*
Mouse	4–10 mg/kg SC, PO	(1–)5 mg/kg SC, PO	100–200 mg/kg SC, IM, PO QID	0.03–0.1 mg/kg SC QID*	Max. 10 mg/kg SC	Max. 5 mg/kg SC
Hamster	4–10 mg/kg SC	(1–)5 mg/kg SC, PO BID*	100–200 mg/kg SC, IM, PO QID	0.03–0.1 mg/kg SC QID*	Max. 4 mg/kg SC*	Max. 5 mg/kg SC*
Rat	4–10 mg/kg SC	1 mg/kg SC, PO	100–200 mg/kg SC, IM, PO QID	0.03–0.1 mg/kg SC QID*	Max. 4 mg/kg SC*	Max. 5 mg/kg SC*

IV intravenously, IM intramuscularly, SC subcutaneously, PO orally, BID 2 × daily, TID 3 × daily, QID 4 × daily, q4 every 4 h, Max. maximum, * no reliable data available

- Although, for example, mice and hamsters are completely different species, they are often grouped together as "small rodents" or "small mammals" for convenience – as is also done in part of this book
- The evaluation of pain is not easy with dogs, cats or horses. With small mammals it is even more difficult – despite tools such as facial expression, abnormal or nest-building behaviour

In general, analgesics should also be used preventively and multimodally in small mammal species.

The use of the NSAID **meloxicam** has proven particularly effective in small mammals because there is an oral formulation that can also be easily administered by the owner at home. **Buprenorphine** as a partial μ opioid receptor agonist is not as effective as a pure μ agonist, but is popular in small mammals because of its relatively long duration of action. Local anaesthetics are still used rarely in small mammals. This is probably due to statements in older textbooks that they have a severe toxic effect on rodents. However, this has turned out to be unsubstantiated and in mice, for example, **lidocaine** up to 10 mg/kg and **bupivacaine** up to 5 mg/kg can be used safely and efficiently, even in combination.

Different analgesics can be used depending on the indication (▶ Table 9.2). More detailed information on the respective analgesics can be found in the chapter "Drugs" (p. 63).

9.3.9 Postoperative pain management concepts: Horse

Perioperative pain management in horses is partly discussed in the chapters "Species anaesthesia" (p. 219) and "Colic in horses" (p. 336). Various analgesic combinations are available as **continuous rate infusions (CRI) postoperatively** or for the treatment of pain due to other causes. The combinations are **listed in the order of analgesic effect**, i.e. as a therapeutic approach for mild to severe pain. The lidocaine used is, of course, without added vasoconstrictive agents.

Dosage

1. Ketamine + Lidocaine CRI
- **Lidocaine** 1.5–2 mg/kg/h (initial bolus: 1.3–2 mg/kg over 10–15 min IV)
- **Ketamine** 0.2–0.6 mg/kg/h (initial bolus: 1 mg/kg over 30 min IV)

Dosage

2. Ketamine + Lidocaine + Detomidine CRI

- **Ketamine** 0.4–0.8 mg/kg/h (initial bolus: 1 mg/kg over 30 min IV)
- **Lidocaine** 1.5–2 mg/kg/h (initial bolus: 1.3–2 mg/kg over 10–15 min IV)
- **Detomidine** 0.002–0.004 mg/kg/h

Dosage

3. Morphine + Lidocaine + Ketamine (MLK) CRI

- **Morphine** 0.02 mg/kg/h (initial bolus 0.1 mg/kg over 10 min IV)
- **Lidocaine** 1.5–2 mg/kg/h (initial bolus: 1.3–2 mg/kg over 10–15 min IV)
- **Ketamine** 0.4–0.8 mg/kg/h (initial bolus: 1 mg/kg over 30 min IV)

Dosage

4. "Pentafusion": Ketamine + Morphine + Lidocaine + Detomidine + Acepromazine CRI

- Mix **Lidocaine** 3 mg/kg AND **Ketamine** 0.6 mg/kg in 1 l NaCl 0.9%
- Mix **Morphine** 0.025 mg/kg AND **Detomidine** 0.004 mg/kg AND **Acepromazine** 0.002 mg/kg in a second bag of 1 l NaCl 0.9%

Both mixtures should be administered separately at a CRI of 70 ml/h each.

Ketamine and morphine should not be used at these doses for longer than 48 h due to accumulation. However, both drugs can of course be continued at lower doses (e.g. in chronic laminitis, fractures).

With each administration of continuous rate infusions, the **effect must be monitored regularly and the dose adjusted** as needed. In addition, NSAIDs and non-pharmacological analgesic therapies (p. 469), e.g. application of crushed ice, can and should be used (if the patient's condition and illness permit).

9.3.10 Literature

[1] Dalla Costa E, Minero M, Lebelt D, Stucke D, Canali E, Leach MC. Development of the Horse Grimace Scale (HGS) as a pain assessment tool in horses undergoing routine castration. PLoS ONE 2014; 9: e92281

[2] Deutsche Interdisziplinäre Vereinigung für Schmerztherapie (DIVS) e. V. S3-Leitlinie Behandlung akuter perioperativer und posttraumatischer Schmerzen. Köln: Deutscher Ärzte-Verlag 2008

[3] Holton L, Reid J, Scott EM, Pawson P, Nolan A. Development of a behaviour-based scale to measure acute pain in dogs. Vet Rec 2001; 148: 525–531

[4] Matsumiya LC, Sorge RE, Sotocinal SG, Tabaka JM, Wieskopf JS, Zaloum A, King OD, Mogil JS. Using the mouse grimace scale to reevaluate the efficacy of postoperative analgesics in laboratory mice. J Am Assoc Lab Anim Sci 2012; 51: 42–49

[5] Valverde A, Gunkel CI. Pain management in horses and farm animals. J Vet Emerg Crit Care 2005; 15: 295–307

[6] Woolf CJ und Chong MS. Preemptive analgesia – treating postoperative pain by preventing the establishment of central sensitization. Anesth Analg 1993; 77: 362–379

9.4 Local anaesthesia

9.4.1 General considerations

Local anaesthesia, when used correctly, can perfectly complement general anaesthesia or be used generally as excellent analgesic option for pain conditions (▶ Table 9.3). The effect is based on interrupting the transmission of the pain stimulus by preventing depolarisation at the nerve cell membrane. Local analgesic treatment can be performed in many different ways with varying efficacy:

- **Topical application** of local anaesthetics: Application or spraying onto the skin or mucous membrane
- **Infiltrative administration**: Injecting tissues in an untargeted way, blocking nerve conduction
- **Regional anaesthesia**: Targeted injection next to one or more nerves
- **Central administration**: Injection into the epidural or spinal space

Table 9.3 Effect of local anaesthetics depending on conditions

Good effect	Poor effect
Thin nerves	Thick nerves
Healthy tissue	Inflamed tissue
Low vascularisation	Strong vascularisation
Vasoconstriction	Increased tissue perfusion
Correct dosage	Insufficient dosage
Correct local anaesthetic	Unfamiliarity with anatomy

Lidocaine gel and EMLA cream

These two topically applied local anaesthetic formulations should be available in your practice:

- **Lidocaine gel** is always practical when mucous membranes "need" local analgesia, e.g. when placing a urinary catheter, during rhinoscopy or as protection in wounds before clipping (the gel then has an additional analgesic effect and is washed off after clipping).
- **EMLA cream** as a eutectic mixture of lidocaine and prilocaine has a local anaesthetic effect on the skin if enough time is given for it to take effect. EMLA cream is used, for example, before placing IV catheters in puppies, cats or rabbits.

Drugs that can be used are primarily:
- **Local anaesthetics** without addition of vasoconstrictor, e.g.
  - Lidocaine (p. 108) 2% SC, IM, IV, tissue, epidural; max. dose 4–8 mg/kg/24 h
  - Bupivacaine (p. 76) 0.5% SC, IM, tissue, epidural; max. dose 2 mg/kg/24 h
  - Ropivacaine (p. 137) 0.5% or 0.75% SC, IM, tissue, epidural; max. dose 2–3 mg/kg/24 h
- **Opioids** without addition of preservative, e.g.
  - Morphine (p. 123), especially intraarticular, epidural/spinal
  - Methadone (p. 119) epidural/spinal
  - Buprenorphine (p. 77), especially for local anaesthesia in the head region
- **Ketamin** (p. 105) epidural/spinal

Other drugs (e.g. **alpha2 agonists**) can also be used. Often, the best and longest lasting effect is achieved with a combination of drugs.

General indications

The use of local anaesthetics is useful before surgical (painful) interventions, as a diagnostic procedure and for the treatment of other types of pain of various causes. In short: Perfect analgesia (almost) without side effects! This technique is particularly suitable for patients who require a (cardiovascular) protective, balanced anaesthesia.

Most disadvantages or side effects can be avoided by proper technique, correct use of material and drug as well as knowledge of the anatomy (▶ Table 9.4).

Table 9.4 Advantages and disadvantages of local anaesthesia

Advantages	Disadvantages
Excellent analgesia	Danger of nerve injury
Dose reduction of further anaesthetics, therefore less (cardiovascular) side effects	Knowledge of anatomy and pharmacology necessary
Simple techniques available	Equipment required (nerve stimulator, ultrasound, spinal cannulas)
Cost-effective	Risk of overdose
Faster recovery phase	Technique must be mastered

II

General contraindications

- Skin infection or pyoderma at the injection site
- Coagulopathy
- Bacteraemia, sepsis
- If clean or sterile conditions cannot be created

Technique – general

In principle, the administration of local anaesthetics can be performed blindly based on anatomical landmarks and/or under control with a nerve stimulator and/or under ultrasound guidance. Especially with the technically more demanding regional anaesthesia techniques, such as the nerve block of the femoral and sciatic nerve, the combined approach with nerve stimulator and ultrasound seems to produce the most reliable results.

However, the following **basic rules** always apply:
- Work cleanly
- Use sterile material (cannulas, syringes)
- Use sterile drugs
- Monitoring for undesirable side effects
- Animal under sedation or general anaesthesia
- Always aspirate before injection and ensure that you do not administer IV
- For central local anaesthesia techniques:
  - Clip the puncture site
  - Surgical cleaning and disinfection
  - Work under sterile conditions (drape, sterile glove)

Potential side effects of local anaesthetics

- Blockade of efferent motor nerves, causes muscle paralysis or weakness (sometimes also desired)
- Local irritation of the tissue, delayed wound healing demonstrated in vitro
- Damage to nerves (temporary or permanent) due to mechanical injury, sloppy work or inflammation
- CNS symptoms in case of overdose or hypersensitivity: fine tremor, restlessness, seizures, depression, coma
- Cardiovascular side effects: bradycardia, vasodilatation, hypotension, risk of death

Good to know

Overdose of local anaesthetics
In case of overdose, central nervous effects are usually noticed first. These often occur before the cardiovascular effects!
   Therapy in case of overdose:
1. **Stop administration** of local anaesthetics immediately
2. If possible, call an experienced anaesthetist
3. Give **100% oxygen**, slight hyperventilation
4. If necessary, administer **shock therapy and fluids**
5. Titrate necessary **drugs** according to effect
   a) CNS symptoms: **Midazolam** or **Diazepam** IV
   b) Vasovagal response: **Noradrenalin** or **Ephedrine**
   c) Bradycardia: **Atropine** or **Glycopyrrolate**
   d) Severe CNS or cardiovascular symptoms as quasi-antidote after overdose of bupivacaine:
      - 1.5 ml/kg lipid solution 20% bolus slowly IV, THEN
      - 0.1 ml/kg lipid solution 20% over 30 min IV

Different local anaesthetics can be used (▶ Table 9.5). Onset and duration of effect may vary.

Owner education

The owner should always be educated about pain management and consent should be obtained for local anaesthetic techniques. The benefits of good analgesia should be emphasised:
- Ask the owner: Do ask for a local analgesia injection at the dentist before treatment?

Table 9.5 Overview of onset and duration of action of various local anaesthetics (according to Labelle and Clark-Price, 2013)

Local anaesthetic	Onset of effect (min)	Duration of effect (min)	Administration
Lidocaine	5–15	30–120	Topical, infiltration, regional, systemic
Procaine	5–15	30–120	Infiltration, regional
Mepivacaine	5–30	90–180	Infiltration, regional
Bupivacaine	15–45	180–360 (–480)	Infiltration, regional
Ropivacaine	15–45	180–360 (–480)	Infiltration, regional
Proparacaine	<1	5–25	Topical cornea
Tetracaine	<1	5–30	Topical cornea

- Less general anaesthetics are needed, therefore a lighter anaesthesia stage is possible
- Pain relief even in the recovery phase
- However, also be honest about possible side effects!

Why local anaesthesia?

The main goal for the patient is to be pain-free postoperatively! This reduces suffering, the animals eat and move again faster and generally have a faster/better recovery phase.

In addition, there is evidence from human medicine that the use of local anaesthesia reduces chronic pain syndromes and the incidence of wound infections. Overall, respiratory and cardiovascular complications are less frequent.

9.4.2 Small animals

In dogs and cats, but also in small mammals, with a little practice, it is relatively easy to perform various local blocks that cause excellent analgesia when carried out correctly. Especially for small dogs, cats or small mammals, it is recommended to use one of the two local anaesthetics (LA) lidocaine 2% (p. 108) or bupivacaine 0.5% (p. 76). Cats are more sensitive to toxic side effects of local anaesthetics, so particular attention should be paid to the dose in these animals. Ropivacaine 0.75% (p. 137) is particularly well suited for neuroaxial and regional anaesthesia of the limbs as it causes differential blockade (more sensory than motor blockade).

Local anaesthesia for procedures on the head

Targeted local anaesthesia provides reliable analgesia in the area of the head in order to carry out procedures in the oral cavity or dental treatment, rhinoscopy, wound care or other operations without pain. It is worth having a cat or dog skull for anatomical comparison in order to reliably find the anatomical landmarks.

Again, always aspirate before injecting, if blood is aspirated, re-position the cannula. If blood is aspirated again, the procedure should be aborted.

Rostral part of the maxilla: Infraorbital nerve (n. infraorbitalis)

▶ **Sensory blockade**
- Teeth in the maxilla rostral to the infraorbital foramen (from P3)
- Skin, mucosa and gingiva in the upper jaw rostral to the infraorbital foramen
- Upper lip
- Parts of the nasal cavity and dorsum of the nose

▶ **Approach and localisation in the dog**
- 22–25 G, 2.5 cm cannula
- Palpation of the infraorbital foramen in the dog approx. 1 cm above the distal root of P3
- Puncture through the skin or with the lip raised through the mucosa (▶ Fig. 9.2)
- Advance the cannula approx. 1 cm rostral to the foramen, under the mucosa into the hole; be careful in brachycephalic dogs, do not advance!
- The further you can advance the needle (without resistance) into the hole, the larger the desensitised area will be; caution eyeball! Again, do not advance in brachycephalic dogs!
- Injection volume depending on the size of the dog from 0.2–0.5 ml LA after aspiration

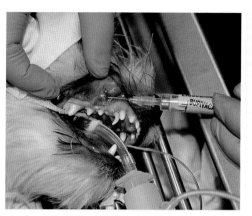

Fig. 9.2 Local anaesthesia of the infraorbital nerve in dogs for extraction of a persistent canine tooth.

II

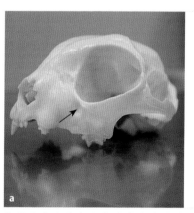

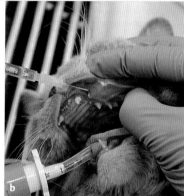

Fig. 9.3 Local anaesthesia of the infraorbital nerve in the cat.
a Anatomical localisation of the infraorbital foramen in the cat skull.
b Injection of local anaesthetics at the infraorbital nerve in the cat.

▶ Approach and localisation in the cat
- 25 G, 1.5 cm cannula
- Locate the infraorbital foramen directly ventral to the orbit
- **Do not advance the cannula** into the hole, as there is a risk of puncturing the eyeball, as the infraorbital foramen is directly adjacent to the orbit (▶ Fig. 9.3a)
- Injection volume of 0.2–0.3 ml LA relatively superficially in the mucosa above the foramen (▶ Fig. 9.3b)

Entire upper jaw: Maxillary nerve (n. maxillaris)

Anatomically, the nerve at this level is the caudal portion of the infraorbital nerve, but it is often referred to as the maxillary nerve. There are different approaches to anaesthetise the maxillary nerve caudal to the pterygopalatine fossa: from intraoral or extraoral, i. e. through the skin (dog and cat), as well as via the infraorbital canal as when anaesthetising the infraorbital nerve (p. 418). The approach via the infraorbital canal is used rather rarely and should only be performed in dogs, otherwise the eyeball may be punctured. To deposit LA up to the maxillary nerve, a larger volume must be used. The highest success rate seems to be achieved with an intraoral access using a bent cannula (90° angle).

▶ Sensory blockade
- All teeth in the upper jaw, adjacent gingiva, mucosa and bone
- Maxillary sinus
- Roof of the mouth, hard and partly soft palate
- Skin including nose up to the medial septum

▶ Approach and localisation in dogs and cats
- **Intraoral approach**, can be done from laterally (▶ Fig. 9.4) or ventrally with a bent cannula:
  - 22–25 G, 1.5–2.5 cm cannula
  - Insert the cannula caudal to the last molar a few millimetres vertically from ventral to dorsal

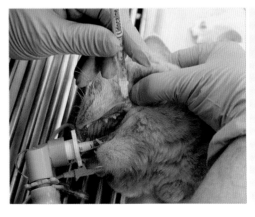

Fig. 9.4 Local anaesthesia of the maxillary nerve in the cat.

- **Extraoral approach** (dog):
  - ○ 22–25 G, 2.5 cm cannula
  - ○ The ventral rim of the zygomatic arch is palpated
  - ○ At the most rostral point, at the border of the last molar, the cannula is inserted at a slight angle towards rostral and ventral
  - ○ It is advanced a few millimetres and LA (0.2–0.5 ml) is injected after aspiration

Rostral part of the mandible: Mental nerve (n. mentalis)

▶ Sensory blockade
- All structures rostral to the (medial) mental foramen
- Incisors
- Lips

▶ Approach and localisation in dogs and cats
- 22–25 G, 2.5 cm cannula
- Palpation of the medial mental foramen (cannot really be palpated in the cat) on the lateral side of the rostral mandible just below the mesial root of P2 (dog) or medial to the labial frenulum (dog and cat)
- In small dogs and cats, it is sufficient to deposit approx. 0.2–0.3 ml LA above the hole (▶ Fig. 9.5); the foramen is so small that you can hardly insert a cannula

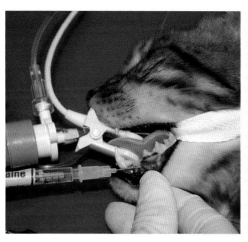

Fig. 9.5 Local anaesthesia of the medial mental foramen in the cat.

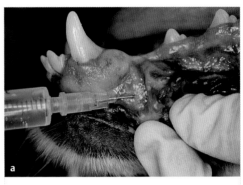

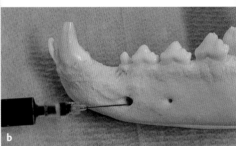

Fig. 9.6 Local anaesthesia of the mental nerve in dogs.
a Approach.
b Anatomical localisation of the mental foramen.

- In larger dogs, the cannula can be advanced a few millimetres into the hole from rostral to caudal and then the LA (0.3–0.5 ml) injected after aspiration (▶ Fig. 9.6)

Entire body of the mandible: Inferior alveolar nerve (n. alveolaris inferior)

The inferior alveolar nerve, which originates from the mandibular nerve, can again be accessed from intra- or extraorally. In smaller animals, the extraoral approach is easier.

▶ Sensory blockade
- All teeth in the lower jaw, adjacent gingiva and bone
- Skin over the entire quadrant

▶ **Approach and localisation in dogs and cats**
- **Intraoral approach** (▶ Fig. 9.7):
  - ○ 22–25 G, 1.5–2.5 cm cannula
  - ○ Intraoral palpation of the mandibular foramen on the medial side of the mandibular ramus with one finger
  - ○ Leave the fingertip "lying" over the hole
  - ○ Advance the cannula along the periosteum until the tip of the cannula lies in the mucosa under the fingertip
  - ○ After aspiration, inject a volume of 0.2–0.5 ml, a bubble should form under the fingertip in the mucosa
- **Extraoral approach** (well suited for small animals, ▶ Fig. 9.8):
  - ○ 22 G, 2.5 cm cannula or longer for larger animals

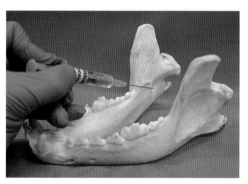

Fig. 9.7 Local anaesthesia of the inferior alveolar nerve in dogs (intraoral approach).

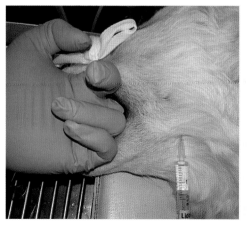

Fig. 9.8 Local anaesthesia of the inferior alveolar nerve in dogs (extraoral approach).

◦ Again, palpate the mandibular foramen intraorally with one finger and leave the fingertip over it

◦ Insert a cannula from the outside on the medial side of the most ventral point of the mandible and slide the cannula in the mucosa along the bone until it lies under the fingertip (**caution**: do not poke yourself!), then proceed as described above

Local anaesthesia for enucleation: Retrobulbar block

The retrobulbar block is not without risk but, if performed correctly, can provide excellent analgesic care for the patient during and after this painful procedure.

▶ Sensory blockade
• Eyeball, partially eyelids (some tone may be maintained)
• Parts of the skin or tissue around the eye

▶ Risks
• Puncture of the eyeball, optic nerve or vessels
• Haemorrhage
• Injection of LA into the cerebrospinal fluid surrounding the optic nerve
• Triggering the oculo-cardiac reflex

▶ Approach and localisation in dogs and cats
• There are several ways to access the retrobulbar space
• An injection via the dorso-lateral approach is often used
• 22 G, 2–3 inch spinal cannula (1 inch = 2.54 cm), cannula should be bent (▶ Fig. 9.9a)
• Volume of LA should be adjusted to the size of the animal: Cat and small dog approx. 0.5–2 ml LA, large dog up to 5 ml LA; maximum dose should be calculated as always
• The upper eyelid is pulled slightly upwards and the cannula is inserted through the conjunctiva at the dorso-lateral orbital rim
• Cannula is pushed along the bony orbit to above and behind the eyeball (▶ Fig. 9.9b)
• Stop in time to avoid puncturing the nerve sheath around the optic nerve
• Aspirate – if blood or cerebrospinal fluid is aspirated, the procedure should be aborted! Inject slowly while monitoring vital signs.
• Another option is the **peribulbar block**, which is associated with fewer risks, but large volumes of LA are injected into the conjunctiva.

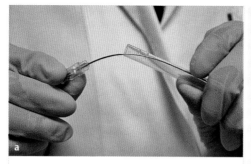

Fig. 9.9 Retrobulbar block in the cat.
a Pre-bending the spinal cannula.
b Advancing on the dorso-lateral orbital rim.

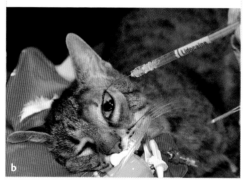

Limbs

There are many simple, but also technically more demanding ways of administering local anaesthesia to parts of the limb. A few of them are described below:

- Intraarticular administration
- Regional anaesthesia: Ring block, brachial plexus block, femoral and sciatic nerve block
- Central anaesthesia: Epidural or spinal anaesthesia (discussed separately below as this type of local anaesthesia not only affects the limbs)

Intraarticular administration

Before or after arthroscopy and arthrotomy, local injection of opioids (usually **morphine** 0.1 mg/kg) can provide analgesia. The use of local anaesthetics (especially **bupivacaine**) is controversially discussed as study results indicate that chondrocytes can be damaged by high-dose, high-concentration LA administered continuously. However, a diluted single injection in a low dose is still considered harmless.

If drugs are injected intraarticularly preoperatively, care should be taken to ensure absolute sterility and a sufficiently long exposure time before washing them out of the joint with irrigation solution. Otherwise, injection after closure of the joint capsule is recommended.

Distal forelimb, hindlimb or tail: Ring block

The ring block is a simple local analgesia technique for performing procedures on the distal limb or distally on the tail.

▶ Sensory blockade
- Distal to the ring block if injection is without gaps

▶ Approach and localisation
- The injection site should be clipped, washed and disinfected
- Using a thin cannula (22–25 G), LA is injected into the subcutaneous tissue forming a ring around the limb (proximal to the site to be operated on, ▶ Fig. 9.10)

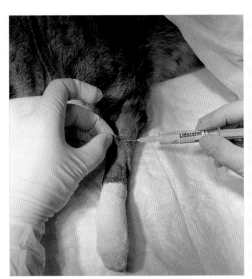

Fig. 9.10 Ring block of the distal forelimb of a cat.

- If the maximum calculated dose is not sufficient in terms of volume, it can be diluted with 0.9% NaCl
- Aspirate prior to each injection and, of course, never inject into vessels or infected or tumorous tissue

Forelimb distal to the elbow: Brachial plexus block

The brachial plexus is composed of the ventral branches of C6, C7, C8 and Th1. The most important nerves from cranial to caudal are: Suprascapular nerve, axillary nerve, musculocutaneous nerve, radial nerve, median nerve and ulnar nerve. The brachial plexus is most easily and traditionally located with a nerve stimulator and an insulated cannula; depending on the equipment available, the plexus can also be located with better reliability using ultrasound.

▶ **Sensory blockade**
- Distal humerus
- Elbow joint and all distal structures if the plexus has been completely desensitised

▶ **Risks**
- Incomplete effect if the nerve bundle has only been partially desensitised
- Puncture of the axillary artery and vein, haemorrhage
- Infection in case of unsterile procedure

▶ **Approach and localisation**
- First, locate the most important anatomical landmarks: Shoulder joint, acromion, greater tuberosity of the humerus and the jugular vein (▶ Fig. 9.11a)
- Prepare a 22 G, 50 mm (cats and small dogs) or 100 mm (large dogs) insulated cannula for the nerve stimulator
- Patient in lateral position, the limb to be anaesthetised is on top
- Puncture site medial to the shoulder joint should be clipped, washed and disinfected, the entire site should be sterile
- After flushing the injection line, connecting the electrical line and connecting the neutral electrode, the cannula is inserted and slowly advanced caudally towards the middle of the scapula (▶ Fig. 9.11b)
- The nerve stimulator is switched on with a low mA value; the closer the tip of the cannula is to the nerve, the lower the current required to trigger depolarisation (if the tip of the cannula is in the nerve, depolarisation is no longer triggered)

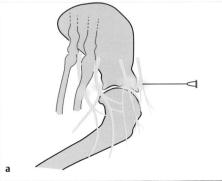

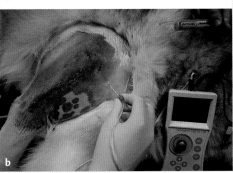

Fig. 9.11 Local anaesthesia of the brachial plexus in dogs.
a Schematic overview. (Source: Graphic designer: Attilio Rocchi)
b Performing local anaesthesia of the brachial plexus in dogs with the aid of a nerve stimulator.

- Stimulation of each individual nerve causes a characteristic muscle contraction: e.g. extension of the elbow = radial nerve, flexion of the elbow = musculocutaneous nerve; if the nerve response is observed, the local anaesthetic (e.g. bupivacaine 0.5%, volume depending on the calculated dose) can be injected after aspiration; it can be combined with e.g. dex-/medetomidine (1–5 µg for each ml LA)

Block of the femoral and sciatic nerve

Nerves can be desensitised with local anaesthetics via different approaches and different procedures. Depending on which approach is chosen, the desensitised area varies and the time and equipment required changes depending on the procedure. In practice, it is worth choosing a simple approach, which is sufficient for most surgeries in the knee joint and distally. The **femoral nerve** can be reached paravertebrally or with a lateral preiliac or inguinal approach. The

inguinal approach is described below, which may also desensitise the **saphenous nerve**. The sciatic nerve can be desensitised laterally proximally or medially – the **lateral medial sciatic block** is described below.

The following local anaesthetics are commonly used for desensitisation: Lidocaine 2% (p. 108) with a fast onset and relatively short duration of action, bupivacaine 0.5% or 0.25% (p. 76) with a somewhat slower onset but longer duration of action, or ropivacaine 0.75% (p. 137) or less concentrated with differential blockade, therefore less motor block. If alpha2 agonists (e.g. dexmedetomidine [p. 86]) are added, the duration of action can be prolonged to an average of 14 hours. The recommended volume should not exceed 0.1 ml/kg, the maximum dosages of LA should be observed.

▶ Sensory and motor blockade (when using LA)
- Block of the **femoral nerve** and possibly the **saphenous nerve** desensitises the following structures:
  - Femur starting from the middle of the diaphysis distally
  - Knee joint, medial side of joint capsule and adjacent soft tissues
  - Skin of dorso-medial tarsus and first phalanges
- Block of the **sciatic nerve** desensitises the following structures:
  - Parts of the knee joint and adjacent soft tissues
  - Limb distal to the knee joint

Desensitisation of both nerves allows a (mostly) non-painful procedure to be performed on the entire limb distal to the middle of the femur. The same precautions and contraindications apply as for central anaesthesia.

▶ Possible complications/risks
- Puncture of arteries or veins, haemorrhage, formation of a haematoma
- Incomplete desensitisation (caudo-medial and cranio-lateral part of the thigh and cranio-lateral part of the knee are partially innervated by other nerves)
- Nerve injury
- Infection in case of unsterile work
- Intoxication in case of overdose of local anaesthetic

Careful!

Avoiding nerve damage with local anaesthesia
Before any injection near nerves, the correct position of the cannula tip must be checked. There are several strategies to avoid nerve damage.

Ultrasound:
- During the injection of LA, if the cannula tip is positioned correctly, displacement of the nerve by the injected volume can be detected
- Around the nerve, the so-called **donut sign** becomes visible: The nerve is surrounded by fluid

Nerve stimulator
- The closer the tip of the cannula is to the nerve, the lower the current required (e.g. 0.2 mA) to trigger depolarisation. However, if the tip of the cannula lies **in the nerve**, depolarisation is **no longer triggered**
- Below 0.26–0.3 mA, one should probably no longer continue nerve stimulation, as then there is a risk of being in the nerve sheath and damaging the nerve
- In general, **no resistance** should be felt when injecting LA

▶ **Approach and localisation.** The combined technique using a nerve stimulator and ultrasound is described below. The advantage is greater safety, as nerves can be localised and structures visualised. During injection of LA, the correct position and distribution of the LA can be controlled by ultrasound.

- **Femoral (and saphenous) nerve block – inguinal approach**
  - The anaesthetised patient should be in lateral position with the leg to be treated facing up- and backwards
  - The area around the injection site (medial and cranial thigh) is clipped, washed and disinfected; overall sterile conditions must be ensured, ideally a sterile drape is used
  - The positive electrode of the nerve stimulator is attached over the knee joint of the leg to be desensitised and the injection line of the cannula (22 G, 50 mm) is flushed with LA
  - The nerve stimulator is switched on with a low current (e.g. 0.4 mA)
  - Position the ultrasound probe so that the nerve bundle consisting of the femoral and saphenous nerves can be located in the inguinal region near the femoral artery
  - The cannula is inserted cranially of the ultrasound probe and advanced through the belly of the sartorius muscle in a caudo-dorsal direction

- The iliac facia must be pierced ("pop") to ensure distribution of LA around the nerve bundle; vessels must be visualised continuously to avoid accidental puncture
- Once the cannula tip is positioned adjacent to the nerve bundle, the current should be increased to 0.5 mA to confirm the correct position (outside vessels or nerves) via muscle contraction
- The injection site should be as proximal as possible to where the femoral nerve exits the greater psoas to increase the chances of desensitising the saphenous nerve as well
- After aspiration, injection can be started; if the procedure is correct, the LA will appear on the ultrasound image, distributed around the nerve bundle

- **Sciatic nerve block – lateral medial approach**
  - The anaesthetised patient should lie relaxed in lateral position with the leg to be treated on top (▶ Fig. 9.12)
  - The area around the puncture site (caudal thigh) is clipped, washed and disinfected; sterile work must be ensured, ideally a sterile drape is also used

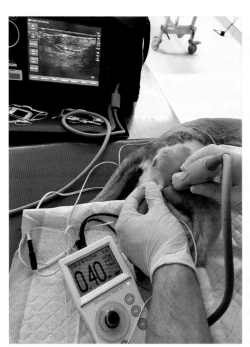

Fig. 9.12 Ultrasound and nerve stimulator-guided local anaesthesia of the sciatic nerve.

- The nerve stimulator is prepared (if not already done so) in the manner described above
- Localisation of the insertion site: The ultrasound probe is positioned directly below the greater trochanter (*trochanter major*) and the ischial tuberosity (*tuber ischiadicum*) in a caudo-cranial direction; the sciatic nerve can be identified as a small hyperechogenic "double disc" or recumbent figure of eight medial to the biceps femoris muscle and cranial to the semitendinosus muscle
- The nerve stimulator cannula is advanced in a caudo-cranial direction through the semitendinosus muscle medial to the fascia of the biceps femoris muscle
- The tip of the cannula should always remain visible and should be carefully inserted through the nerve sheath around the sciatic nerve
- The current should now be increased to about 0.5 mA to confirm the correct cannula position by characteristic muscle contractions
- After aspiration, start injecting; if the procedure is correct, the LA will appear on the ultrasound image, distributed around the nerve bundle

It is worthwhile to look at more detailed and illustrated descriptions of the different procedures and approaches, as the possibilities are almost endless and would go beyond the scope of this book. All those interested are recommended to read the excellent literature on nerve stimulator and ultrasound-guided local anaesthesia in dogs and cats.

Thorax: Intercostal block

The intercostal block is relatively easy to perform and can be used for analgesic management of a thoracotomy, for the placement of a thoracic drain or for rib fractures. Due to the fact that the nerves overlap and thus supply several ribs, two intercostal spaces each cranial and caudal to the incision site should always be blocked in addition to the affected intercostal space, i.e. 5 intercostal spaces in total (▶ Fig. 9.13). Respiratory function does not seem to be affected by desensitisation.

▶ **Approach and localisation**
- The intercostal nerves are located at the caudal edge of each rib in a bundle with arteries and veins
- As always, the maximum dose of LA (p. 413) should be calculated for each patient; as it may be useful to repeat the block possibly at the end of surgery, the volume should be divided and diluted with 0.9% NaCl if required

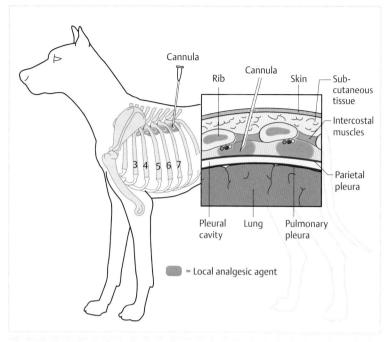

Fig. 9.13 Schematic illustration of the intercostal block.

- Puncture sites are clipped, washed and disinfected; overall, sterile work must be ensured, as accidental intrathoracic puncture cannot be ruled out
- The patient lies on his side, the intercostal space is palpated and the puncture is made in the centre (injection site in the cat is a few millimetres deep, in obese dogs much deeper)
- It is essential to aspirate now! If air is aspirated, you have punctured too deeply into the pleural space or the lung (this should not happen!), then withdraw the cannula and aspirate again
- If no more air or blood can be aspirated, inject slowly

This block can be performed through the skin as described or, for example, during a thoracotomy directly under visualization: The intercostal nerves are located directly under the parietal pleura. An ultrasound-guided technique may be helpful.

Depending on the size of the animal, the maximum dose determines the total volume. Dividing by 5 results in the volume of LA per intercostal space.

Epidural/spinal anaesthesia

Epidural anaesthesia in small animals can be easily learned with some commitment and good instructions. With this technique, effective analgesia of the caudal half of the body can be achieved. In small animals, local anaesthetics are usually administered in the lumbosacral space, i.e. between the vertebral bodies L7 and S1, as this is where the largest "gap" between the vertebral bodies is.

Anatomically, it should be noted that in **dogs** the spinal cord usually ends at the level of L6 or L7, so spinal administration is rather unlikely (▶ Fig. 9.14). In the **cat**, on the other hand, the spinal cord ends between L7 and S3, so penetration of the dura mater and therefore spinal administration must be expected (▶ Fig. 9.15).

Good to know

What to do if epidural suddenly becomes spinal?
In cats in particular, it is possible that the tip of the cannula is (accidentally) placed in the spinal space after puncture of the lumbosacral space. This can be recognised by the aspiration of cerebrospinal fluid. When this happens, the dose calculated for epidural administration should be reduced to ⅓ and injected slowly. The anterior half of the animal's body should be kept slightly elevated.

▶ Sensory and motor blockade (when using LA)
- Hip and hindlimb
- (Partly) abdomen and abdominal organs
- Tail and perineum
- (Partly) genital organs

▶ Potential complications/risks
- Puncture of the lateral venous plexus and haemorrhage (rather negligible at the level of the cauda equina) or accidental intravenous application
- Infection when working with contaminated material
- **When using local anaesthetics:**
  ○ Persistent motor block for hours or days, in very rare cases longer

II

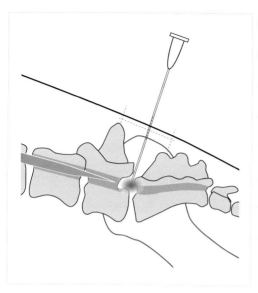

Fig. 9.14 Epidural anaesthesia dog. Anatomical cross section. (Source: Graphic designer: Attilio Rocchi)

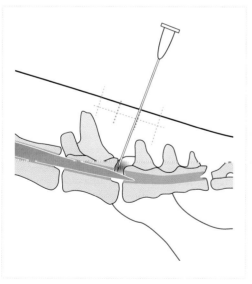

Fig. 9.15 Epidural/spinal anaesthesia cat. Anatomical cross section. (Source: Graphic designer: Attilio Rocchi)

○ Hypotension and bradycardia if LA migrates too far cranially and sympathetic parts of spinal nerves from T5 to L3 are blocked, leading to severe vasodilatation

○ Respiratory depression

▶ **Contraindications**
- Skin infection/pyoderma especially at the injection site
- Coagulopathy
- Discospondylitis, arthrosis at the puncture site
- Altered anatomy that prevents reliable detection of localisation
- Infection, bacteraemia, sepsis
- Hypovolaemia (if local anaesthetics are used, which may migrate cranially and cause vasodilatation)
- If sterile conditions cannot be achieved

▶ **Approach and localisation**
- The anaesthetised patient should be positioned perfectly straight in sternal position, the hind legs can either be positioned crouched or pulled cranially (opens the lumbosacral space); lateral position is also possible e.g. in case of fractures of the hind legs, but may make palpation of midline more difficult and possibly falsify the tests for correct cannula position (loss of resistance tests)
- First, palpate the most important anatomical landmarks (▶ Fig. 9.16): Lumbosacral space between the spinous process (*proc. spinosus*) of L7 and the sacral crest (*crista sacralis mediana*) of S1 and the iliac wings on the right and left

Fig. 9.16 Epidural anaesthesia in a dog.
a Position the dog straight in the sternal position.
b Palpation of the intervertebral space L7–S1.
c Controlled advancement of the spinal cannula until just before the yellow ligament.
d After removing the stylet, check that the cannula is correctly positioned using the hanging drop technique: Insert a drop of 0.9% NaCl into the cone of the spinal cannula.
e Advancing the cannula into the spinal canal.
f When the cannula enters the spinal canal, the fluid is sucked in by the vacuum (= hanging drop technique).
g Attach syringe with drugs and aspirate.
h Slow injection of drugs.

II

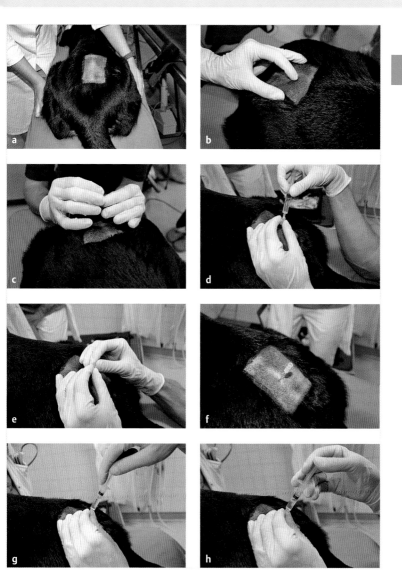

- The puncture site is clipped, washed and disinfected; the entire procedure must be performed in a sterile manner
- In the dog, the puncture site is exactly in the middle of the lumbosacral space, in the cat at the junction from the caudal to the middle third of the space (i.e. slightly further caudally than the middle of the space, ▸ Fig. 9.14, ▸ Fig. 9.15)
- The spinal cannula is inserted sterilely and as smoothly as possible at a perpendicular angle to the skin and advanced, the bevel pointing in the direction in which it is to be injected (e.g. tail amputation: caudally); the stylet can be held in the cannula with the index finger
- The cannula is advanced through
  - Skin
  - Subcutaneous tissue (no resistance)
  - Interspinosal ligament (*lig. interspinosum*) (slight resistance)
  - Yellow ligament (*lig. flavum*) (you feel a stronger resistance, "pop"), then the cannula is in the epidural space; if pushed further (in the cat), the tip of the cannula may be in the spinal space
- If the tip of the cannula hits bone (= ventral spinal canal), pull the cannula back a little
- As soon as you are sure that you are in the epidural space, aspirate; if there is no blood or cerebrospinal fluid, inject slowly
- Usually, local anaesthetics sink downwards following gravity, regardless of the position of the animal; if one side in particular is to benefit from the local block, it must be immediately placed downwards and left there for some time (approx. 5–10 min); if an even distribution is desired, the patient should either remain in sternal position or be placed in dorsal recumbency
- In principle, when using LA, the thorax and head should be positioned slightly higher compared to the rest of the body to avoid too much migration cranially (can lead to severe hypotension and apnoea, among other things)

Good to know

This is how I recognise that I am in the epidural space!
Compared to the surrounding tissue, the epidural space offers very little resistance to injection of air or fluids (loss of resistance). On the contrary, there is (usually) even a vacuum. There are two common ways of testing this loss of resistance to ensure that the tip of the cannula is in the epidural space.

Hanging drop technique
Before inserting the cannula through the yellow ligament (*lig. flavum*) (it takes some practice to identify the right moment), pull the stylet and drip sterile 0.9% NaCl into the cone of the spinal cannula (▶ Fig. 9.16). Then advance the cannula through the yellow ligament. The moment you reach the epidural space, the drop is literally sucked in. This only really works when the patient is in sternal position. In some patients, the test does not work even though you have actually placed the cannula correctly.

Loss of resistance test
Sterile 0.9% NaCl and a little air is drawn into a syringe. To check the correct position of the cannula, the syringe is placed firmly on the spinal cannula and aspirated (▶ Fig. 9.16). If no blood is aspirated, inject carefully. The air should not compress and the air-fluid interface should literally "flee" from the plunger of the syringe.

▶ **Which drugs?** Various anaesthetics can be used as a single injection. The choice must be made on the basis of indication and follow-up care. Often it is a good idea to combine two or even more drugs in order to take advantage of all good properties. In general, only drugs that **do not contain preservatives** should be used. Some examples are given below:

- **Lidocaine 2%**
  - Up to 4 mg/kg, a volume of 0.2 ml/kg (large dogs) to 0.3 ml/kg (small dogs and cats) should not be exceeded; this also applies when combined with other drugs
  - Onset of action after 5 min, duration of action up to 120 min
  - Sensory and motor blockade
- **Bupivacaine 0.5%**
  - 0.2–1 mg/kg, a volume of 0.2 ml/kg (large dogs) to 0.3 ml/kg (small dogs and cats) should not be exceeded; this also applies when combined with other drugs
  - Onset of action after 10–20 min, duration of action 3–4 h
  - Sensory and motor blockade

- **Ketamine**
  - 1 mg/kg
  - Onset of action after 10–30 min, duration up to 2 h
- **Morphine**
  - 0.1 mg/kg
  - Onset of action after 30–60 min, duration 6–24 h
  - Bladder control for 24 h after epidural injection (urinary retention)
  - Side effects: Pruritus, nausea, vomiting possible
- **Methadone**
  - 0.1–0.3 mg/kg
  - Onset of action after 30–40 min, duration 8–12 h
- **Medetomidine**
  - 0.005–0.01 mg/kg
  - Onset of action after 20–30 min, duration 2–6 h
  - Systemic side-effects (p. 111) possible

Local anaesthetics can be combined very well with opioids and opioids with ketamine or dex-/medetomidine.

Castration

In **male small animals**, local anaesthesia of the spermatic cord with nerve plexus is very easy to perform. Once the local anaesthetic is properly injected, only light general anaesthesia is required to enable painful procedures and to allow the recovery phase to be calm and pain-free. Contraindication is pathologically (tumorous, inflammatory) altered testicular tissue.

▸ Desensitised area
- Testicular parenchyma
- Spermatic cord with nerve fibres of the testicular plexus

▸ Approach
- Hair removal (plucking or clipping), cleaning and disinfection of the surgical area with iodine solution
- 22–26 G 2.5 cm cannula
- Calculate the maximum volume of LA, i. e. lidocaine (p. 108) or bupivacaine (p. 76), draw up this amount or less
- Use thumb and forefinger to fix the testes, in small mammals identify the fat body
- After aspiration, inject one third of the amount of LA centrally into the testicular parenchyma of each testicle so that the testicle feels tight

- The LA diffuses to the spermatic cord; it can take a few minutes – wait!
- In addition, infiltrate the incision line subcutaneously with the remaining third of the LA

In **female small animals**, infiltration of the incision line is one way to provide local analgesia. Infiltration of the mesovarium with lidocaine during surgery appears to have little effect on vital signs and potential reduction of the inhalation anaesthetic. The benefit therefore seems limited.

Literature

[1] Arnholz M, Hungerbühler S, Weil C, Schütter AF, Rohn K, Tünsmeyer J, Kästner SBR. Ultraschallgesteuerte Nervenblockade des Nervus femoralis und ischiadicus im Vergleich zur Epiduralanästhesie bei orthopädischen Eingriffen am Hund. Tierärztl Prax 2017; 45(K): 5–14

[2] Beckman BW, Legendre L. Regional nerve blocks for oral surgery in companion animals. Compend Contin Ed Pract Vet 2002; 24: 439–444

[3] Branson KR, Ko JC, Tranquilli WJ, Benson J, Thurmon JC. Duration of analgesia induced by epidurally administered morphine and medetomidine in dogs. J Vet Pharmacol Therap 1993; 16: 369–372

[4] Bubalo V, Moens YP, Holzmann A, Coppens P. Anaesthetic sparing effect of local anaesthesia of the ovarian pedicle during ovariohysterectomy in dogs. Vet Anaesth Analg 2008; 35: 537–542

[5] Burford JH, Corley KT. Morphine-associated pruritus after single extradural administration in a horse. Vet Anaesth Analg 2006; 33: 193–198

[6] Chu CR, Izzo NJ, Papas NE, Fu H. In vitro exposure to bupivacaine 0.5% is cytotoxic to bovine articular chondrocytes. Arthroscopy 2006; 22: 693–699

[7] Cruz ML, Luna SPL, Clark RMO, Massone F, Castro GB. Epidural anaesthesia using lignocaine, bupivacaine or a mixture of lignocaine and bupivacaine in dogs. Vet Anaesth Analg 1997; 24: 30–32

[8] Dogan N, Erdem AF, Erman Z, Kizilkaya M. The effects of bupivacaine and neostigmine on articular cartilage and synovium in the rabbit knee joint. J Int Med Res 2004; 32: 513–519

[9] Huuskonen V, Hughes JM, Estaca Bañon E, West E. Intratesticular lidocaine reduces the response to surgical castration in dogs. Vet Anaesth Analg 2013; 40: 74–82

[10] Leibetseder EN, Mosing M, Jones RS. A comparison of extradural and intravenous methadone on intraoperative isoflurane and postoperative analgesia requirements in dogs. Vet Anaesth Analg 2006; 33: 128–136

[11] Lemke KA, Dawson SD. Local and regional anesthesia. Vet Clin North Am Small Anim Pract 2000; 30: 839–857

[12] Olbrich VH, Mosing M. A comparison of the analgesic effects of caudal epidural methadone and lidocaine in the horse. Vet Anaesth Analg 2003; 30: 156–164

[13] Oliver JA, Bradbrook CA. Suspected brain stem anesthesia following retrobulbar block in a cat. Vet Ophthalmol 2013; 16: 225–228

[14] Pascoe PJ, Dyson DH. Analgesia after lateral thoracotomy in dogs. Epidural morphine vs. intercostal bupivacaine. Vet Surg 1993; 22: 141–147

[15] Quandt JE, Rawlings CR. Reducing postoperative pain for dogs: Local anesthetic and analgesic techniques. Comp Cont Ed Vet Med 1996; 18: 101–111

[16] Scarda RT, Tranquilli WJ. Local and regional anesthetic and analgesic techniques: Dogs. In: Lumb & Jones' Veterinary Anesthesia. Tranquilli WJ, Thurmon JC, Grimm KA (Ed.). 4th edition. Ames: Blackwell Publishing 2007; 561–593

[17] Snyder LBC, Snyder CJ. Effect of buprenorphine added to bupivacaine infraorbital nerve blocks on isoflurane minimum alveolar concentration using a model for acute dental/oral surgical pain in dogs. J Vet Dent 2016; 33: 90–96

Comment: Pretty cool: If you add buprenorphine to bupivacaine for the dental block, the analgesic effect seems to be prolonged up to three days!

[18] Thompson SE, Johnson JM. Analgesia in dogs after intercostal thoracotomy. A comparison of morphine, selective intercostal nerve block, and interpleural regional analgesia with bupivacaine. Vet Surg 1991; 20: 73–77

9.4.3 Horses

Many dental, ophthalmic and obstetric procedures can be performed under sedation. Well-placed local blocks are extremely helpful for a safe procedure free of pain.

Here, too, the general rule is: A perfectly placed local anaesthetic is of no use if you do not wait for the effect of the local anaesthetic! So: Perform local analgesia techniques in good time before starting the painful intervention.

Local anaesthesia for procedures on the head

As in small animals, the most reliable analgesia for procedures on teeth, the eye and the rest of the head is obtained by specific local anaesthesia of the supplying nerves. Of course, after a unilaterally applied local anaesthetic, only the ipsilateral side is affected by analgesia. Horses may react by thrashing their heads or walking forward, especially if the nerve is accidentally touched directly. For this reason, sedation (p.226) of the animal is always recommended. A schematic overview of the local blocks on the horse's head described below can be found in ▶ Fig. 9.17.

Rostral part of the upper jaw: Infraorbital nerve (n. infraorbitalis)

▶ Sensory blockade
- Depending on penetration depth and distribution, the sensory blockade affects the rostral part of the maxilla
- Incisors of the maxilla
- Premolars of the maxilla up to, in the optimal case, molars 1 and 2 with adjacent gingiva
- Upper lip, bridge of the nose almost to the medial canthus of the eye

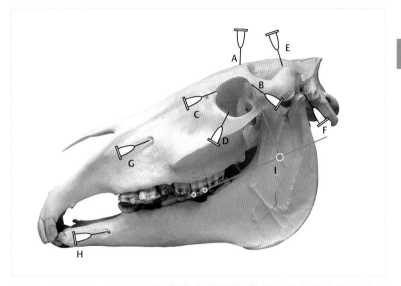

Fig. 9.17 Schematic overview of all described local blocks on the horse's head.
A: *n. frontalis,* **B:** *n. lacrimalis,* **C:** *n. infratrochlearis,* **D:** *n. zygomaticus,*
E and **F:** *n. auriculopalpebralis,* **G:** *n. infraorbitalis,* **H:** *n. mentalis;* **I:** *n. alveolaris inferior*
(medial side of the mandible)

▶ **Approach and localisation**
- 20 G, 5 cm cannula
- Palpation using the "3-finger technique" from the front: Right hand for the left side of the head and vice versa, thumb in the nasoincisive notch (*incisura nasoincisiva*), middle finger rostrally on the facial crest (*crista facialis*), push the levator labii superioris muscle (*m. levator labii superioris*) upwards with the index finger and palpate the infraorbital foramen (*for. infraorbitale,* ▶ Fig. 9.18a)
- Cannula can be advanced 5–8 cm into the foramen, then approx. 5 ml local anaesthetic is applied after aspiration (▶ Fig. 9.18b). Defensive reactions are to be expected in animals that are only lightly sedated. If you do not advance into the canal, but apply rostral to the foramen, only the skin and muscles of the dorsum of the nose, the upper lip and the nostrils will be desensitised

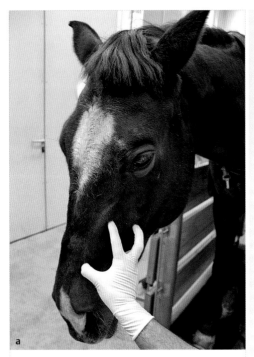

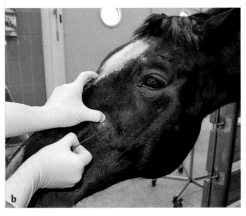

Fig. 9.18 Local anaesthesia of the infraorbital nerve (*n. infraorbitalis*) in horses.
a 3-finger technique.
b Advancing the cannula.

Entire maxilla: Maxillary nerve (n. maxillaris)

The maxillary nerve in horses is injected extraorally, i.e. through the skin from the lateral side. There is a traditional approach, the Palatine Bone Insertion (PBI) in the pterygopalatine fossa (*fossa pterygopalatina*) and a newer technique, the Extraperiorbital Fat Body Insertion (EFBI) technique.

▶ Sensory blockade
- With the newer technique, the following structures are desensitised:
  - All teeth in the upper jaw including the gingiva
  - Mucosa of the maxillary and paranasal sinus
  - Roof of the mouth and parts of the soft palate
  - Skin including nostril up to the medial canthus of the eye

▶ Approach and localisation
- Access from the lateral side through the aseptically prepared and locally anaesthetised skin (▶ Fig. 9.19)
- **Palatine Bone Insertion (traditional approach)**
  - 22 G, longer than 10 cm spinal cannula
  - Vertical insertion ventral to the lateral canthus of the eye directly at the ventral edge of the zygomatic arch (*arcus zygomaticus*)
  - Advance at a slight angle cranially until you hit bone after approx. 5–7 cm
  - If bony resistance is felt after a few cm, the tip of the cannula is on the mandibular branch or rostrally on the zygomatic arch; the cannula is then withdrawn slightly, the position corrected and advanced again

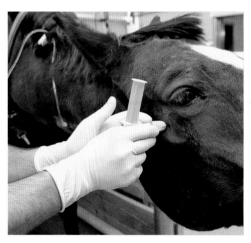

Fig. 9.19 Local anaesthesia of the maxillary nerve (*n. maxillaris*) in horses.

445

- ○ After aspiration, apply approximately 10–20 ml (2 ml/100 kg body weight) LA
- ○ This now obsolete technique is well tolerated by sedated animals, but can be associated with complications (severe haemorrhage, retrobulbar haematoma, circulatory collapse, blindness)
- **Extraperiorbital Fat Body Insertion (new technique)**
  - ○ 22 G, 7.5 cm spinal cannula
  - ○ Vertical insertion ventral to the lateral canthus of the eye directly at the ventral edge of the zygomatic arch just as in the traditional technique, but the cannula is not advanced as far
  - ○ After about 3–3.5 cm depth of penetration, the cannula penetrates the deep fascia of the masseter muscle; then the cannula is advanced about 1.5–2 cm into the extraperiorbital fat body
  - ○ After aspiration, apply approx. 10 to max. 20 ml (2 ml/100 kg body weight) of LA
  - ○ The safety of this local anaesthetic technique is increased by performing the procedure under ultrasound guidance

Rostral part of the mandible: Mental nerve (n. mentalis)

▶ **Sensory blockade**
- The following structures are desensitised with this block:
  - ○ All structures rostral to the mental foramen
  - ○ Incisors of the lower jaw
  - ○ Lips
  - ○ Oral mucosa
  - ○ Skin of the chin

▶ **Approach and localisation**
- 22 G, 2.5 cm cannula
- Lies in the middle of the diastema in the mandible
- The tendon of the depressor labii inferioris muscle *(m. depressor labii inferioris)* must be pushed dorsally
- After aspiration, administer approx. 5 ml of LA directly at the exit point of the nerve from the mental foramen

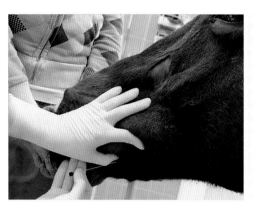

Fig. 9.20 Local anaesthesia of the mental nerve in horses.

Extended rostral portion of the mandible: Mental nerve (n. mentalis), XL block

▶ Sensory blockade
- Same as mentalis block and additionally teeth up to the 3rd premolar, with a bit of luck up to the 1st molar

▶ Approach and localisation
- 20–22 G, 7.5–10 cm spinal cannula (longer cannula!)
- Enter the mental foramen and advance in a ventro-medial direction (▶ Fig. 9.20)
- Administer approx. 10 ml of LA after aspiration

As a rule, horses react violently to this procedure and should therefore be deeply sedated. There is also a risk of tissue injury or haemorrhage. As an alternative, desensibilisation of the inferior alveolar nerve is recommended.

Entire body of the mandible: Inferior alveolar nerve (n. alveolaris inferior)

The mandibular nerve enters the mandibular foramen and continues rostrally within the mandible as inferior alveolar nerve to the mental foramen. This nerve is desensitised at the level of the mandibular foramen. It does not seem to make any difference whether one punctures at a vertical or caudal angle.

▶ **Sensory blockade**
- Entire mandibular branch, teeth of the mandible
- Skin
- Mucous membrane
- Lower lip

▶ **Approach and localisation**
- 18–20 G, 15 cm spinal cannula
- When proceeding vertically, insert at the deepest point of the medial side of the mandible
- Advance vertically (slightly caudally) medially along the mandibular ramus
- The mandibular foramen is located at the intersection of an imaginary extension of the mandibular occlusal surfaces caudally and a second imaginary line vertically downwards from the lateral corner of the eye (▶ Fig. 9.21)
- Administer 10–20 ml LA after aspiration

When injecting large volumes bilaterally, tongue injuries may occur due to desensitisation of the lingual nerve. The owner must be informed! As a precau-

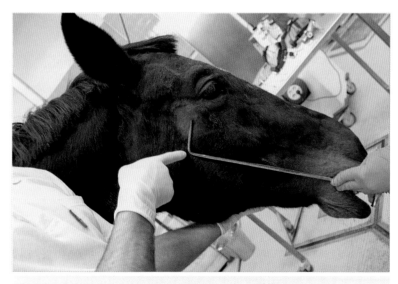

Fig. 9.21 Marking the anatomical localisation of the inferior alveolar nerve (*n. alveolaris inferior*) in the horse.

tion, no food should be offered for 4–5 h after the procedure. An **intraoral approach** (as in small animals) with a slightly curved long spinal cannula has only recently been described in horses. This approach requires smaller volumes, which may reduce the risk of tongue injury.

Local anaesthesia for eye procedures

Local anaesthesia of the eye can have two objectives: On the one hand, a motor blockade (e.g. akinesia of the upper eyelid) and, on the other hand, a sensory blockade in order to be able to perform surgical procedures or examinations without pain. It can enable surgery on the sedated animal or serve as additional analgesia in the horse under general anaesthesia to reduce the dose and therefore the side effects of the general anaesthetic.

Auriculopalpebral (n. auriculopalpebralis) block

This is one of the most commonly performed regional anaesthesia techniques on the horse's eye. In painful processes, blepharospasm is so pronounced that examination or treatment is often not possible. Desensitisation of the purely motor auriculopalpebral nerve, which runs dorsal to the zygomatic arch, results in akinesia of the upper and partly of the lateral lower eyelid.

▶ Motor blockade
- Upper eyelid
- Partial lateral lower eyelid

▶ Approach and localisation
- 22 G, 1.5–2.5 cm cannula
- **1st option**
  - Localisation is 1.5–2 cm below the highest point of the caudal part of the dorsal edge of the zygomatic arch
  - Nerve runs parallel to the zygomatic bone and is easy to palpate; lift the skin slightly, puncture subcutaneously with the cannula directed towards the floor and advance to the upper rim of the zygomatic arch (▶ Fig. 9.22)
  - Aspirate and inject 2.5–5 ml local anaesthetic
- **2nd option**
  - Locate the nerve near the base of the ear and caudal to the mandibular ramus
  - Inject 2.5–5 ml local anaesthetic after aspiration
  - Seems to result in more pronounced akinesia

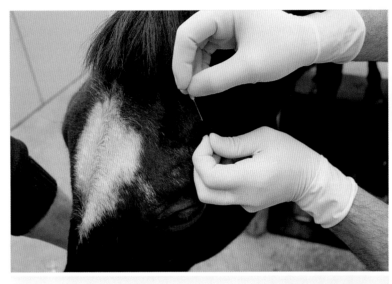

Fig. 9.22 Local anaesthesia of the auriculopalpebral nerve (*n. auriculopalpebralis*) in horses.

Good to know

Note!
- This is a motor blockade, sensory function and therefore pain perception is fully preserved!
- Best used in combination with sedation and sensory blockade (e.g. topically on the cornea and/or the frontal nerve in the supraorbital foramen)
- Protect eye from dust, sun and dehydration until motor function is fully restored

Local anaesthesia of the eyelids

Upper, lower and third eyelids are predominantly innervated by four sensory nerves that can be selectively desensitised.

▶ Sensory blockade
1. **Supraorbital or frontal nerve** (*n. supraorbitalis* or *frontalis*) innervates parts of the forehead and the medial ⅔ of the upper eyelid
2. **Lacrimal nerve** (*n. lacrimalis*) innervates the lateral canthus, the lateral third of the upper eyelid, the lacrimal gland and the conjunctiva
3. **Infratrochlear nerve** (*n. infratrochlearis*) innervates the medial canthus, the third eyelid, the lacrimal gland and the conjunctiva
4. **Zygomatic nerve** (*n. zygomaticus*) innervates the lateral ⅔ of the lower eyelid, skin and conjunctiva in this area

If all four nerves are desensitised, the entire eyelids and the surrounding tissue are anaesthetised.

▶ **Approach and localisation.** Each of these four nerves can be desensitised with 2 to max. 5 ml of local anaesthetic using a 22–25 G, 1.5–2.5 cm cannula (▶ Fig. 9.17).
1. **Supraorbital nerve**: Originates in the supraorbital foramen, should be palpated approx. 5–7 cm dorsal to the medial canthus of the eye in the zygomatic process of the frontal bone; do not insert the cannula deeper than approx. 1 cm into the hole, aspirate and inject
2. **Lacrimal nerve**: Subcutaneous insertion in the lateral canthus, directed medially just below the orbital rim, advance, aspirate, inject
3. **Infratrochlear nerve**: Insert cannula at the palpable small bony prominence above the medial canthus, aspirate, inject
4. **Zygomatic nerve**: Inject subcutaneously after aspiration at the lateral edge of the bony orbit, exactly where the supraorbital part of the zygomatic arch rises upwards

Local anaesthesia of the eyeball and orbit: Retrobulbar block

For corneal procedures, paracentesis of the anterior or posterior chamber for diagnostic purposes or enucleation, local anaesthesia of the sensory and motor nerves supplying eyeball and orbit is recommended. This technique can be performed dorsally or laterally (modified Peterson block "borrowed" from bovine medicine). The dorsal approach is often preferred and therefore discussed here. Deep sedation (p. 226) is important for procedures on a standing horse.

▶ Desensitised area
• All structures supplied by the nerves that emerge from the optic canal (oculomotor nerve, trochlear nerve, optic nerve, maxillary nerve and parts of the trigeminal nerve, among others)

- Sensory and motor blockade
- Does not desensitise the eyelids

▶ **Sensory blockade**
- Eyeball and orbit

▶ **Approach and localisation (dorsal approach)**
- 22 G, 10–12 cm spinal cannula
- Clip and disinfect the puncture site with iodine solution, good sedation/fixation of the horse
- Insert perpendicular to the ground with the head in a normal, relaxed position
- Puncture site approx. 1.5 cm caudal to the centre of the zygomatic process of the frontal bone in the direction of the last premolar in the upper jaw of the opposite side (▶ Fig. 9.23)
- The eyeball rotates dorsally as soon as the cannula touches the fascia surrounding the dorsal muscle cone
- The eyeball rotates back to its central position the moment you pierce the fascia and muscle
- Aspiration and injection of 10–12 ml LA in the retrobulbar fat body in the area around the optic nerve

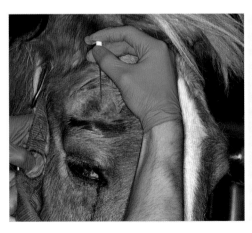

Fig. 9.23 Retrobulbar block in the horse. Dorsal approach.

Caudal epidural anaesthesia

This local anaesthesia technique is easy to perform and provides pain relief for tenesmus caused by painful processes in the perineum, anus, rectum and vagina, during difficult births, for correction of uterine torsion, fetotomy and other obstetric procedures. Caudal epidural anaesthesia can also provide adequate analgesia during surgical procedures such as tail amputation, correction of a recto-vaginal fistula, rectal prolapse or Caslick surgery.

▶ Sensory and motor blockade
- Anus
- Perineum
- Vulva, vagina
- Parts of urethra, bladder and rectum

▶ Approach and localisation
- 18–20 G, 5–7.5 cm spinal cannula
- Localisation between the 1st (Co1) and 2nd caudal vertebrae (Co2), localised by moving the tail up and down: It is the first movable caudal vertebral joint, as the sacrococcygeal joint is often fused
- Lowest point when tail is held all the way up (▶ Fig. 9.24)
- Approx. 5 cm cranial from the base of the tail hair, exactly in the centre
- Work cleanly, in a sterile manner (shave, disinfection, sterile gloves, etc.), as infection can ascend in the spinal canal
- Before epidural injection, anaesthetise subcutaneously with a few ml of LA
- Insert at right angle to the skin, resistance increases when pushing through the yellow ligament (*lig. flavum*) (popping sensation); the skin can be pre-cut with a scalpel if necessary
- Advance until you reach the bottom of the canal (3–7.5 cm depending on the horse), then pull back about 0.5 cm
- Aspirate; no blood should appear; if blood is aspirated, pull out the cannula and reposition a new cannula
- Check correct cannula position; no resistance should be felt when injecting test dose, further testing under epidural/spinal anaesthesia in small animals (p. 434)
- Inject slowly, pull out cannula

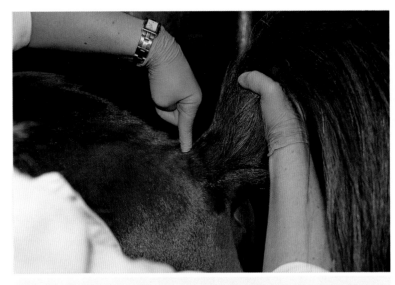

Fig. 9.24 Caudal epidural anaesthesia in the horse. Palpation of the injection site.

Good to know

Note!
In horses, the spinal cord and meninges end approximately in the middle of the sacrum, so a spinal injection is impossible with caudal epidural anaesthesia!

▶ **Which drugs?** The choice must be made based on indication. It is often a good idea to combine two or even more drugs to take advantage of the desired properties. Drugs **should not contain any preservatives**. Some examples are given below:

- **Lidocaine 2%**
  - 0.2 mg/kg
  - Onset of action after 5–15 min, duration of action 60–90 min, possibly up to 120 min
  - Total volume of 6–8 ml (500 kg horse) should not be exceeded, otherwise there is a risk of ataxia and going down

- **Bupivacaine 0.5%**
  - 0.06 mg/kg
  - Onset of action after 10–30 min, duration of action up to 4 h
  - Total volume not more than 6–8 ml
- **Xylazine**
  - 0.2 mg/kg diluted to 6–8 ml in 0.9% NaCl (or e.g. local anaesthetic)
  - Onset of action after 10–30 min, duration up to 2.5–5 h
  - Minimal sedation, ataxia, cardiovascular and respiratory depression
- **Ketamine**
  - 1 mg/kg
  - Onset of action after 10–30 min, duration up to 2 h
  - Ataxia is possible
- **Morphine**
  - 0.1 mg/kg
  - Onset of action after 4–6 h (!), duration 8–18 h
  - Sedation, ataxia possible
- **Methadone**
  - 0.1 mg/kg
  - Onset of action after 15 min, duration up to 5 h
  - No sedation or ataxia

Castration of the stallion: Testicular plexus

Local anaesthesia of the testicles is very easy to perform and allows either castration in the sedated stallion while standing or serves as excellent analgesia for the animal under general anaesthesia. In addition to perioperative analgesia, the recovery phase will also be pain-free and therefore calmer.

Contraindication is pathologically (tumorous, inflammatory) altered testicular tissue.

▶ Desensitised area
- Testicular parenchyma
- Spermatic cord with nerve fibres of the testicular plexus

▶ Approach and localisation
- Two different approaches are described, with a combination of the two techniques seemingly giving the best result
  - **Injection into the spermatic cord** (15–30 ml per testicle with a 3 cm, 20 G cannula) while gently pulling the testicle to expose the spermatic cord

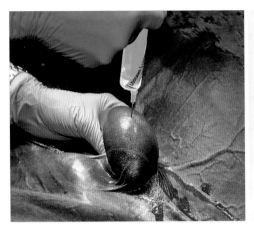

Fig. 9.25 Parenchymal injection of local anaesthetic for castration of the stallion.

○ **Injection into the testicular parenchyma** (15–30 ml per testicle with a longer 18–20 G cannula) after aspiration (▶ Fig. 9.25); diffuses from the pampiniform plexus to the spermatic cord after a few minutes
• For both techniques, the **incision line should also be infiltrated** with 5–10 ml local anaesthetic

Good to know

Note!
Injecting into the spermatic cord can cause a haematoma, which can lead to problems when applying the emasculator.

Literature

[1] Bardell D, Iff I, Mosing M. A cadaver study comparing two approaches to perform a maxillary nerve block in the horse. Equine Vet J 2010; 42: 721–25
[2] Caldwell FJ, Easley KJ. Self-inflicted lingual trauma secondary to inferior alveolar nerve block in 3 horses. Equine Vet Educ 2012; 24: 119–123
[3] Derossi R, Miguel GL, Frazilio FO, Nunes DB, Kassab TA. L-Bupivacaine 0.5% vs. racemic 0.5% bupivacaine for caudal epidural analgesia in horses. J Vet Pharmacol Ther 2005; 28: 293–297
[4] Eberspächer-Schweda E. Sedierung und Lokalanästhesie bei Eingriffen am Kopf des Pferdes. Pferdespiegel 2017; 2: 50–59
[5] Gilger B. Equine Ophthalmology. 2nd ed. Maryland Heights: Saunders Elsevier 2010

[6] Harding PG, Smith RL, Barakzai SZ. Comparison of two approaches to performing an inferior alveolar nerve block in the horse. Aust Vet J 2012; 90: 146–150

[7] Karpie JC, Chu CR. Lidocaine exhibits dose- and time-dependent cytotoxic effects on bovine articular chondrocytes in vitro. Am J Sports Med 2007; 35: 1622–1627

[8] Labelle AL, Clark-Price SC. Anesthesia for ophthalmic procedures in the standing horse. Vet Clin North Am Equine Pract 2013; 29: 179–191

[9] O'Neill HD, Garcia-Pereira FL, Mohankumar PS. Ultrasound-guided injection of the maxillary nerve in the horse. Equine Vet J 2014; 46: 180–4

[10] Robinson EP, Natalini CC. Epidural anesthesia and analgesia in horses. Vet Clin North Am Equine Pract 2002; 18: 61–82

[11] Searle D, Dart AJ, Dart CM, Hodgson DR. Equine castration: review of anatomy, approaches, techniques and complications in normal, cryptorchid and monorchid horses. Aust Vet J 1999; 77: 428–434

[12] Skarda RT, Muir WW3rd. Analgesic, hemodynamic, and respiratory effects of caudal epidurally administered xylazine hydrochloride solution in mares. Am J Res 1996; 57: 193–200

[13] Vogt C. Lehrbuch der Zahnheilkunde beim Pferd. Stuttgart: Schattauer, 2011

9.4.4 Ruminants

Many surgical procedures in ruminants are performed standing with or without sedation under local anaesthesia. It should be noted that the approved local anaesthetic drugs sometimes only have a duration of action of up to 90 minutes, after which analgesia is no longer guaranteed. It may be necessary to inject additional anaesthetics or to ensure analgesia with other methods. However, even after the injection of LA, the effect must be waited for (usually 5–10 min) before starting the painful procedure.

The stress response in cattle is significantly reduced if, in addition to local anaesthesia, animals are sedated with e.g. xylazine and an NSAID is administered for longer-lasting analgesia.

Local anaesthesia for procedures on the head

The most common painful procedures performed on the head are dehorning and enucleation.

Dehorning in cattle: Zygomatic nerve (n. zygomaticus)

Two branches of the zygomatic nerve supply the horn and the base of the horn: The zygomaticotemporal branch and the cornual branch. In older animals, a skin branch caudal to the horn must also be desensitised.

▶ Sensory blockade
• Horn
• Horn base

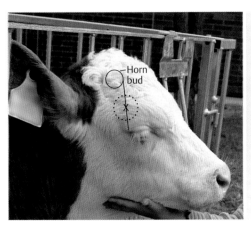

Fig. 9.26 Local anaesthesia for dehorning in calves.

▶ **Approach and localisation**
- 18–22 G, 2.5–4 cm cannula
- In calves, the nerve runs from the horn bud towards the lateral edge of the orbit: Palpate the bony edge; the injection site is halfway between the horn bud and the lateral corner of the eye, ventral to the bony edge (▶ Fig. 9.26)
- The nerve is located about 1 cm deep in smaller cattle, in large animals up to 2.5 cm deep
- Injection of 5–10 ml local anaesthetic after aspiration

In addition, a longer acting analgesic agents (e.g. ketoprofen) should be administered.

Dehorning in the goat: Zygomaticotemporal nerve (n. zygomaticotemporalis) and infratrochlear nerve (n. infratrochlearis)

In contrast to cattle, two different nerves must be desensitised with local anaesthetic in goats: Both horn branches of the zygomaticotemporal nerve (A) and the infratrochlear nerve (B) (▶ Fig. 9.27).

▶ **Sensory blockade**
- Horn
- Horn base

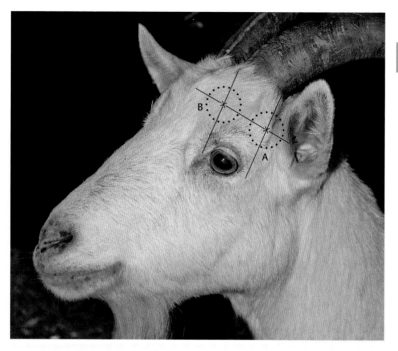

Fig. 9.27 Local anaesthesia for dehorning in goats. A: Zygomaticotemporal nerve, B: Infratrochlear nerve.

▶ Approach and localisation

- 20–22 G, 2.5 cm cannula
- The **zygomaticotemporal nerve** (A) lies midway between the lateral horn base and lateral canthus (▶ Fig. 9.27); insertion close to the caudal edge of the supraorbital process, approx. 1–1.5 cm deep
- The **infratrochlear nerve** (B) lies midway between the medial corneal base and the medial canthus (▶ Fig. 9.27); insertion dorsally and parallel to the dorso-medial edge of the orbit
- It is best to inject in a linear fashion, as the nerves branch out
- Injection of approx. 5 ml local anaesthetic after aspiration, calculate maximum dosages in small animals

A ring block around the base of the horn is recommended for kids.

Enucleation in cattle: Peterson or retrobulbar block

Either the Peterson or the retrobulbar block can be used for enucleation. The Peterson block is technically more demanding but apparently less risky than the retrobulbar block (penetration of the eyeball, orbital haemorrhage, damage to the optic nerve, injection into the optic nerve sheath). In both blocks, the oculo-cardiac reflex (p. 297) can be triggered (vagally mediated severe brady-cardia), in which case the manipulation must be stopped immediately and possibly atropine 0.005 mg/kg IV administered.

▶ Sensory blockade
- As in the horse, all structures supplied by the cephalic nerves C3 to C7 are anaesthetised: Eyeball and entire orbit
- Sensory and motor blockade (immobilisation of the eyeball)
- Does not desensitise the eyelids

▶ Approach and localisation
- (A) **Peterson Block** (▶ Fig. 9.28)
  - First inject a small depot of local anaesthetic (2 ml) into the notch where the frontal bone meets the zygomatic arch

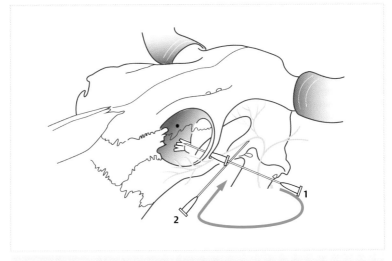

Fig. 9.28 Schematic of the Peterson block in cattle.

- Pre-insert a large 14 G cannula (as a guide cannula) as far as possible cranially and ventrally in this notch
- Enter horizontally and slightly caudally with an 18 G, 12 cm cannula through the guide cannula until you meet the coronoid process of the mandible
- Move cranially until you can push slightly medially past the bone in a caudoventral direction
- When you hit bone, pull back slightly, aspirate carefully and inject about 15 ml of local anaesthetic
- To further anaesthetise the auriculopalpebral nerve, withdraw the cannula until the tip is just under the skin, change direction caudally and inject another 10 ml of LA after about 5–7 cm

- **(B) Retrobulbar block**
  - 18 G, 15 cm cannula, bent to a semicircle (▶ Fig. 9.9)
  - 4-point block with puncture at each of the dorsal, ventral, medial and lateral rims of the orbit
  - Push away the eyeball with one finger, puncture the conjunctiva and advance along the orbital wall
  - Depth approx. 8–9 cm
  - Once the cannula is placed retrobulbar, gently aspirate and inject 5–10 ml LA

Claw surgery: Intravenous regional anaesthesia

Intravenous regional anaesthesia (IVRA) is also called BIER block after its first describer August Bier. It is an excellent method for the analgesic treatment of painful procedures on the distal limb or claw in cattle, small ruminants and pigs. The IVRA is ideally performed in lateral position or, in the case of standing animals, also on the raised leg.

- **Advantages**
  - No exact anatomical knowledge required
  - Only one injection (reduces tissue trauma and risk of contamination)
  - Fast
  - Reduces bleeding in the surgical area
- **Disadvantages**
  - The block inexplicably does not work in about 5–10% of all animals
  - Haemorrhages that have not been stopped only become apparent when the tourniquet is removed

▶ Sensory and motor blockade
- Limb distal to the tourniquet

▶ **Approach and localisation**

- A catheter can be placed before the tourniquet is applied or a cannula can be placed after the tourniquet is applied (puncture sites, see ▶ Table 9.6)
- Catheterise a vein of the distal limb after clipping and disinfection as close as possible to the surgical site; of course, it must be a different access than the one through which infusion solution and drugs may be given
- If necessary, create an area free of blood by wrapping the limb from distal to proximal
- Attach the Esmarch tourniquet proximally or distally to the carpus or tarsus or proximally to the elbow, depending on the location (▶ Fig. 9.29a)

Table 9.6 Puncture sites of the superficial veins for intravenous regional anaesthesia on the front- and hindlimb in cattle. The volume refers to a 2% solution of an approved local anaesthetic in cattle (approx. 500 kg), e.g. procaine.

Vein	Site of injection	Volume
Frontlimb		
Common dorsal digital vein III (*v. digitalis dorsalis communis III*)	Dorsal, exactly axially at the level of the fetlock joint	20 ml
Common palmar digital vein II/IV (*v. digitalis palmaris communis II/IV*)	Palmar, from medial (II) or lateral (IV), the cannula is advanced dorsally of the dewclaw into the depression between the medial interosseous muscle (*m. interosseus medius*) and the metatarsal bone	20 ml
Radial vein (*v. radialis*)	Medial to the accessory carpal bone (*os carpi accessorium*), subcutaneous in the area of the carpal tunnel	40 ml
Hindlimb		
Common dorsal digital vein III (*v. digitalis dorsalis communis III*)	Dorsal, exactly axial at the level of the fetlock joint	20 ml
Common plantar digital vein II/IV (*v. digitalis plantaris communis II/IV*)	Plantar, from medial (II) or lateral (IV) the cannula is advanced dorsally and proximally of the dewclaws into the depression between the interosseus medius muscle (*m. interosseus medius*) and the metatarsal bone	20 ml
Lateral saphenous vein (*v. saphena lateralis*)	On the lateral side of the tarsus	40 ml

From: Erkrankungen der Klauen und Zehen des Rindes, Eds: Fiedler, Maierl, Nuss, 2004, Schattauer

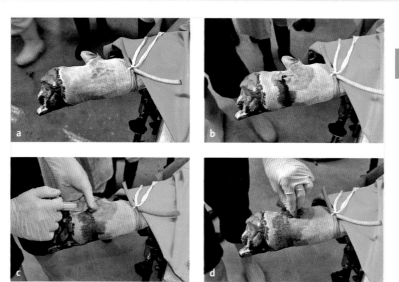

Fig. 9.29 Intravenous regional anaesthesia of the limb in cattle.
a Attaching the tourniquet.
b Insertion of the cannula.
c Lidocaine injection.
d Compression of the puncture site.

- If not catheterised but to be injected via the cannula, insert cannula now after having clipped and disinfected (▶ Fig. 9.29b)
- Rapid injection of 2% lidocaine: 20–40 ml (bovine), 3–5 ml (small ruminants, pigs) **without added adrenalin** (▶ Fig. 9.29c)
- If the cannula or catheter is withdrawn now, compress the puncture site with your finger and massage it to prevent haematoma formation (▶ Fig. 9.29d)
- Onset of action after 5–10 min, duration of action until tourniquet is removed, sometimes up to 30 min longer

Good to know

Using the Esmarch's tourniquet
- Leave in place for at least 20 min to avoid lidocaine intoxication
- If it is necessary to open the tourniquet earlier, open slowly and in small steps to prevent local anaesthetic from flooding too quickly into the systemic circulation
- A tourniquet hurts! Ideally, one has a 2nd tourniquet that can be placed in the anaesthetised area after injection of the LA. The first tourniquet can then be removed
- The tourniquet should be on the limb for a maximum of 60–90 minutes, otherwise there is a risk of ischaemia and therefore long-term damage to the tissue

Abdominal wall/flank

Various local anaesthesia techniques can be used for laparotomy:
- **Line block**, i.e. local anaesthesia of the incision line
- **Inverted L block**, in which a line anaesthesia of the supplying nerves is performed
- Proximal or distal **paravertebral anaesthesia**

Described below are the line and inverted L block.

Line block

▶ Sensory blockade
- Infiltrated area
- **Advantages**
  - Very easy to perform
  - No exact anatomical knowledge necessary
- **Disadvantages**
  - Very large volumes of LA required, potentially leading to intoxication, haematoma formation and wound healing problems
  - Deeper layers are insufficiently desensitised and still sensitive to pain
  - No muscle relaxation

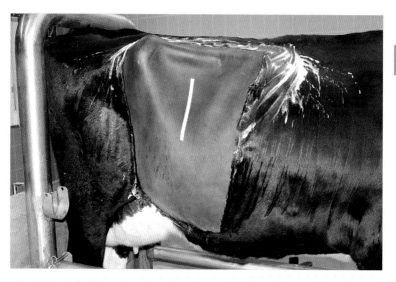

Fig. 9.30 Localisation of the incision line for local anaesthesia for a laparotomy (right side).

▶ Approach and localisation
- In the planned incision line (▶ Fig. 9.30) subcutaneous depots are first injected at a depth of approx. 2 cm (2.5–8 cm, 18 G cannula)
- Subsequently, the underlying layer is infiltrated through the anaesthetised skin to a depth of approx. 5–7 cm
- A total of approx. 50–100 ml of an approved 2% LA, e.g. procaine, can be used

Inverted L block

▶ Sensory blockade
- Flank region caudal to the last rib and ventral to the transverse processes of the lumbar vertebrae by desensitisation of the ventral branches of the 13th thoracic and the 1st to 4th lumbar spinal nerves
- **Advantages**
  - ○ Relatively easy to perform
  - ○ No LA in the incision line

465

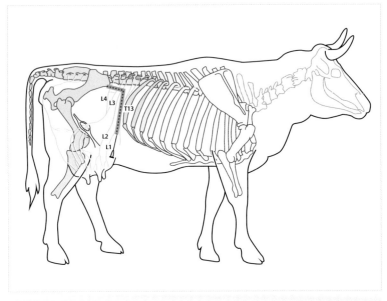

Fig. 9.31 Inverted L block of the abdominal wall.

- **Disadvantages**
  - Very large volumes LA necessary
  - Somewhat more time consuming
  - Deeper layers are inadequately desensitised and are still sensitive to pain

- ▶ **Approach and localisation**
- Procedure as for the line block
- Localisation is a few cm caudally and along the last rib to the level of the costal cartilage, then a few cm ventrally of the transverse processes to the 4th lumbar vertebra (▶ Fig. 9.31)
- A total of approx. 100 ml of LA can be injected in the adult animal

Caudal or lumbosacral epidural anaesthesia

As in the horse, this technique is very useful for inducing sensory and motor blockade for procedures involving the anus, vulva, vagina and penis, as well as for tenesmus and vaginal or uterine prolapse. In **cattle**, not only the caudal epidural (between S5 and Co1 or Co1 and Co2, i.e. the first two caudal vertebrae) but also the lumbosacral epidural anaesthesia is easy to perform.

▶ **Approach and localisation**
- 18–20 G, 5–7.5 cm (spinal) cannula
- Localisation between sacrum and 1st caudal vertebra (Co1) or Co1 and Co2; locate by moving the tail up and down (▶ Fig. 9.32a) or palpation of the lumbosacral space as a depression between the last lumbar vertebra and the sacrum (▶ Fig. 9.32b)
- Clip, disinfect, put on gloves, work in a sterile manner
- In awake animals, anaesthetise locally with a few ml subcutaneously before epidural injection
- Insert at a right angle to the skin; when advancing, resistance increases when pushing through the yellow ligament (*lig. flavum*) (popping sensation)
- Advance until you reach the floor of the canal (caudally approx. 2–4 cm), then retract approx. 0.5 cm
- Aspirate; no blood should appear; if it does, reposition the cannula
- Check for correct cannula position; no resistance should be felt when injecting test dose, further tests see epidural/spinal local anaesthesia in small animals (p. 434)
- Inject slowly, withdraw cannula

Good to know

Note!
Spinal cord and meninges end at about at the level of L6 in cattle, so a spinal injection is unlikely with lumbosacral injection, and impossible with caudal epidural anaesthesia.

In cattle, for a **caudal epidural anaesthesia**, 1 ml of 2% of an LA per 100 kg can be administered at a rate of max. 1 ml/s. This causes analgesia of the perineum, inner thigh and tail and up to the middle of the sacrum.

With the combination of 0.03 mg/kg **xylazine** plus 2% **procaine** or **lidocaine** at 5 ml, analgesia extends further cranially after a few minutes and lasts up to 2 h.

When using the **lumbosacral approach**, LA should be avoided in order to prevent the animal from going down. **Alpha2 agonists**, **ketamine** or **opioids** can be used without obtaining motor blockade.

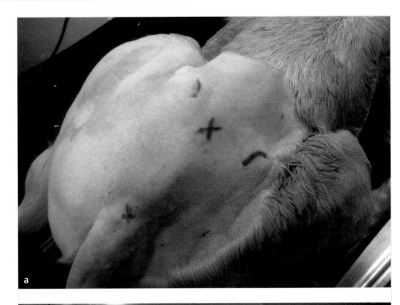

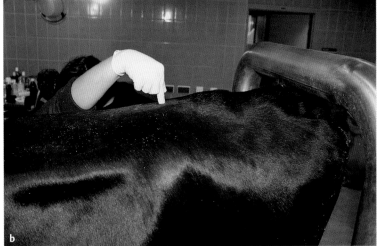

Fig. 9.32 Epidural anaesthesia in cattle.
a Localisation of the lumbosacral space (x cranial) and the sacrococcygeal puncture site (x caudal) in calves.
b Palpation of the lumbosacral space in adult cattle.

Literature

[1] Bier A. Über einen neuen Weg Localanästhesie an den Gliedmassen zu erzeugen. Arch Klin Chir 1908; 86: 1007–1016

[2] Fehlings K. Intravenöse regionale Anästhesie an der V. digitalis dorsalis communis III – eine brauchbare Möglichkeit zur Schmerzausschaltung bei Eingriffen an den Vorderzehen des Rindes. Dtsch Tierärztl Wschr 1980; 87: 4–7

[3] Pearce SG, Kerr CL, Bouré LP, Thompson K, Dobson H. Comparison of the retrobulbar and Peterson nerve block techniques via magnetic resonance imaging in bovine cadavers. J Am Vet Med Assoc 2003; 223: 852–855

[4] Scarda RT. Local and regional anesthetic and analgesic techniques: Ruminants and swine. In: Lumb & Jones' Veterinary Anesthesia. Thurmon JC, Tranquilli WJ, Benson GJ (Ed.). Philadelphia: Lippinkott Williams & Wilkins 1996; 479–514

9.5 Non-pharmacological analgesic treatment options

In addition to analgesic therapy with medication, there are a number of helpful methods that can alleviate acute postoperative or chronic pain. Relatively easy methods can also be used in the daily routine to support treatment.

It is known that the sensation of pain can be modulated at the level of the spinal cord and brain. Through this **modulation**, the degree of pain can be attenuated or intensified. A simple example: Emotions can influence pain perception. Bad smells, fear or cold increase pain sensation. Happiness, a feeling of well-being or good smells dull the sensation of pain. From these findings it is easy to deduce how the environment should be designed for a patient suffering from pain.

Physical therapies include treatment with cold or heat. Cold packs (cool packs, crushed ice or similar ► Fig. 9.33) can be applied to painful (surgical) areas. **Cryotherapy** has an analgesic effect and reduces oedema and inflammation.

In contrast, **heat therapy** (heat lamp, hot packs) can be helpful for chronic pain. It relieves pain and promotes blood circulation. In addition, the warmth can increase the sense of well-being.

The use of **gentle surgical techniques** and **short operating times** also reduce pain in the post-operative phase. **Careful handling of the tissue** or **small skin incisions** (e.g. in laparoscopic surgery) or a skin suture that is not too tight can contribute significantly to a quick recovery.

In addition to analgesic care, ideal **postoperative management** also includes
• Well-fitting bandages that do not compress or constrict and are changed regularly

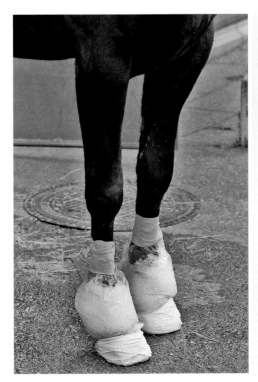

Fig. 9.33 Inflammation and pain relief with cryotherapy for severely painful laminitis in horses.

- Cleanliness (cleaning behaviour is often impaired by neck collars, especially important in cats)
- For dogs, going outside regularly to urinate and defecate

The more complex procedures, which can be carried out after additional training or by a specialist, include **physiotherapy**, **transcutaneous electrical nerve stimulation** (TENS), **acupuncture** and more.

9.5.1 Literature

[1] Van Eps AW, Orsini JA. A comparison of seven methods for continuous therapeutic cooling of the equine digit. Equine Vet J 2016; 48: 120–124
[2] Villemure C, Slotnick BM, Bushnell MC. Effects of odors on pain perception: deciphering the roles of emotion and attention. Pain 2003; 106: 101–108

10 Cardiopulmonary resuscitation (CPR) in small animals

The necessary equipment for cardiopulmonary (and cerebral) resuscitation should be available in an easily accessible place:

Endotracheal tubes of all sizes; **laryngoscope**, **stylet**; **oxygen** source, **AMBU bag**; **venous catheters**; **emergency drugs** and dosage lists; **monitoring** equipment: **electrocardiography** (ECG), **pulse oximeter**, **capnograph**, **thermometer**; **thoracotomy** and **tracheostomy set**.

In an **emergency**, the following procedure is recommended:

- Short medical history, usefulness of CPR and explanation of consequences, prognosis and costs to the owner
- Check consciousness. Pay attention to eyes!
- Call for help (minimum 2 persons, best 4–5 persons), ideally you would have 5 persons who take over the following tasks:
  - Cardiac massage
  - Ventilation
  - Monitoring (pulse, record keeping)
  - IV catheter placement, drawing up and administering drugs, start infusion
  - Owner contact, alternating with person performing cardiac massage
- **One person must be in charge!**
- Note the time
- Briefly check respiration and pulse
  - **Caution:** Do **not** reach into the mouth when the animal is fighting to breath!
  - Do not "waste" too much time for pulse search, maximum 10 s

Start resuscitation according to the A – B – C scheme: A for **A**irways, B for **B**reathing, C for **C**irculation in patients with obvious respiratory problems (e.g. brachycephalic patient). Start with C – A – B scheme in all other patients with cardiovascular arrest of unknown origin.

10.1 Airways

Are the airways open? Secure the airway by orotracheal intubation. If there is a foreign body or similar in the airway that cannot be removed: Tracheotomy!

- VERY IMPORTANT: Check the correct position of the endotracheal tube in the trachea: Visualisation using the laryngoscope, potentially bilateral auscultation as described under "Airway management" (p. 153).

- Inflate the cuff and tie the tube well (behind the ears)
- Possibly place a large IV catheter percutaneously in the trachea as a temporary solution until tracheotomy and administer oxygen through it

10.2 Breathing

Ventilating the patient by intermittent positive pressure ventilation (p. 370), IPPV

- Oxygen flow 100–200 ml/kg/min with anaesthesia machine or AMBU bag via the endotracheal tube
- Frequency: 8–12×/min
- Depth of breath (= maximum pressure on bag) is clinically guided by chest excursion – it should look physiological; if manually ventilated via anaesthesia machine, pressure manometer can be used as a guide: Peak inspiratory pressure should not exceed 10–15 cmH$_2$O. For more details see chapter on "Manual positive pressure ventilation" (p. 371).

10.3 Circulation

Feel pulse on femoral artery for 5 s, cardiac auscultation bilaterally for 5 s.
- No pulse palpable or no heartbeat audible:
  - Cardiac massage: Right or left lateral position or dorsal recumbency for barrel-shaped thorax; hard surface underneath (▶ Fig. 10.1)
  - Good position of the resuscitator is important: Arms stretched out, with the upper body leaning over the patient
  - Depth of compression about ⅓ of the width of the chest, completely release pressure in between compressions
  - Frequency: 100–120×/min (depending on the size of the patient)

10.3.1 Cardiac pump

- **Cat, small dogs** (< 10 kg): Compression of the thorax over the heart with one hand: Take the thorax like a tennis ball between the thumb and the remaining 4 fingers and compress
- **Medium-sized dogs:** Careful compression of the thorax over the heart with both hands

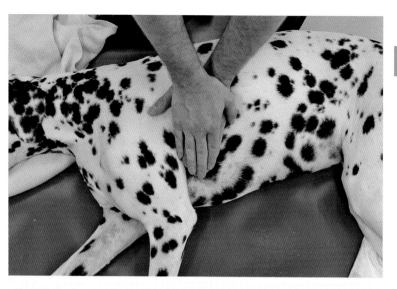

Fig. 10.1 Cardiac massage in a large dog.

10.3.2 Thoracic pump

- **Large dogs** (> 25 kg): At the level of the widest thoracic extension: Compression with both hands (▶ Fig. 10.1)
- In **narrow chested breeds** (e. g. greyhounds) also heart pump; works similarly to small dogs and cats by (almost) directly compressing the heart through the chest wall; is sometimes also more effective

If possible, replace the persons performing CPR every 2 minutes or earlier if necessary.

Never interrupt cardiac massage – if something absolutely has to be interrupted, it is ventilation. It is better that there is always a little oxygen circulating than that there is a lot of oxygen in the lungs and it is not transported further.

Caution

Complications during resuscitation

During resuscitation, complications may arise due to the pressure applied externally to the thorax or abdomen and positive pressure ventilation:

- **Rib fractures**: Are very painful, but as long as the ribs do not impale the lung tissue, they are negligible in this situation
- **Spontaneous pneumothorax**: Quick diagnosis is important (often the first thing noticed is the increasing rigidity of the thorax and problems with manual ventilation), the thoracic wall should be opened immediately

Signs of effective CPR:

- **Peripheral pulse** (femoral artery, dorsal pedal artery) present
  - Not easy to palpate during CPR, but still do not waste too much time looking for it
- **Capnography**: $etCO_2$ increases (**caution**: Hypo-/hyperventilation!); $etCO_2$ is a reliable outcome parameter; if the value remains in the single digits despite resuscitation efforts, the prognosis is very poor
- **SpO_2 increases** (**caution**: False measurement due to rhythmic movement of chest compression; this is falsely "recognised" by the device as a pulse)
- **Pupils** slowly **narrowing** again, eyes rotate down from central position
- **Cranial reflexes** (palpebral reflex, corneal reflex) are **present** again
- **ECG** (usually only can be read during pauses) returns to **normal**

Good to know

Avoid hyperventilation

One of the most common mistakes in resuscitation is that the patient is severely hyperventilated. In the heat of the moment, too deep breaths are given too fast. Under clinical conditions, care must be taken to maintain normal respiratory rate and depth.

A **resuscitation cycle lasts 2 minutes**, then **STOP CPR** and do a brief **evaluation**

- Evaluation: ECG, auscultation, pulse palpation: Duration approx. 10 s
- If no action is noticeable on the part of the patient, i.e. no improvement or significant deterioration, the next cycle follows with 2 min

10.3.3 Open cardiac massage

Must be discussed with the owner! Involves a long, costly and labour-intensive convalescence phase.

- Consider if external cardiac massage is unsuccessful after 3–5 minutes
- Localisation of the skin incision is on the left side in the 5th intercostal space (behind the shoulder blade, at the level of the elbow, cranial to the rib) above the heart
- Open the thorax and the pericardium (**note**: From now on **pneumothorax**!)
  - Patient must be intubated beforehand!
  - Do **not** perform ventilation during thoracic incision to avoid lung injury
  - Pay attention to the phrenic nerve when opening the pericardium!
- Milk out the heart from the tip towards the base
- Caution: Do not rotate the heart, vessels will also be rotated!
- Further indications for open cardiac massage:
  - Fluid in the pericardium
  - Fluid in the thorax
  - Obese animals
  - Open abdomen or thorax during surgery
  - Patient anatomy (very large dogs where external heart massage is inevitably difficult)

10.4 Emergency drugs

Depending on the cause of respiratory and circulatory arrest, appropriate medication has to be administered (▶ Table 10.1).

First choice route of administration: Intravenous (IV) via the largest possible venous access

Second choice route of administration: Intraosseous (IO), especially for small patients or unsuccessful attempts to catheterise the veins

- If circulation is poor, cut down is necessary (cephalic vein, jugular vein). Always cut down diagonally (not transversely, not longitudinally) over the vessel
- Always flush (IV and IO) medications (5–50 ml) so that they also reach the heart!
- If neither IV nor IO access is available, **intratracheal administration** is the **third choice**:
  - Dose must be increased approx. 5 ×
  - Dilute with infusion solution (amount depending on the size of the animal)
  - With feeding tube via endotracheal tube into the trachea
  - Suitable for adrenalin and atropine, among others

Table 10.1 CPR emergency drugs and dosages listed according to body weight

Drug (concentration)	Body weight (kg)	2.5	5	10	15	20	30	40	50	70
	Dose (mg/kg)	ml	ml	ml	ml	ml	ml	ml	ml	ml
Adrenaline (1:1000; 1 mg/ml) Low dose	0.01	0.03	0.05	0.1	0.15	0.2	0.3	0.4	0.5	0.7
Adrenaline (1:1000; 1 mg/ml) High dose	0.1	0.25	0.5	1	1.5	2	3	4	5	7
Atropine (0.5 mg/ml)	0.04	0.2	0.4	0.8	1.1	1.5	2.2	3	3.7	5.2
Lidocaine 2% (20 mg/ml)	2	0.25	0.5	1	1.5	2	3	4	5	7

CRP Cardiopulmonary resuscitation

10.4.1 Which drug is administered when?

- In **asystole** or **pulseless electrical activity** (i. e. you can still see activity on the ECG but can no longer feel a pulse) = circulatory arrest: Administration of low dose **adrenalin** (0.01 mg/kg) IV after every 2nd resuscitation cycle (i. e. every 4 min, max. 3 times in total)
  - If no spontaneous cardiac activity after a total of 10 minutes, increase dose to 0.1 mg/kg **adrenalin** IV
  - Administer **atropine** (max. 2 doses in total, 0.04 mg/kg IV) alternating with adrenalin
- In case of refractory **ventricular tachycardia** or **ventricular fibrillation**: If defibrillation is not possible or unsuccessful: **Lidocaine** 2 mg/kg IV
- Bicarbonate administration (p. 392) and electrolyte correction (p. 386) should only be done once an appropriate blood gas analysis is available

> 30 min CPR without success: Reconsider the sense of it!

10.5 ECG and other monitoring

Continuous monitoring of vital parameters and assessment of the success of resuscitation efforts.

Arrest rhythms (p. 354) that can be detected with the ECG and appropriate therapy:
- **Asystole:** Adrenalin + /– atropine
- **Pulseless electrical activity:** Adrenalin + /– atropine
- **Ventricular fibrillation:** Defibrillation
- **Pulseless ventricular tachycardia:** Defibrillation, if unsuccessful: Lidocaine

Possible post-arrest rhythms (p. 354):
- **Bradycardia**: Atropine
- **Escape rhythm**: Try atropine
- **Ventricular tachycardia**: Lidocaine

In addition to the electrical activity at the heart (ECG), oxygen saturation of the arterial blood (pulse oximeter), blood pressure, respiratory gases and temperature should also be monitored. Deviations from normal values should be treated.

10.6 Fluids

If hypovolaemia (e.g. due to blood loss, prolonged vomiting/diarrhoea) or massive vasodilation is suspected, bolus infusion therapy with crystalloid and colloid solutions is indicated.

- Start with 20–30 ml/kg **crystalloid solution** (e.g. Ringer's solution, Sterofundin ISO) over 10–15 min IV, then re-evaluate. Repeat if necessary
- If the patient remains hypotensive, additional **colloid solutions** can be administered: 2–5 ml/kg as a bolus over a few minutes, can be repeated (also as a continuous drip) up to max. 30 ml/kg/24 h
- In principle, the cat requires smaller infusion volumes than the dog, as it has a smaller blood volume
- If possible, infusion solutions should be warmed up to body temperature
- In case of cardiogenic shock, (aggressive) infusion therapy is not indicated!

Careful!

In shock patients, infusion of 5% glucose solution is not recommended!
The 5% glucose in the solution are immediately metabolised by the body and free water remains. This leads first to pathological hyperglycaemia, which worsens the prognosis, especially in shock patients with unstable circulation, and second free water dilutes electrolytes such as Na, K and Cl, among others, which can have far-reaching consequences (e.g. hyponatraemia can lead to swelling of brain cells with subsequent life-threatening increase of intracranial pressure).

Infusion of 5% glucose solution is to be reserved for a few clinical indications. In cases of hypoglycaemia, therapy should be infusion of a balanced electrolyte solution to which glucose has been added.

▶ Successful CPR
- Often the underlying problem remains; always consider the usefulness of CPR and discuss it with the owner (risk-benefit analysis)
- Continue oxygen therapy, continue positive pressure ventilation if necessary
- Close monitoring of the cardiovascular situation (ECG, blood pressure, urine production)
- Close monitoring of the neurological status
- Ensure close monitoring of blood values like glucose, lactate, electrolytes, blood gases, etc.
- Resuscitated patients remain intensive care patients for at least 24 h

▶ **Write a protocol**
- Who was involved?
- What was administered or performed and when?
- Who determined death and when?
- Ideally, discuss the protocol with the team afterwards and ask yourselves what you could do better next time

10.7 Literature

[1] Balakrishnan A. Resuscitation Strategies for the Small Animal Trauma Patient. Vet Clin North Am Small Anim Pract. 2020; 50: 1385–1396
[2] Edwards TH, Rizzo JA, Pusateri AE. Hemorrhagic shock and hemostatic resuscitation in canine trauma. Transfusion. 2021; 61 Suppl 1: S264–S274
[3] Fletcher DJ, Boller M, Brainard BM, Haskins SC, Hopper K, McMichael MA, Rozanski EA, Rush JE, Smarick SD. RECOVER evidence and knowledge gap analysis on veterinary CPR. Part 7: Clinical guidelines. J Vet Emerg Crit Care 2012; 22: 102–131
[4] Fletcher DJ, Boller M. Updates in small animal cardiopulmonary resuscitation. Vet Clin North Am Small Anim Pract 2013; 43: 971–987
[5] Hoehne SN, Kruppert A, Boller M. Kardiopulmonale Reanimation in der Kleintierpraxis [Small animal cardiopulmonary -resuscitation (CPR) in general practice]. Schweiz Arch Tierheilkd. 2020; 162: 735–753
[6] Hofmeister EH, Brainard BM, Egger CM, Kang S. Prognostic indicators for dogs and cats with cardiopulmonary arrest treated by cardiopulmonary cerebral resuscitation at a university teaching hospital. J Am Vet Med Assoc. 2009; 235: 50–57
[7] Schmittinger CA, Astner S, Astner L, Kössler J, Wenzel V. Cardiopulmonary resuscitation with vasopressin in a dog. Vet Anaesth Analg. 2005; 32: 112–114

11 Euthanasia

The following chapter describes euthanasia methods for small mammals, as well as small and large animals kept as companion animals. What is not covered in this chapter is the decision-making and decision criteria for or against euthanising an animal. Nor will it discuss at what point euthanasia is justified or when it constitutes an unjustified killing. The focus should be on the ideal procedure and methods to make this traumatic event as gentle, calm and stress-free as possible for everyone involved: Patient, owner and veterinarian!

11.1 Eu thanatos (gr.) = the good death

The aim of euthanasia should be to end the life of a single living being as free of pain, as respectfully and aesthetically pleasing as possible, in order to minimise suffering and pain.

Good to know

The approach must be adapted to the situation
If it is a **geriatric, sick animal**, time should be taken together with the owner to make the decision calmly and subsequently to carry out euthanasia calmly.

However, if the animal is **severely injured and in pain**, euthanasia should be carried out quickly as soon as the decision has been made.

11.2 Owner conversation

In the context of euthanising an animal, time and cost should ideally be irrelevant. The animal (and owner) should be treated with care and respect. This also applies to the already dead animal body, at least as long as the owner is present. The conversation should always be friendly, reassuring and empathetic. The owner should be reassured that the decision makes sense and each step of the euthanasia process should be explained in detail.

- The owner must be aware that the animal may react in the course of euthanasia (movement, vocalisation) and be able to understand and interpret these reactions. A detailed explanation in advance is important: Even if the animal moves, unconsciousness and therefore insensibility is guaranteed: "It may not look nice, but it is no longer anything that the animal feels or is bothered by". Muscle twitching is a physiological phenomenon of dying, also contractions of the diaphragm that look like the animal is gasping for air

- Written consent from the owner should be obtained before euthanasia. If this is not possible, e.g. in the case of an emergency euthanasia after an accident, a second veterinarian should examine the injured animal and record the findings that led to the decision for euthanasia
- It must be clarified: Should a post-mortem examination/obduction be carried out? And: What should be done with the body of the animal?

11.3 How to carry out euthanasia

The "technical" aspects of euthanasia are practically always the same, regardless of the animal species, but must be individually adapted depending on the situation or circumstances. The description below refers to gentle euthanasia of individual pets with owners.

- Decision for euthanasia
- Owner conversation
- Deep sedation, possibly IM, to allow calm placement of IV catheter. Allow animal to fall asleep in the presence of the owner
- Placement of IV catheter (with the exception of small mammals). Can also take place before sedation if reasonable and possible. It is essential to check that the IV catheter is 100% in place!
- Give the owner time to say goodbye; some owners want euthanasia done as quickly as possible – individual decision
- Induce deep anaesthesia, IV whenever possible, in exceptional cases e.g. small mammals also IM or IP possible
- Euthanasia with an approved drug formulation ideally IV (exception in small mammals it is also possible to use intraperitoneal or intracardiac route of administration)
- Reliable confirmation of death
- Professional disposal of the animal body
- Euthanasia should ultimately "feel" more like a ceremony than a medical act for the owner

11.3.1 Euthanasia in small animals

Ideally, euthanasia can be carried out calmly in the familiar surroundings and without strangers. Once the decision to euthanise has been made and owner conversation has been completed, the process of euthanasia can begin.

Animal species in which placement of an IV catheter is not possible

If the animal species is one in which an IV catheter cannot be routinely placed – e.g. guinea pigs (p. 200), ferrets (p. 206), small rodents (p. 213) – initial sedation makes very little sense. Deep anaesthesia can be induced directly via SC, IM or IP injection, depending on the species. Sufficient time should be allowed for the anaesthetic drugs to take maximum effect.

Euthanasia is performed by injection of an approved euthanasia drug, usually **pentobarbital** or the mixed drug **T61**. Recommended routes of administration for animals without IV catheters are intraperitoneal, for deeply anaesthetised animals also intracardiac. The dosage must be adjusted according to the type of administration, e.g. for IP injection the dose should be tripled compared to IV administration.

SC or IM injection is not recommended. Injection into organs with low absorption capacity such as liver or kidney is not recommended but seems to work well clinically if done correctly. Intrapulmonary injection is also discouraged in part because of the potential for coughing, gasping and respiratory distress. According to AVMA guidelines, intrapulmonary, SC and IM application are even not accepted methods!

Animal species in which placement of an IV catheter is possible

When dealing with a species in which it is possible to place an IV catheter (e.g. **dog**, **cat**, **rabbit**), deep sedation should first be induced by IM injection, e.g. with **acepromazine** in combination with **butorphanol**, both in rather **high doses**. The injection is not painful, the volume is small and acepromazine even has an antiemetic and anxiolytic effect – properties that are desirable in this situation. Deep sedation with alpha2 agonists is rather not recommended in this particular case, as vasoconstriction may complicate IV catheterisation.

Deep sedation – IM and in the owner's presence if possible – before IV catheterisation and induction of anaesthesia before actual euthanasia are extremely important! It keeps the situation calm, there is no need for restraint and the owner gets time and opportunity to see their pet peacefully fall asleep. Nothing is more traumatic and worse for the owner than having to watch three people forcefully restrain their animal in the last seconds of its life, only to need two attempts to place the IV catheter in the desperately resisting animal!!! This situation must be avoided at all costs!!

After deep sedation, an **IV catheter** should be placed in the lateral or medial saphenous vein on the **hindlimb**, if possible, so that drugs can be administered as far away from the head (and the owner) as possible. In very calm or sick animals, the placement of the IV catheter is of course also possible without prior sedation. The correct placement of the catheter should be checked in any case before the injection. At this point at the latest, the animal should be placed lovingly on a blanket or in its basket. The owner should (again) be given the opportunity to say goodbye to his animal (without the veterinarian being present) if desired.

Following this, general anaesthesia should be induced quickly and reliably, e.g. by IV injection of **propofol** in a high dose. After the onset of unconsciousness, wait a short time so that the anaesthetics can exert the maximum effect.

Then the preparation for euthanasia, usually **pentobarbital** or the mixed preparation **T61** can be administered strictly IV, as the preparations containing pentobarbital are strongly alkaline and tissue irritating. Dose recommendations of the individual drug preparation must be followed carefully.

Small things in dealing with the already sedated, anaesthetised or even deceased small animal that make all the difference are
- Place the animal in its usual basket or on a blanket
- Cover the body, but leave the head free and cover injuries, catheters and tubes
- Position the body in a physiological position
- Close the eyes if possible, put the tongue in the mouth

Death (p. 484) of the animal must be reliably confirmed.

11.3.2 Euthanasia in horses and other large animals

Ideally, euthanasia takes place in familiar surroundings and there is another person available besides the owner who can hold and control the animal by the halter or lead rope, if necessary. When the decision for euthanasia has been made and conversation with the owner has been completed, the animal can be sedated.

If an IV catheter is already in place or can be placed without stress, it is possible to administer sedation IV specific to the individual animal and species. The correct placement of the IV catheter should be checked again before the injection. If the animal is stressed or defensive or if excessive restraint would be necessary (e.g. in **pigs**), it is recommended to administer the sedation IM first and to place the IV catheter without stress only after the sedative drug has taken effect.

If the animal is deeply sedated, general anaesthesia should be induced. In large animals such as **horses**, it is important that a 2nd person prevents the animal from falling over backwards and going down uncontrollably by restraining the head. The procedure is identical to the induction of anaesthesia for surgical procedures and subsequently allows a calm and controlled euthanasia.

After the onset of unconsciousness and positioning of the animal in lateral recumbency, another 1–2 min should be waited so that the anaesthetics can exert a maximum effect. Then the euthanasia preparation, usually **pentobarbital** or the mixed preparation **T61** can be administered quickly and strictly IV. Dose recommendations in the instructions for use must be followed carefully. Preparations containing pentobarbital are highly alkaline and tissue irritating. They can cause severe pain and therefore reactions if administered paravenously. Therefore, the correct placement of the IV catheter should be checked again before injection and any other method of administration should be rejected. When using the auricular vein (e.g. in **pigs**, **small ruminants**, **South American camelids**), highly concentrated pentobarbital products should be diluted with NaCl 0.9%. The deeper the anaesthesia before euthanasia, the fewer reactions the animals show in the course of euthanasia. **Horses** in particular may continue to show deep breaths for several minutes after the onset of unconsciousness and only lightly anaesthetised, which is usually disturbing for the owner.

The death of the animal must be reliably confirmed. The removal of the dead animal body should be planned and organised in advance. After confirmation of death and before transport, the horseshoes should be removed.

11.4 Confirmation of death

Cardiac arrest should occur within 2 min after IV injection of the euthanasia drug. With other modes of administration, the onset of death may take longer. If death does not occur after a reasonable period of time, the IV catheter should be checked again, and a second dose administered in any case. A combination of criteria is used to reliably confirm death. These include:

- Absence of pulse
- Absence of breathing
- Loss of reflexes, such as corneal or interdigital reflexes
- Absence of breath sounds or heart sounds by auscultation
- Mucous membranes turning grey
- Eyeballs soften and yield to pressure

Ten minutes after the initial confirmation of death, heart and lungs should be auscultated again to confirm cardiac and respiratory arrest again.

11.5 Literature

[1] Binder R. Euthanasie von Heimtieren – das Tierschutzrecht zwischen Lebensschutz und Leidverkürzung. Wien Tierärztl Monat – Vet Med Austria 2018; 105: 119–28

[2] Buck-Werner ON, Von Rechenberg B. Euthanasie des Hundes und Besitzerbetreuung. In: Kohn B, Schwarz G (Ed.): Praktikum der Hundeklinik. 12th ed, Enke in Georg Thieme Verlag KG, Stuttgart 2018, 1327–1333

[3] Fürst A. Euthanasie – Sanftes Hinscheiden des Pferdes. Hundkatzepferd 2013; 2: 20–22

[4] Leary S, Underwood W, Anthony R, Cartner S, Corey D, Grandin T, Greenacre C, Gwaltney-Brant S, McCrackin MA, Meyer R, Miller D, Shearer J, Yanong R, Golab GC, Patterson-Kane E. AVMA Guidelines for the euthanasia of animals: 2013 edition. 2013; 1–102

[5] Niggemann JR, Eberspächer-Schweda E. Akzeptierte und empfohlene Euthanasiemethoden – ein Überblick für die Kleintierpraxis. Wien Tierärztl Monat – Vet Med Austria 2018; 105: 139–47
Comment: This review article (in German) provides additional information on the euthanasia of birds, reptiles, fish, invertebrates, pregnant animals, foetuses and neonates.

[6] Payne SA, Langley-Evans A, Hillier R. Perceptions of a "good" death: A comparative study of the views of hospice staff and patients. Palliative Med 1996; 10: 307–12

[7] Tritthart A. Euthanasie von Klein- und Heimtieren – wodurch ist das tierärztliche Handeln legitimiert? Wien Tierärztl Monat – Vet Med Austria 2018; 105: 111–7

485

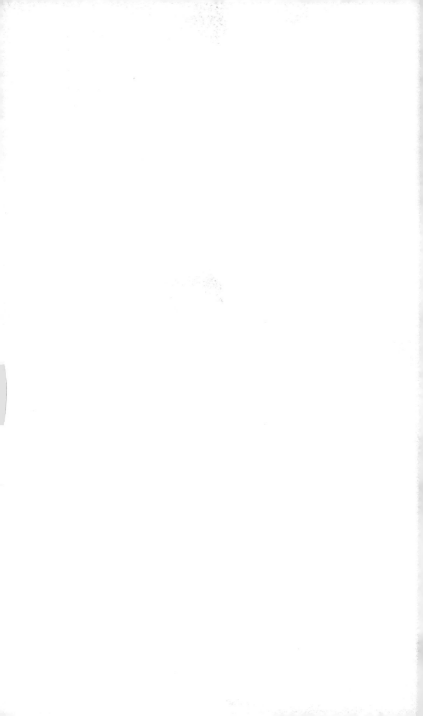

Part III
Appendix

12 List of abbreviations

2,3-BPG	2,3-Biphosphoglycerate
ACE	Angiotensin converting enzyme
ACT	Activated clotting time
ADH	Anti-diuretic hormone
AMBU	Artificial Manual Breathing Unit
Aqua dest.	Distilled water
ASA	American Society of Anesthesiologists
AST	Aspartate-aminotransferase
AV block	Atrio-ventricular block
AVA	Association of Veterinary Anaesthetists
BE	Base excess
BGA	Blood gas analysis
BID	Lat. bis in die; twice a day (treatment times)
BW	Body weight
Ca	Calcium
CK	Creatine kinase
Cl	Chloride
cmH$_2$O	Centimetre water column
CNS	Central nervous system
CO$_3^{2-}$	Carbonate
COHb	Carboxyhaemoglobin
COX	Cyclooxygenase
CPP	Cerebral perfusion pressure
CPR	Cardio pulmonary resuscitation
CRI	Continuous rate infusion
CT	Computer tomography
CVP	Central venous pressure
DCM	Dilated cardiomyopathy
DLVOTO	Dynamic left ventricular outflow tract obstruction
DM	Diabetes mellitus
ECG	Electrocardiogram
etCO$_2$	Endtidal carbon dioxide
ETT	Endotracheal tube
EU	European Union
FiO$_2$	Fraction of inspired oxygen
Fr	French (1 Fr equals about ⅓ mm)
G	Gauge, gage (= size specification for e.g. IV catheters; the larger the G, the smaller the catheter)

GABA	Gamma-aminobutyric acid
H⁺	Hydrogen ions
H_2CO_3	Carbonic acid
Hb	Haemoglobin
HCM	Hypertrophic cardiomyopathy
HCO_3^-	Hydrogen carbonate
Hct	Haematocrit
HES	Hydroxyethylstarch
HR	Heart rate
HYPP	Hyperkalaemic periodic paralysis
ICP	Intracranial pressure
ID	Inner diameter
IO	Intraosseous
IOP	Intraocular pressure
IP	Intraperitoneal
IPPV	Intermittent positive pressure ventilation
IU	International unit
K	Potassium
KCl	Potassium chloride
LA	Local anaesthesia, local anaesthetic, local analgesia
LED	Light-emitting diode
MAC	Minimum alveolar concentration
MAP	Mean arterial pressure
MDR1-gene	Multiple drug resistance1-gene
mEq	Milliequivalent
mmHg	Millimetre mercury column
mmol	Millimole
MRT	Magnetic resonance tomography
N	Nitrogen
N_2O	Nitrous oxide
Na	Sodium
NaCl	Sodium chloride
NMDA	N-Methyl-D-Aspartate
NSAID	Non-steroidal anti-inflammatory drug
OD	Outer diameter
p_aCO_2	Arterial partial pressure of carbon dioxide
p_aO_2	Arterial partial pressure of oxygen
pCO_2	Partial pressure of carbon dioxide
PCV	Pressure controlled ventilation
PEEP	Positive endexpiratory pressure
pO_2	Partial pressure of oxygen

PDA	Persistent ductus arteriosus
PEA	Pulseless electrical activity
PO	Lat. per os; orally, oral administration
PR	Pulse rate
PSS	Portosystemic shunt
PT	Prothrombin time
PTT	Partial thromboplastin time
PVC	Polyvinylchloride
Q	Perfusion
QID	Lat. quarter in die; four times a day (therapy times)
RR	Respiratory rate
SAC	South American camelid
SAM	Systolic anterior motion
SDMA	Symmetric dimethylarginine (sensitive and early marker of declining glomerular filtration rate in dogs and cats)
SID	Lat. semel in die; once a day (therapy times)
SpO$_2$	Oxygen saturation (of haemoglobin in the arterial blood)
Tab	Tablet
TID	Lat. ter in die; three times a day (therapy times)
TIVA	Total intravenous anaesthesia
TP	Total protein
V	Ventilation
V/Q	Ventilation - perfusion
VAA	Fully antagonisable anaesthesia
VCV	Volume controlled ventilation
VES	Ventricular extrasystoles
vs.	Lat. versus, versus
µg	Microgram

13 Further reading

The following textbooks are recommended for further study of veterinary anaesthesiology and perioperative management. The list is not complete, but is intended to be a start and a stimulus for in-depth study.

It should be emphasised again at this point that anaesthesiology is a discipline whose teaching opinion and implementation is to a large extent country-specific on the one hand and dependent on the "teachers of teachers" on the other. Many roads lead to good anaesthesia! It is therefore absolutely necessary to accept and allow other and differing teaching opinions, as long as they are not obviously contraindicated, outdated or harmful to patients.

[1] Martin L. All you really need to know to interpret arterial blood gases (English). 2nd edition, Philadelphia: Lippincott Williams & Wilkins 1999
Comment: The book that at last explains in an understandable way how to interpret blood gases correctly. A must-have for anaesthetists and intensive care specialists.

[2] Duke-Novakovski T, de Vries M, Seymour C. BSAVA Manual of Canine and Feline Anaesthesia and Analgesia (English). 3rd edition, Shurdington, Cheltenham, UK: British Small Animal Veterinary Association 2016
Comment: Is useful to get an overview. Is quite good to read up on case-related anaesthesia management.

[3] Muir WW, Hubbell JAE. Equine Anesthesia – Monitoring and Emergency Therapy (English). 2nd edition, St. Louis: Saunders Elsevier 2008
Comment: This is the "bible" for equine anaesthetists. Detailed and well described. Belongs in the bookshelf of the large animal anaesthetist.

[4] Boron WF, Boulpaep EL. Medical physiology (English). 3rd edition, Philadelphia: Saunders Elsevier 2016
Comment: Explains all the important physiology for medical professionals in an understandable way and with great graphics.

[5] West JB, Luks AM. West's Respiratory physiology – the essentials (English). 10th edition, Philadelphia: Lippincott Williams & Wilkins 2015
Comment: Very good book, perfect for learning and teaching respiratory physiology, inexpensive, concise. A must-have for anaesthetists to understand the basics.

[6] Silverstein DC, Hopper K. Small Animal Critical Care Medicine (English). 3rd edition, London, UK: Elsevier 2022
Comment: The absolute favourite book on emergency and intensive care medicine. Every topic is discussed in a compact and understandable way.

[7] Campoy L, Read MR. Small Animal Regional Anesthesia and Analgesia (English). 1st edition, Ames, IA: John Wiley & Sons 2013
Comment: All local blocks in small animals are described in a practical way. Gives a good overview of the options!

[8] Otero PE, Portela DA. Manual of Small Animal Regional Anesthesia – Illustrated anatomy for nerve stimulation and ultrasound-guided nerve blocks (English) 2nd edition, Buenos Aires, Argentina: 5 m Publishing 2019
Comment: All local blocks in small animals are described in detail in a practical, extensively illustrated manner. Anyone who wants to use local anaesthesia (including nerve stimulator and ultrasound-guided local anaesthesia) should have this book for reference!

[9]   Dorsch JA, Dorsch SE. Understanding Anesthesia Equipment (English). 5th edition, Philadelphia: Lippincott Williams & Wilkins 2007

       Comment: The all-encompassing knowledge of anaesthesia equipment in one book. It answers all the questions you didn't even know you had.

[10] Dugdale, A, Beaumont G, Bradbrook C, Gurney M. Veterinary Anaesthesia – Principles to Practice (English). 2nd edition, Ames, IA: John Wiley & Sons 2020

       Comment: This book was written from former study materials for the diplomate exam. Very profound, but compact and competently presented. Recommended!

[11] Grimm KA, Lamont LA, Tranquilli WJ, Greene SA, Robertson SA. Veterinary Anesthesia and Analgesia – The Fifth Edition of Lumb and Jones (English). 5th edition, Ames, IA: John Wiley & Sons 2015

       Comment: The "bible" for veterinary anaesthetists. The 5th edition is completely revised and extremely well done. Should be on the bookshelf of every veterinarian.

Index

A

Index